KU-575-846

Exercise for Prevention and Treatment of Illness

Exercise for Prevention and Treatment of Illness

Linn Goldberg, MD
Associate Professor of Medicine
Director, Human Performance Laboratory
Division of General Internal Medicine
Oregon Health Sciences University
Portland, Oregon

Diane L. Elliot, MD
Professor of Medicine
Associate Director, Human Performance Laboratory
Division of General Internal Medicine
Oregon Health Sciences University
Portland, Oregon

 F. A. Davis Company • Philadelphia

F. A. Davis Company
1915 Arch Street
Philadelphia, PA 19103

Copyright © 1994 by F.A. Davis Company

All rights reserved. This book is protected by copyright. No part of it may be reproduced, stored in a retrieval system, or transmitted in any form or by any means, electronic, mechanical, photocopying, recording, or otherwise, without written permission from the publisher.

Printed in the United States of America

Last digit indicates print number: 10 9 8 7 6 5 4 3 2 1

Developmental Editor: Bernice M. Wissler
Production Editor: Arofan Gregory
Cover Design By: Steven R. Morrone

As new scientific information becomes available through basic and clinical research, recommended treatments and drug therapies undergo changes. The authors and publisher have done everything possible to make this book accurate, up to date, and in accord with accepted standards at the time of publication. The authors, editors, and publisher are not responsible for errors or omissions or for consequences from application of the book, and make no warranty, expressed or implied, in regard to the contents of the book. Any practice described in this book should be applied by the reader in accordance with professional standards of care used in regard to the unique circumstances that may apply in each situation. The reader is advised always to check product information (package inserts) for changes and new information regarding dose and contraindications before administering any drug. Caution is especially urged when using new or infrequently ordered drugs.

Library of Congress Cataloging in Publication Data

Exercise for prevention and treatment of illness / [edited by]
  Linn Goldberg, Diane L. Elliot.
      p.   cm.
    Includes bibliographical references and index.
    ISBN 0-8036-4163-X
    1. Exercise therapy.   2. Medicine, Preventive.   I. Goldberg,
Linn.   II. Elliot, Diane L.
    [DNLM: 1. Exercise Therapy.   2. Exercise.   3. Preventive Medicine.
  WB 541 E935 1944]
  RM725.E915 1994
  615.8′2 — dc20
  DNLM/DLC
  for Library of Congress   93-46467
                                                                          CIP

Authorization to photocopy items for internal or personal use, or the internal or personal use of specific clients, is granted by F.A. Davis Company for users registered with the Copyright Clearance Center (CCC) Transactional Reporting Service, provided that the fee of $.10 per copy is paid directly to CCC, 27 Congress St., Salem, MA 01970. For those organizations that have been granted a photocopy license by CCC, a separate system of payment has been arranged. The fee code for users of the Transactional Reporting Service is: 8036-4163/94 0 + $.10.

We dedicate this book to our wonderful families who make our lives joyful, entertaining, and complete.

L.G. To Herman and Anita, Jack and Helen, Gabe, Andrew, Aaron, Michael, Alex, and especially Marsha (Misha)

D.L.E. To Jean, Tom, Molly, Britt, and Lauren

Preface

· ·

The use of exercise to prevent and treat disease is an ancient concept, yet only recently has scientific evidence supported its widespread benefit. Physical activity is important for "healthy" individuals, as it decreases mortality and increases well-being. Its role among those with various problems, including risk factors for heart disease and osteoporosis, has been advocated by national health organizations. In addition to its beneficial effect on disease prevention (primary prevention), exercise inhibits or delays clinical presentation of medical problems (secondary prevention) and can improve functional capacity or even reverse illness (tertiary prevention).

This book is intended for health care providers and for those who teach and practice preventive medicine. Our hope is that it provides a clinically useful guide to prescribing exercise. The contributors to the text are experts in their respective fields and include educators, researchers, and practicing clinicians. In each chapter, extensively referenced background information is provided, along with specific guidelines for physical training. Case vignettes illustrate many of these clinical concepts and assist readers' retention and application of the information. The book can be read as a review of exercise recommendations for individuals with illness, or referred to when seeing a specific patient for whom exercise is to be prescribed.

Exercise is a unique intervention. Unlike some pharmacologic therapies, its impact on one risk factor or disease process is not offset by adverse effects or other risk factors. We are certain that if the effects of exercise could be bottled, it would be the most widely prescribed medication.

Linn Goldberg, MD
Diane L. Elliot, MD

Acknowledgments

. . . .

We would like to thank our contributors for their participation, expertise, and willingness to align their chapters to the style we specified, as well as their patience in completion of this multiauthored text. We also appreciate the tolerance of our family, friends, and local colleagues, who have encouraged and supported us during the longer-than-expected process. Finally, we are grateful to our editors, Bernice Wissler and Linda Weinerman, for their interest, lasting support, and attention to detail that the final stages of editing required.

Contributors

· ·

ALAN F. BARKER, MD
Associate Professor of Medicine
Medical Director of Respiratory Care
  Services
Acting Head, Pulmonary and Critical Care
Oregon Health Sciences University
Portland, Oregon

CHARLES C. BENIGHT, PhD
Assistant Professor of Clinical Psychology
University of Colorado at Colorado
  Springs
Colorado Springs, Colorado

ROBERT M. BENNETT, MD
Professor of Medicine
Chairman, Division of Arthritis and
  Rheumatic Diseases
Oregon Health Sciences University
Portland, Oregon

CAROL S. BURCKHARDT, RN, PhD
Associate Professor of Nursing
Assistant Professor of Medicine (Research)
Oregon Health Sciences University
Portland, Oregon

RICHARD M. BUTLER, DO
Associate Professor of Medicine
Michigan State University College of
  Osteopathic Medicine
Director of Ambulatory Training
Mount Clemens General Hospital
Mount Clemens, Michigan

BARBARA N. CAMPAIGNE, PhD
Assistant Professor of Pediatrics
Division of Cardiology
Children's Hospital Medical Center
Cincinnati, Ohio

SHARON R. CLARK, PhD, FNP
Associate Professor of Nursing
Assistant Professor of Medicine (Research)
Oregon Health Sciences University
Portland, Oregon

MARK R. COLVILLE, MD
Associate Professor of Surgery
Division of Orthopedics
Oregon Health Sciences University
Portland, Oregon

RICHARD A. DEYO, MD, MPH
Professor, Departments of Medicine and
  Health Services
Director, Robert Wood Johnson Clinical
  Scholars Program
University of Washington
Seattle, Washington

DIANE L. ELLIOT, MD
Professor of Medicine
Associate Director, Human Performance
  Laboratory
Division of General Internal Medicine
Oregon Health Sciences University
Portland, Oregon

LINN GOLDBERG, MD
Associate Professor of Medicine
Director, Human Performance Laboratory
Division of General Internal Medicine
Oregon Health Sciences University
Portland, Oregon

SIG-LINDA JACOBSON, MD
Assistant Professor of Medicine
Department of Obstetrics and Gynecology
Oregon Health Sciences University
Portland, Oregon

**TERENCE KAVANAGH, MD, FRCPC,
  DPhysMed (Lond.), FACC, FCCP**
Medical Director and Chief Executive
  Officer
Toronto Rehabilitation Centre
Associate Professor, Department of
  Medicine
University of Toronto
Toronto, Ontario

MARK J. MORTON, MD
Associate Professor of Medicine
Division of Cardiology
Oregon Health Sciences University
Portland, Oregon

ERIC S. ORWOLL, MD
Chief, Endocrinology and Metabolism
Portland Veterans Administration
  Medical Center
Associate Professor of Medicine
Oregon Health Sciences University
Portland, Oregon

PATRICIA PAINTER, PhD
Transplant Exercise Physiologist
University of California at San Francisco
  Transplant Service
Stanford University Center for Research
  in Disease Prevention
Moffitt Hospital
San Francisco, California

MARILYN S. PAUL, BA
Research Assistant
Division of Cardiology
Oregon Health Sciences University
Portland, Oregon

FELIX J. ROGERS, DO
(Clinical) Professor of Medicine
Michigan State University College of
  Osteopathic Medicine
Down River Cardiology Consultants
Trenton, Michigan

C. BARR TAYLOR, MD
Professor
Department of Psychiatry and Behavioral
  Sciences
Stanford University School of Medicine
Stanford, California

MARYL L. WINNINGHAM, PhD
Assistant Professor
University of Utah College of Nursing
Salt Lake City, Utah

THANK YOU FOR YOUR BUSINESS!

Thank you for your order from AnybookUK. We value your business and
hope that you were pleased. If so, please leave positive feedback for us;
if not, please contact us first so that we can make it right!
Customer Service : anybookuk@bellsouth.net

ORDER# 736-8824774-8849807   12.10.07

Exercise for Prevention and Treatment of Illness
[Paperback] by Goldberg, Linn

ISBN   080364163X   PRICE 25.75

SKU   VI-080364163X

BUYER   jane.silk@btinternet.com

TO REORDER YOUR UPS DIRECT THERMAL LABELS:

1. Access our supply ordering web site at **UPS.COM®** or contact UPS at 800-877-8652.

2. Please refer to label #0211790801 when ordering.

Contents

. . . .

PART I

Epidemiologic and Physiologic Considerations

CHAPTER 1

EXERCISE IN HEALTHY INDIVIDUALS

RICHARD M. BUTLER, DO, and FELIX J. ROGERS, DO

PHYSICAL ACTIVITY AND
  CORONARY HEART DISEASE
  Cross-Sectional Studies
  Longitudinal Studies
PRESCRIBING EXERCISE
  PROGRAMS
  Pre-Exercise Evaluation
  Exercise testing

*Components of the Exercise
  Prescription*
Risks During Exercise
  Cardiovascular risks
  Musculoskeletal injuries
  Environmental stresses
  Implementing exercise
  programs

Over the past several years, there has been increasing interest in prescribed exercise for the promotion and maintenance of health. A large body of scientific information now exists supporting the prescription of physical activity for many clinical situations. This information has resulted in the United States Public Health Service declaring ". . . physical fitness and exercise to be 1 of 15 priority areas in which improvement is expected to lead to substantial reduction in premature morbidity and mortality."[1]

Primary care providers are in an excellent position to encourage patients to become more active. It is important that clinicians develop an understanding of the benefits of regular physical activity and become its proponents for their patients. In this chapter we review data supporting the clinical application of exercise for health maintenance and promotion, focusing on its role in the primary prevention of coronary heart disease (CHD). In addition, we outline the principles of exercise prescription and suggest methods by which physicians may successfully promote and maintain exercise programs.

Acknowledgment:
We wish to thank Richard Frankel, PhD; Marlene Woo, PA-C, and Joyce Mooty, RD, for their editorial assistance.

Physical Activity and Coronary Heart Disease

Most members of western industrialized societies remain sedentary in their occupations and leisure time. Stephens, Jacobs, and White[2] concluded that fewer than 20% of U.S. adults engage in enough regular physical activity. Approximately 40% of the adult population perform some degree of moderate exercise; the remaining 40% are completely sedentary. Similar trends have been reported in school-age children.[3]

Although a sedentary lifestyle may affect several aspects of health, it is the relationship to coronary heart disease that has received the most study. It has been hypothesized that a sedentary lifestyle may independently contribute to the development of coronary heart disease. To evaluate this relationship, numerous epidemiologic studies have been conducted. The majority of these studies have been observational. These studies evaluate relationships among naturally occurring events within a population, using either cross-sectional or longitudinal designs.[4]

Cross-sectional studies are performed by identifying a random sample of individuals free of CHD within a population. These individuals are evaluated for the presence of coronary heart disease risk factors and range of physical activity. Multivariant analysis is used to determine if increased levels of physical activity are independently correlated with more favorable coronary risk profiles.

Longitudinal investigations also begin by evaluating coronary risk factors and physical activity in a random sample of individuals free of CAD. The sample is followed to determine if physical activity level at baseline independently predicts the development of coronary risk factors or active coronary heart disease.

Numerous methods have been used to quantify physical activity levels. Techniques include standardized questionnaires or structured interviews during which participants recall past and present leisure-time activity levels or total activity levels. Individuals also may be stratified by job classification and energy expended at work. In addition, objective measures of physical fitness obtained during exercise testing have been used.

Conclusions from observational studies are limited, because they may reflect healthier individuals selecting more active lifestyles, rather than exercise causing improved levels of health. However, well-performed observational studies incorporate design techniques that control for these and other possible sources of bias, improving the strength of the observed relationships.[5] Much of the support for the beneficial effects of physical activity has come from observational investigations.

CROSS-SECTIONAL STUDIES

Table 1–1 presents the results of cross-sectional studies evaluating the association of physical activity and coronary risk profile. The studies are organized according to the method used to assess physical activity. All studies using questionnaires to assess leisure-time activity have found a more favorable risk profile in active individuals,[6-8] although this association accounted for only a small amount of the variability in coronary risk profile in one study.[6] In contrast, questionnaire assessment of occupational activity was either not associated with the coronary risk profile,[7] or inversely correlated with increased levels of cigarette smoking and systolic blood pressure.[8]

Investigators using both exercise testing and questionnaires have generally found that reports of habitual activity correlate positively with measures of physical fitness. Questionnaire assessment of leisure-time activity or combined leisure-time and occupational activity appear most strongly correlated with physical capacity.[9-12] Questionnaires derived only from occupational activity are not as strongly correlated with measures of physical abilities.[9,13]

Ten cross-sectional studies[9-18] evaluating the relationship of objective measures of physical fitness to coronary risk profile have found a beneficial association with at least two coronary risk factors. Increased physical fitness appeared most consistently associated with lower blood pressure and lower percentage of body fat, and was variably related to the serum lipid profile.

The relationship of physical fitness to cigarette smoking is inconsistent. Three studies[9,16,17] have found a negative correlation between physical fitness and cigarette smoking; four have found either no relationship[11,15] or increased levels of smoking among those with greater physical fitness.[10,12]

In summary, cross-sectional studies appear to support the hypothesis that individuals who report increased exercise during leisure time or demonstrate higher levels of physical fitness have a more desirable coronary risk profile. However, questionnaire assessment of only occupational activity does not appear to have this association.

LONGITUDINAL STUDIES

Table 1–2 summarizes the results of longitudinal studies evaluating the relationship of physical activity and cardiovascular health. The studies are organized by outcome measure and method of physical activity assessment. Investigators have found that increased physical fitness[19] or increased levels of reported daily activity[20] are associated with a lower risk for the future development of hypertension in previously normotensive individuals. Paffenbarger and coworkers[20] found that the protective benefit of increased physical activity appeared greatest in those reporting participation in vigorous activities such as running or swimming, even for individuals who were overweight.

Longitudinal studies[11,21-23a] also have found that increased physical fitness is associated with a decreased incidence of future coronary heart disease. Two separate investigations,[24,25] which used job classification to quantify activity levels, have found that individuals who spend less energy on the job are at a greater risk for future coronary heart disease. However, when recall questionnaires are used to classify occupational activity, this beneficial association is not confirmed.[23,26,27]

Other studies[23,28,29] have evaluated leisure-time activity with recall questionnaires. Two separate groups of investigators[28,29] have found that self-reports of increased participation in leisure-time physical activity are associated with reduced risk of fatal and nonfatal coronary events. In contrast, another group[23] does not observe this relationship.

Of the investigators using questionnaires to assess total daily activity, all[30-33] have found a beneficial association between increasing habitual activity and decreased risk of future coronary heart disease among several different

Table 1–1 CROSS-SECTIONAL STUDIES EVALUATING THE ASSOCIATION OF PHYSICAL ACTIVITY AND CORONARY RISK PROFILE

Author	Subjects	Assessment		Results Increased Activity Level Associated with				
				Total Chol	HDL	Obesity	BP	Smoking
Folsom et al[6]	1,616 M/F age 25–74 Minnesota Heart Survey	Questionnaire Leisure-time activity		0	↑	↓	↓*	↓
Hickey et al[7]	15,171 M age 25–74 Irish Heart Foundation	Questionnaire Leisure-time and occupational activity	LTA:	↓	NA	↓	↓	↓
			OA:	0	NA	0	0	0
Bjartveit, Foss, and Gjervig[8]	57,859 M/F age 35–49 in 3 Norwegian counties	Questionnaire Leisure-time and occupational activity	LTA:	↓	NA	0	0	↓
			OA:	0	NA	0	↑	↑
Leon et al[9]	175 M age 36–59	Max GXT plus questionnaire Leisure-time and occupational activity	PWC:	0	NA	↓	0	↓
				PWC + correlated with LTA; not with OA.				
Crow et al[10]	12,860 M age 35–57 MRFIT study	Submax GXT plus questionnaire Leisure-time activity	PWC:	0	NA	↓	↓	↑
				PWC + correlated with LTA.				
Sobolski et al[13]	2,565 M age 40–55 Belgian and Slovakian workers	Submax GXT plus questionnaire Leisure-time and occupational activity	PWC:	↓	↑	↓	↓	0
				PWC + correlated with LTA and OA (association with OA was weak).				

Study	Population	Test						
Ekelund et al[11]	4,276 M age 30–69 Lipid Research Clinics	Submax GXT plus questionnaire Total activity	PWC:	↓ (↓LDL) (↓TG) PWC + correlated with questionnaire activity score.	↑	0	↓	0
Gordon et al[12]	6,238 M age 34–60 Lipid Research Clinics	Submax GXT plus Questionnaire Total activity	PWC:	0 PWC + correlated with questionnaire activity score.	↑	NA	↓	↑
Cooper et al[14]	3,000 M mean age 45	Max GXT	PWC:	↓ (↓TG)	NA	↓	↓	NA
Patton and Vogel[15]	360 M age 17–35 Military personnel	Max GXT	PWC:	↓↑†	NA	↓	0	0
Brown, Myles, and Allen[16]	250 M age 18–50 Canadian Forces personnel	Submax GXT	PWC:	↓	NA	↓	↓	↓‡
Gibbons et al[17]	1,700 F age 18–65	Max GXT	PWC:	0 (↓Chol/HDL) (↓TG)	↑	NA	↓	→ (weak)
Sedwick et al[18]	1,500 M/F age 20–65	Submax GXT	PWC: M:	↓ (↓TG)	NA	NA	↓	NA
			F:	0	NA	NA	↓	NA

*Female only.

†Age 26–35 only.

‡Age < 30 only.

Key: Chol = cholesterol, HDL = high-density lipoprotein, BP = blood pressure, M = male, F = female, 0 = no association, ↑ = increased, ↓ = decreased, LTA = leisure-time activity, NA = not addressed in this study, OA = occupational activity, Max GXT = maximal graded exercise testing, PWC = physical working capacity, + = positively, Submax GXT = submaximal graded exercise testing, LDL = low-density lipoprotein, TG = triglycerides.

Table 1-2 LONGITUDINAL STUDIES EVALUATING THE ASSOCIATION OF PHYSICAL ACTIVITY AND CARDIOVASCULAR HEALTH

Author	Subjects/Duration	Assessment	Results
			Incidence of Hypertension
Blair et al[19]	6,039 M/F age 20–65/ 1–12 yr (median, 4 yr)	Max GXT	↓PWC: 1.52 times ↑risk; ↓PWC plus baseline BP in upper range of normal: 4 times ↑risk
Paffenbarger et al[20]	14,998 M alumni age 35–74/6–10 yr	Questionnaire of daily activity	2 h/wk vigorous sports: 35% ↓incidence*
			Incidence of Coronary Heart Disease
Peters et al[21]	2,779 M age 35–55/mean, 4.8 yr	Submax GXT	Lower ½ PWC: 2 times ↑risk
Ekelund et al[11]	4,275 M age 30–69/mean, 8.5 yr	Submax GXT	↓PWC: 2.8 times ↑risk
Blair et al[22]	10,244 M (mean age, 41 yr) 3,120 F (mean age, 50 yr)/mean, 8 yr	Max GXT	↓PWC: 8 times ↑risk CHD death in M; 9 times ↑risk CHD death in F
Sobolski et al[23]	2,363 M age 40–55/5 yr	Submax GXT and Questionnaire of occupational and leisure-time activity	↓PWC: ↑risk; LTA: Not related† OA: Not related
Paffenbarger and Hale[24]	6,351 M longshoremen age 35–74/22 yr	Job classification	Jobs expending < 1,800 kcal/d: 50% ↑in CHD death 3 times ↑in sudden death
Brunner et al[25]	10,517 M/F Israeli kibbutzniks age 40–64/15 yr	Job classification	2–3.5 times ↑risk

Study	Population/Duration	Method	Activity Type	Findings
Keys[26]	12,763 M in 7 countries/10 yr	Questionnaire	Occupational activity	OA: Not associated
Punsar and Karvonen[27]	1,711 M in eastern Finland age 40–59/10 yr	Questionnaire	Occupational activity	OA: Not associated
Morris et al[28]	17,944 M civil servants in Britain age 40–65/8.5 yr	Questionnaire	Leisure-time activity	LTA: *Vigorous LTA* had 40% ↓risk of fatal MI, and 50% ↓risk of nonfatal MI
Slattery, Jacobs, and Nichaman[29]	3,043 M railroad workers/17–20 yr	Questionnaire	Leisure-time activity	↓LTA: 1.39 times ↑risk of CHD death in most sedentary compared to most active men
Kannel and Sorlie[30]	3,320 M/F in Framingham study age 35–64/14 yr	Questionnaire	Total activity	↓TA: ↑risk in men No association in women
Garcia-Palmieri et al[31]	8,793 M in Puerto Rico age 45–64/8.25 yr	Questionnaire	Total activity	↓TA: ↑risk
Paffenbarger et al[32]	16,936 Harvard alumni age 35–74/12–16 yr	Questionnaire	Total activity	TA: Expending < 2,000 kcal/wk: 31% ↑risk for CHD mortality
Leon et al[33]	12,138 M in MRFIT study age 35–57/7 yr	Questionnaire	Total activity	TA: Engaging in 30–60 min/d of light to moderate activity: 36% ↓CHD mortality

* Strongest benefit seen in overweight individuals.
† Those reporting vigorous activity had half the incidence of CHD, but results were not statistically significant.
Key: M = male, F = female, Max GXT = maximal graded exercise testing, ↓ = decreased, PWC = physical working capacity, ↑ = increased, BP = blood pressure, Submax GXT = submaximal graded exercise testing, CHD = coronary heart disease, LTA = leisure-time activity, OA = occupational activity, MI = myocardial infarction, TA = total activity

male populations. However, a beneficial effect was not observed in women by the only investigators to include them in their analysis.[30] Clearly more data are needed to determine the role of physical activity in the maintenance of women's health.

To summarize, most, but not all, epidemiologic investigations have confirmed a beneficial association between increased reports of habitual activity or direct measures of physical fitness and cardiovascular health. When only occupational activity is assessed by questionnaires, however, both cross-sectional and longitudinal studies have not documented a beneficial association. In contrast, investigators using job classification to assess occupational activity have confirmed a beneficial association. These data may allow insight as to how much activity seems necessary. Although a beneficial effect of low-level activities such as gardening and walking[34] has been observed, a more consistent relationship appears when individuals report participation in more vigorous activities such as running, swimming, and cross-country skiing.[20,23,32,33] It is important to note, however, that lower-level activities do appear to confer beneficial effects.[35]

Prescribing Exercise Programs

Aerobic exercise is associated with numerous benefits. In addition to a more desirable cardiovascular risk profile and lower incidence of coronary heart disease (as discussed in Chapters 2 and 3), regular physical activity may also promote improved psychological well-being.[36-38] However, health care professionals do not often counsel their patients on the benefits of regular exercise. Those physicians who do attempt to implement exercise programs often give incomplete and inaccurate information to patients.[39,40] An understanding of the components of an exercise prescription and strategies for implementation facilitates successful promotion of physical activity.

PRE-EXERCISE EVALUATION

Before encouraging sedentary individuals to become more active, it is important to identify those who may be at increased risk for adverse cardiovascular responses during exercise. The American College of Sports Medicine[41] has developed a classification system that can be used to identify such individuals. The three risk categories shown in Table 1–3 have been proposed based on patient age and the presence of underlying coronary risk factors or active CHD. The age cutoffs identify individuals within each group who should be evaluated by a physician prior to beginning an exercise program. Individuals below the age cutoffs should be at low risk for adverse events during exercise. They need only receive initial instruction regarding the principles of exercise prescription and then may proceed to unsupervised exercise.

An alternative approach to identifying higher-risk individuals has been developed by Chisholm and associates.[42] These authors have developed a self-administered set of seven questions known as the Physical Activity Readi-

Table 1–3 **INDIVIDUALS WHO SHOULD UNDERGO PRE-EXERCISE EVALUATION* PRIOR TO BEGINNING AN EXERCISE PROGRAM**

Risk Category†	Age
Apparently healthy individuals‡	
Men	≥45
Women	≥50
Higher-risk individuals§	
Men	≥35
Women	≥40
Individuals with disease¶	All ages

* The pre-exercise evaluation should include a directed assessment for abnormalities of the cardiopulmonary, peripheral vascular, musculoskeletal, and metabolic or endocrine systems (see text).
† Adapted from the American College of Sports Medicine.[41]
‡ Without *coronary risk factors*: hypertension, diabetes mellitus, family history of coronary artery disease prior to age 50, obesity, smoking, increased cholesterol, and sedentary lifestyle.
§ With one or more known *coronary risk factors* (see above).
¶ With known cardiac or pulmonary disease or symptoms suggestive of cardiopulmonary disease.

ness Questionnaire (Table 1–4). This questionnaire can be easily displayed in a physician's office or other community settings. Individuals who respond yes to any question should consult a physician prior to implementing an exercise program. Those without a positive response should be at low risk and after receiving initial instruction may proceed to unsupervised exercise. The safety of this questionnaire has been validated against objective measures such as resting and exercise electrocardiography.[42]

The pre-exercise evaluation should include a focused history and physical examination. Its purpose is to identify abnormalities in the cardiopulmonary, peripheral vascular, musculoskeletal, and metabolic or endocrine systems that could influence the safety of an exercise program. Previous and current activity levels should be assessed. Use of medications should be reviewed, including use of nonprescription drugs. The current level of alcohol and cigarette consumption should also be noted. The total cholesterol level should be measured for all individuals who have not undergone prior cholesterol screening. Lipoprotein subtype analysis can be performed as recommended by the National Cholesterol Education Program.[43] Patients taking diuretics should have a serum potassium determination. Further laboratory studies are not helpful in the pre-exercise evaluation and are needed only to facilitate diagnosis in

Table 1–4 **THE PHYSICAL ACTIVITY READINESS QUESTIONNAIRE (PAR-Q)**

1. Has your doctor ever said you have heart trouble?
2. Do you frequently have pains in your heart and chest?
3. Do you often feel faint or have spells of severe dizziness?
4. Has a doctor ever said your blood pressure was too high?
5. Has your doctor ever told you that you have a bone or joint problem such as arthritis that has been aggravated by exercise, or might be made worse with exercise?
6. Is there a good physical reason not mentioned here why you should not follow an activity program even if you wanted to?
7. Are you over age 65 and not accustomed to vigorous exercise?

Adapted from Chisholm et al.[42] p. 376.

individuals with abnormal symptoms or physical findings. Resting electrocardiograms (ECGs) are of no value in asymptomatic individuals with normal findings on cardiac examination and should be performed only to aid in the diagnosis of abnormal history and physical examination findings.[44]

Exercise Testing

The use of exercise ECG analysis to screen asymptomatic individuals prior to starting an exercise program is controversial.[45] Although exercise testing has been used to evaluate the cardiovascular response to exercise, measure functional capacity, and establish heart rate parameters to guide the exercise prescription, its main recommended use is to identify individuals who may have latent CHD. Those with undiagnosed CHD, particularly sedentary individuals, appear to be at an increased risk for cardiac events during exertion. One study[46] reported that among sedentary individuals with undiagnosed CHD, primary cardiac arrest was 56 times more likely to occur during exercise than at rest. Although habitually active individuals appeared to have a much lower incidence of cardiac arrest, they too experienced a fivefold increase in risk during activity compared to rest.

However, exercise electrocardiography is limited in its ability to identify asymptomatic individuals who may be at greater risk prior to training. The low prevalence of CHD in asymptomatic populations results in a far greater likelihood that a positive exercise ECG in an asymptomatic individual is due to a false-positive response than to undiscovered CHD. It has been shown that when applied to asymptomatic, low-risk populations, 16 out of 17 abnormal ECG responses will be false positives.[47] For exercise testing to be of value it must be applied to those whose pretest likelihood of CHD is high enough to improve the predictive value of a positive test.

The American College of Sports Medicine[41] recommends that exercise testing be performed on all individuals identified in Table 1–3. An alternative approach to the use of exercise testing is presented in Figure 1–1. Individuals in the "apparently healthy" group, with a normal pre-exercise evaluation, may proceed to unsupervised exercise without testing. If, during initial low-level exercise training, individuals experience any difficulties suggestive of CHD, then a symptom-limited maximal exercise test should be performed. If abnormal symptoms or physical findings suggestive of underlying heart disease are discovered during the pre-exercise evaluation, we recommend performing a symptom-limited maximal exercise test prior to the initiation of training. Exercise testing should be performed for individuals in the "higher-risk" group, with one or more CHD risk factors, if they are age 50 or older. All individuals, regardless of age, who have known CHD or symptoms suggestive of underlying disease also should undergo exercise testing. Further testing, including thallium scintigraphy and coronary angiography, would be performed based on coronary risk stratification.[48]

COMPONENTS OF THE EXERCISE PRESCRIPTION

The prescription for aerobic exercise is divided into five components (Table 1–5): mode, intensity, duration, frequency, and progression of training.

The exercise mode most often recommended is dynamic exercise that uses large muscle groups and can be maintained for a prolonged duration. These

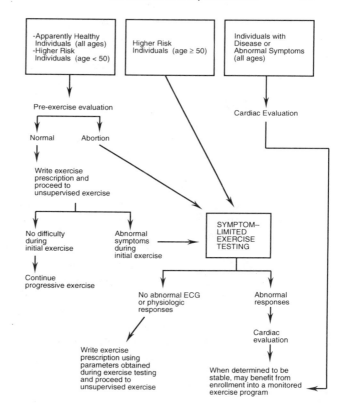

Figure 1–1 Algorithm for the use of exercise testing in pre-exercise evaluation. See Table 1–3 for definitions. (ECG, electrocardiography.)

activities are fueled primarily by aerobic metabolism and include walking, jogging, running, swimming, bicycling, cross-country skiing, and aerobic dance. Exercises that involve both arms and legs, such as use of the Schwinn Airdyne stationary cycle (Schwinn Bicycle Co., Chicago), cross-country skiing simulators, and rowing machines, may be performed by individuals who desire

Table 1–5 **COMPONENTS OF AN EXERCISE PRESCRIPTION**

Component	Comments
Exercise mode	*Aerobic activities* (i.e., walking, running, aerobic dance, bicycling, swimming, cross-country skiing)
	Strength training
Exercise intensity	70% to 85% of MHR
	"Moderate" to "strong" (or 3 to 5) on the Borg scale*
Exercise duration	5 minutes of warm-up exercise at low intensity
	20 to 60 minutes at training heart rate
	3 minutes of cool-down exercise at lower intensity
Exercise frequency	Three to seven sessions spaced throughout the week
Progression of training	*Initial conditioning stage*: First 4 to 6 weeks
	Improvement stage: Week 6 to 6 months
	Maintenance phase: 6 months and on

*See Table 1–6 for Borg[52] scale.
Key: MHR = maximum heart rate (either measured during maximal exercise testing or estimated with the formula 220 − age).
Adapted from the American College of Sports Medicine: *Guidelines for Exercise Testing and Prescription*, ed 4. © Lea & Febiger: Philadelphia; 1988.

improved upper-body aerobic fitness. All individuals should receive instruction on the proper use of the exercise equipment prior to beginning a training program.

Low-impact exercises such as swimming and bicycling are recommended for individuals with conditions, such as obesity or arthritis, that place them at increased risk for musculoskeletal injury (see Chapters 4 and 10). A history of activities the individual enjoys will help guide the choice of mode. An ability to vary the activity also may improve compliance.

Circuit weight training (CWT)[49] is a type of strength (resistive) training available in many health-club settings. CWT differs from traditional, or priority, weight-lifting programs in that the resistance exercises are performed at stations arranged in a circuit. Each station exercises a different muscle group, often alternating between upper and lower body. A single set of 10 to 15 repetitions at a moderate amount of resistance, usually 40% to 60% of maximal exertion, is performed at each station. The exerciser moves from station to station in the circuit in a continuous fashion with minimal rest (15 to 30 seconds) between sets. Two to three circuits are usually completed in a single session. Although free weights can be used, most circuits contain specialized exercise machines. The continuous nature and high number of repetitions involved in CWT may improve both muscular strength and endurance.[49] The lower resistance during CWT may decrease injury risk, making this form of weight lifting more appealing.

Priority, or noncircuit, weight training differs in that fewer repetitions with greater resistance than CWT are performed, resulting in larger increases in strength without affecting aerobic capacity. Although stations are used, as in CWT, training usually consists of exercising at one station with a rest period between sets, without alternating to other stations. Thus training is slower, allowing for more recovery time before repeating an exercise or moving to another station. The weight lifting may be performed in a pyramid fashion, beginning with lower weights (40% to 60% of maximal exertion) and increasing to a higher weight. Alternatively, the amount of weight could be fixed (60% of maximal exertion or greater), without changing the weight after the interval warm-up period. However, the potential for injury is greater with higher levels of resistance.

Aerobic exercise intensity is guided by measuring heart rate or using perceived exertion scales. When using heart rate parameters, the training rate is 70% to 85% of the individual's maximum heart rate. Maximum heart rate can either be measured directly during graded exercise testing or estimated with the formula 220 − age. A recent study[50] using expired gas analysis has confirmed the accuracy of this equation for determining exercise intensity parameters. Patients should be taught to monitor exercise heart rate and should be instructed to alter intensity of exercise to maintain the prescribed range.

An alternative method for setting exercise intensity is to use ratings of perceived exertion. Borg and Linderholm[51] are credited with initial attempts to relate perceived levels of exertion to objective measures of exercise intensity. More recently, a 10-point numerical scale[52] containing parallel verbal descriptions of exertion level has been developed (Table 1–6). Using this scale, most individuals should be directed to exercise at a numerical value of 3 to 5, or a verbal rating of "moderate" to "strong." An advantage of perceived exertion

Table 1–6 **BORG SCALE OF PERCEIVED EXERTION***

Numerical Rating	Verbal Rating
0	Nothing at all
0.5	Very, very weak
1	Very weak
2	Weak
3	Moderate
4	Somewhat strong
5	Strong
6	
7	Very strong
8	
9	
10	Very, very strong
•	Maximal

*See also Borg's 20-point scale, Table 3–6.
Adapted from Borg GA: Psychosocial bases of perceived exertion. *Med Sci Sports Exerc* 1982; 472:194–381; ©Williams & Wilkins.

scales is that individuals may avoid over-exertion by not exceeding a sensation of "strong" work regardless of the heart rate response. In addition, individuals using medications that may alter heart rate response, such as beta-adrenergic blocking agents, may more accurately guide intensity with perceived exertion. An additional rule of thumb is that exercise intensity should be such that an individual is able to carry on a conversation without difficulty during exercise. Finally, heart rate should return to within 10 beats of baseline values within 10 to 15 minutes after stopping exercise.

Exercise duration at the training heart rate should range from 20 to 60 minutes.[41] Each exercise period should begin with gentle stretching of the muscles that will be used during training. Stretching is performed by slowly developing tension across a muscle group and holding the stretch without bouncing motions for 5 to 10 seconds. After stretching, 3 to 5 minutes of low-intensity aerobic exercise is performed before achieving the training heart rate, to begin increasing muscle blood flow and to reduce the possibility of injuries. Exercise sessions should conclude with a cool-down period during which intensity is gradually decreased to prevent venous pooling and post-exercise hypotension. Stretching after exercise will improve flexibility and decrease muscle stiffness.

Exercise frequency should begin with three sessions equally spaced throughout the week. Training frequency can be increased as conditioning occurs.

The final component of an exercise prescription is a schedule for training progression. Three stages are identified (see Table 1–5). The initial conditioning stage is a period of 4 to 6 weeks, during which exercise intensity should be in the lower range of 70% of the maximum heart rate. Exercise duration and frequency should also be set in the lower limits. The next phase of training has been labeled the improvement stage. During this period, the intensity, duration, and frequency of exercise can be increased at 2- to 3-week intervals. As aerobic fitness improves, it will become necessary to perform higher work loads to achieve prescribed training heart rates. By 6 months, individuals have entered the maintenance phase, in which the major emphasis is on continued compliance with the exercise program. Varying activities and attempting to keep exercise enjoyable are essential to long-term compliance.

RISKS DURING EXERCISE

Although numerous benefits can be achieved when one exercises on a regular basis, several risks also are identifiable. Exercise prescriptions can be developed to minimize the potential for injury.

Cardiovascular Risks

Although cardiac arrest during exercise in experienced runners has been reported,[53,54] myocardial infarction and sudden cardiac death during exercise are rare events. Those at greatest risk are habitually sedentary individuals with underlying CHD who quickly progress from rest to highly intense physical work.[46] Habitually active individuals, on the other hand, have a much lower risk of cardiac death during exertion.[46,55]

To minimize the cardiovascular risks, it is important to initiate exercise programs for sedentary individuals with lower-intensity activities, such as walking. Individuals should be instructed to stop exercising if they experience unusual symptoms such as chest discomfort, excessive shortness of breath, leg claudication, or dizziness. These may be warning signs of an impending cardiac event, and the individual should be evaluated by a physician prior to resuming exercise. If these principles and the previous guidelines for pre-exercise evaluation are followed, the cardiovascular risks during exercise should be small.

Musculoskeletal Injuries

Musculoskeletal complaints appear to be relatively common during exercise. In a retrospective survey[56] of men and women runners participating in a 10-km race, it was found that more than one third of respondents had experienced an injury in the previous year. However, most injuries resulted only in a slowing or reduction in weekly running mileage, with approximately 15% reporting that their complaints were severe enough to seek medical attention. A retrospective analysis[57] of aerobic dance injuries over an 18-month period reported that 43% of students and 76% of instructors experienced a musculoskeletal complaint, but most injuries were not severe enough to require cessation of dancing.

In addition to acute injuries, there has been concern that individuals who perform high-impact exercises, such as running for many years, may accelerate degenerative joint disease. A cross-sectional survey[58] found that individuals aged 50 to 72 years who had been running for an average of 11 years reported less musculoskeletal disability and fewer physician office visits than a matched control group. Another study[59] found no greater clinical or radiologic evidence of osteoarthritis in male runners (mean age, 55 years) than in a matched control group of nonrunners. Studies are now evaluating the possibility of long-term musculoskeletal injury in runners,[58] but current evidence does not support this concern.

Several recommendations can be followed to lower the risk of acute musculoskeletal injury. An increase in either the frequency or duration of exercise is associated with a greater incidence of injuries.[56,60] During initial stages of training, patients should limit sessions to three times per week, with durations of 20 minutes at their training heart rate. Increases should be made slowly as fitness is achieved. Using different training modes, as well as alternating high-intensity and low-intensity training sessions, also may assist injury prevention.

Obese individuals and those with arthritis should engage in low-impact activities such as stationary cycling, swimming, or walking programs (see Chapters 4 and 10). Environmental factors such as running surface also are of concern. Running on pavement may lead to more musculoskeletal complaints, and either a softer surface or greater shoe cushion should be recommended.

Accidents can be another cause of injury. Reflective clothing should be worn when exercising in the dark. Bicycling on city streets deserves particular mention. One survey of 1,200 university students found that about one third had experienced a bicycling accident in the previous 3-year period.[61] About two thirds of the accidents resulted in an injury, with approximately one third of those injured seeking medical attention. Head injuries are added risks for bicyclists, and the importance of well-fitting protective headgear should be stressed. In addition, bicyclists should be reminded to ride with the direction of traffic. Appropriate bicycle lighting is necessary during low-light conditions.

Environmental Stresses

Varying environmental conditions may influence the safety of exercise. Of particular importance is heat stress.[62] During exertion, large amounts of heat are generated by active muscles. Since hot and humid environments reduce the body's ability to dissipate heat, exercise during these conditions can increase the risk for heat-related injury. The risk is highest among those in poor physical condition. Physical training in warm temperatures promotes a process known as heat acclimatization. The body's ability to dissipate heat is increased through physiologic adaptations that include shunting of large volumes of blood to cutaneous vessels and increased rates of sweating.

The most common form of exertional heat injury is heat exhaustion, a condition heralded by symptoms of progressive weakness, fatigue, and frontal headache. Findings of the physical examination may include alterations in cognitive ability, as well as hypotension and tachycardia. Progression to heatstroke may occur. Treatment of heat exhaustion includes immediate cessation of exercise and rehydration. If the patient can ingest fluids, then a 0.1% sodium chloride solution (two 10-grain salt tablets in 1 liter of water) can be consumed.[63] For severely affected individuals, particularly if alterations in consciousness are present, IV normal saline solutions should be administered.

Heatstroke is a medical emergency. The classic findings include hypotension with tachycardia and possible shock, vomiting, diarrhea, and impairment of mental functioning. Convulsions and coma can occur. Although the cessation of sweating is an important finding, it has been reported to occur in only 50% of victims.[62] Heatstroke always is accompanied by large increases in core body temperature, from levels of 104° F (40° C) to as high as 112° F (44° C). Laboratory abnormalities include evidence of disseminated intravascular coagulation, decreased blood glucose, and decreased potassium. Rhabdomyolysis elevates muscle enzymes such as creatine kinase. Treatment is directed at rapid lowering of body temperature and fluid replacement. Use of standard rectal thermometers may not accurately document the level of hyperpyrexia, and deep core temperature must be measured 15 to 20 cm from the rectal verge with a thermometer capable of recording extremely high temperatures.

Several factors increase an individual's risk of heat-related injury. These include obesity, a history of burns sustained over a large percentage of body surface area, poor physical condition, and diabetes mellitus with autonomic neuropathies. Additional host factors include salt, water, and potassium depletion. Certain drugs can alter the body's ability to compensate for heat stress. Included are diuretics, anticholinergic agents (such as tricyclic compounds that produce anticholinergic side effects), phenothiazines, haloperidol, and antihistamines.[62] Acute alcohol intoxication also may impair the ability to dissipate heat.

To reduce the risk of heat-related injury, the body must be able to cool itself by sweating. Loose clothing that maximizes the amount of skin exposed to the air should be worn during hot and humid conditions. People should be warned never to exercise in plastic sweat clothing, which does not permit evaporation of water. Maintaining adequate hydration before and during exercise is important. Encourage exercise in the cooler morning and evening hours during hot summer weather. Most importantly, warn people to stop exercising when early symptoms of heat exhaustion, such as progressive muscle fatigue, headache, or nausea, appear.

Implementing Exercise Programs

CASE: J.A., a 47-year-old man, presents with a complaint of an upper respiratory tract infection. He has not seen a physician for several years. After he is evaluated and a treatment plan for his current complaint is recommended, it is suggested that J.A. might benefit from a complete history and physical examination. He is scheduled to return in 2 weeks. Before leaving he has a total cholesterol level drawn.

During the return visit, a review of cardiac risk factors reveals no history of hypertension or diabetes; he is 5 feet 8 inches tall and weighs 185 pounds. He has never smoked, and there is no family history of premature CHD. His total cholesterol level is 245 mg/dL. He lives a sedentary lifestyle and does not engage in regular exercise. J.A. is a salesman for a computer company. The majority of his day is spent behind a desk making phone calls, or in his car. He avoids stair climbing and uses elevators when possible. Review of systems and physical examination are unremarkable.

When asked whether he has ever considered adopting an exercise program, he states that some colleagues at work had recently joined a health club near the office and that he had thought about joining. Using Figure 1–1, it is determined that J.A. could proceed with unsupervised exercise without exercise testing. If he should experience abnormal symptoms during initial training, then exercise testing may be performed.

COMMENT: J.A. has three coronary artery risk factors: obesity, elevated blood cholesterol, and a sedentary lifestyle (see Table 1–3). He is therefore placed into the "higher-risk" category. It is recommended that men older than age 35 in this category undergo a pre-exercise history and physical examination. J.A. may benefit from altering his sedentary lifestyle, as an exercise program could reduce body fat and improve his serum cholesterol level. Aerobic exercise also may improve his ability to handle stress and increase his sense of psychological well-being.

When prescribing a training program, give the patient an early opportunity to describe any thoughts or concerns he may have about exercise. Health care providers can structure encounters to allow patients to express their reactions to recommendations.[64] The patient in this example had thought about exercise. If a patient has never considered adopting an exercise program, it would be appropriate to explore prior experiences, beliefs, and knowledge about exercise. Some individuals will have concerns that exercise could be dangerous and should be avoided. Failing to ask patients to describe their worries regarding treatment recommendations may limit acceptance and adherence.[65]

Health care providers should ask patients about their commitment to adhere to recommendations to exercise. A patient's stated acceptance appears to be a strong predictor of compliance.[66] In addition, it would be helpful to ascertain whether the patient believes that an exercise program will benefit him or her personally. The belief of personal benefit, known as "self-efficacy," is a predictor of acceptance and compliance.[67,68]

In this case, J.A. believes that exercise can improve his heath and agrees to an exercise program. He hopes to lose weight and improve his response to stress at work. He describes his previous exercise experiences. His last exercise participation was in college and included intramural flag football and basketball. He has never been injured. Potential barriers to an exercise program are identified. J.A. works long days and is busy in the evenings at home helping his wife care for their two children. He also travels out of town several times a year and feels this might interrupt an exercise routine. J.A. is asked to describe strategies that would facilitate incorporating exercise into his lifestyle. He is able to identify that his colleagues in the office often use the health club before work or during lunchtime and that if he exercises with them it might facilitate adherence to a program.

This interaction highlights an important concept. The health care provider can encourage a patient to identify potential barriers and facilitators that might influence an exercise program. Because patients must adopt lifestyle changes, they should be encouraged to develop their own strategies to facilitate adherence.[65] If a patient has a difficult time with these questions, do not be too quick to supply answers. It may be appropriate to give the patient more time for further consideration and, if necessary, to set a later date to continue the discussion. The importance of encouraging a patient to develop his or her own strategies cannot be overstated. The health care provider's role is to act as a collaborator and lend guidance to an exercise prescription that will optimize benefits and ensure safety.

Copies of Tables 1–5 and 1–6 can be used as handouts. The types of dynamic, aerobic exercises and CWT programs that the patient would like to try should be reviewed. Circuit weight training performed early in a conditioning program improves muscular strength and may decrease the risk for injury during the initial phases of aerobic conditioning.[69]

J.A. initially sets the intensity of aerobic exercise by monitoring his pulse. Since he is 47 years old, using the formula 220 − age, J.A. calculates his maximum heart rate at 173 bpm. His training heart rate is determined within a range of 70% to 85% of maximum (121 to 147 bpm). In the initial conditioning stage (Table 1−5), his training heart rate is set in the lower range of 70% of maximum, or about 120 bpm.

Another index of appropriate exercise intensity is that it is a level that allows individuals to comfortably carry on a conversation. If the heart rate exceeds 10 beats above resting level 10 to 15 minutes after exercise, then subsequent exercise intensity should be decreased. While the individual learns to guide exercise intensity by monitoring heart rate, a perceived exertion level also can be used to determine intensity, using the numerical or verbal scale supplied in Table 1−6.

During the initial conditioning stage (the first 4 to 6 weeks), J.A. is instructed to exercise at his training heart rate for 20 minutes per session, beginning with three exercise sessions per week. Exercise duration gradually can be increased to 30 to 40 minutes if no adverse complications develop. Also, the patient should cool down after exercise (for example, from running to a slow walk) to prevent possible venous pooling and hypotension.

Table 1−5 is used to described the "progression of training." As J.A. progresses into the improvement stage, both frequency and intensity of training can be increased. During the maintenance phase it is most important to develop strategies to maintain exercise compliance.

Long-term adherence to exercise programs is a difficult problem. About 50% of individuals will discontinue exercise during the first year.[70] It is important for patients to plan and develop strategies to help themselves maintain adherence. Common barriers reported include increased demands at work or home, travel requirements, scheduling conflicts, and personal illnesses.[71] Planning may lessen the impact of these occurrences. Developing a social support system and incorporating a spouse or family members into exercise can improve long-term adherence,[72] as may exercising with colleagues at work. Performing activities that promote feelings of enjoyment and well-being also is a strong motivator for long-term adherence.[72] The principles of facilitating implementation of an exercise program are outlined in Table 1−7.

Summary

Even though the benefits of exercise are becoming widely known, most Americans still remain sedentary. It is estimated that less than 10% of sedentary adults will begin an exercise program in a given year, and long-term adherence remains poor among those who do attempt to exercise regularly.[72] Regular physical activity can play an important role in the promotion and maintenance of health for the majority of individuals in our society. Health care providers should take a proactive role toward exercise. Using the outline provided for the pre-exercise evaluation and exercise prescriptions, safe programs can be designed. Individuals should be encouraged to develop personal-

Table 1–7 **STRATEGIES TO FACILITATE THE IMPLEMENTATION OF EXERCISE PROGRAMS**

Begin by asking whether the patient has ever considered adopting an exercise program. If not, follow with a brief description of the personal benefits that the patient could achieve from such a program.

Allow an early opportunity for the patient to respond to the recommendation. Encourage disclosure from the patient of any possible thoughts or reactions.

Determine if the patient believes that an exercise program will benefit him or her personally (self-efficacy). Help the patient set personal goals for exercise.

Elicit from the patient a statement accepting an exercise program

Make writing an exercise prescription the main agenda for the office visit. If necessary, schedule a separate return visit.

Have the patient develop a list of potential barriers and facilitators to adopting and maintaining compliance with an exercise program. This may need to be a "homework" assignment.

Develop a schedule for return visits to review success and progression of the exercise program.

Encourage the patient to involve other people and incorporate a variety of activities in the exercise regimen. Exercise must be "fun" to promote long-term adherence.

ized routines, with the health care provider acting as a collaborator and guide in the process.

REFERENCES

1. Friedewald WT: Physical activity research and coronary heart disease [editorial]. *Public Health Rep* 1985; 100:115–117.
2. Stephens T, Jacobs DR Jr, White CC: A descriptive epidemiology of leisure-time physical activity. *Public Health Rep* 1985; 100:147–158.
3. Presidents Council on Physical Fitness and Sports: Fitness of U.S. school children deteriorating. *Public Health Rep* 1986; 101: 441–442.
4. Paffenbarger RS Jr: Contributions of epidemiology to exercise science and cardiovascular health. *Med Sci Sports Exerc* 1988; 20:426–438.
5. Curfman GD, Thomas GS, Paffenbarger RS: Physical activity and primary prevention of cardiovascular disease. *Cardiology Clinics* 1985; 3:203–222.
6. Folsom AR, et al: Leisure time physical activity and its relationship to coronary risk factors in a population-based sample: The Minnesota Heart Survey. *Am J Epidemiol* 1985; 121:570–579.
7. Hickey N, et al: Study of coronary risk factors related to physical activity in 15,171 men. *BMJ* 1975; 3:507–509.
8. Bjartveit K, Foss OP, Gjervig T: The cardiovascular disease study in Norwegian counties: Results from first screening. *Acta Med Scand* 1983; 675(suppl):1–184.
9. Leon AS, et al.: Relationship of physical characteristics and life habits to treadmill exercise capacity. *Am J Epidemiol* 1981; 113:653–660.
10. Crow RS, et al: Risk factors, exercise fitness and electrocardiographic response to exercise in 12,866 men at high risk of symptomatic coronary heart disease. *Am J Cardiol* 1986; 57:1075–1082.
11. Ekelund LG, et al.: Physical fitness as a predictor of cardiovascular mortality in asymptomatic North American men: The Lipid Research Clinics Mortality Follow-up Study. *N Engl J Med* 1988; 319: 1379–1384.
12. Gordon DJ, et al.: Smoking, physical activity, and other predictors of endurance and heart rate response to exercise in asymptomatic hypercholesterolemic men: The Lipid Research Clinics Coronary Primary Prevention Trial. *Am J Epidemiol* 1987; 125:587–600.
13. Sobolski JC, et al.: Physical fitness does not reflect physical activity patterns in middle-aged workers. *Med Sci Sports Exerc* 1988; 20:6–13.
14. Cooper KH, et al.: Physical fitness levels vs. selected coronary risk factors: A cross-sectional study. *JAMA* 1976; 236:166–169.
15. Patton JF, Vogel JA: Prevalence of coronary heart disease risk factors in a young military population. *Aviat Space Environ Med* 1980; 51:510–514.
16. Brown TE, Myles WS, Allen CL: The relationship between aerobic fitness and cer-

tain cardiovascular risk factors. *Aviat Space Environ Med* 1983; 54:543–547.

17. Gibbons LW, et al.: Association between coronary heart disease risk factors and physical fitness in healthy adult women. *Circulation* 1983; 67:977–983.

18. Sedgwick AW, et al.: Relationships between physical fitness and risk factors for coronary heart disease in men and women. *Aust NZ J Med* 1984; 14:208–214.

19. Blair SN, et al.: Physical fitness and incidence of hypertension in healthy normotensive men and women. *JAMA* 1984; 252:487–490.

20. Paffenbarger RS Jr, et al.: Physical activity and incidence of hypertension in college alumni. *Am J Epidemiol* 1983; 117:245–257.

21. Peters RK, et al.: Physical fitness and subsequent myocardial infarction in healthy workers. *JAMA* 1983; 249:3052–3056.

22. Blair SN, et al.: Physical fitness and all-cause mortality: A prospective study of healthy men and women. *JAMA* 1989; 262:2395–2401.

23. Sobolski J, et al.: Protection against ischemic heart disease in the Belgian Physical Fitness Study: Physical fitness rather than physical activity? *Am J Epidemiol* 1987; 125:601–610.

23a. Sandvik L, et al.: Physical fitness as a predictor of mortality among healthy middle-aged Norwegian men. *N Engl J Med* 1993; 328:533–537.

24. Paffenbarger RS Jr, Hale WE: Work activity and coronary heart mortality. *N Engl J Med* 1975; 292:545–550.

25. Brunner D, et al.: Physical activity at work and the incidence of myocardial infarction, angina pectoris and death due to ischemic heart disease: An epidemiological study in Israeli collective settlements (Kibbutzim). *J Chron Dis* 1974; 27:217–233.

26. Keys A: *Seven Countries: A Multivariate Analysis of Death and Coronary Heart Disease.* Harvard University Press; Cambridge, Mass., 1980.

27. Punsar S, Karvonen MJ: Physical activity and coronary heart disease in populations from East and West Finland. *Adv Cardiol* 1976;18:196–207.

28. Morris JN, et al.: Vigorous exercise in leisure-time: Protection against coronary heart disease. *Lancet* 1980; 2:1207–1210.

29. Slattery ML, Jacobs DR Jr, Nichaman MZ: Leisure time physical activity and coronary heart disease death: The US Railroad Study. *Circulation* 1989; 79:304–311.

30. Kannel WB, Sorlie P: Some health benefits of physical activity: The Framingham Study. *Arch Intern Med* 1979; 139:857–861.

31. Garcia-Palmieri MR, et al.: Increased physical activity: A protective factor against heart attacks in Puerto Rico. *Am J Cardiol* 1982; 50:749–755.

32. Paffenbarger RS Jr, et al.: Physical activity, all-cause mortality, and longevity of college alumni. *N Engl J Med* 1986; 314:605–613.

33. Leon AS, et al.: Leisure-time physical activity levels and risk of coronary heart disease and death: The Multiple Risk Factor Intervention Trial. *JAMA* 1987; 258:2388–2395.

34. Magnus K, Matroos A, Strackee J: Walking, cycling, or gardening, with or without seasonal interruption, in relation to acute coronary events. *Am J Epidemiol* 1979; 110:724–733.

35. Rippe JM, et al.: Walking for health and fitness. *JAMA* 1988; 259:2720–2724.

36. Farmer ME, et al.: Physical activity and depressive symptoms: The NHANES I Epidemiologic Follow-up study. *Am J Epidemiol* 1988; 128:1340–1351.

37. Blumenthal JA, et al.: Psychological changes accompany aerobic exercise in healthy middle-aged adults. *Psychosom Med* 1982; 44:529–536.

38. Taylor CB, Sallis JF, Needle R: The relation of physical activity and exercise to mental health. *Public Health Rep* 1985; 100:195–202.

39. Hage P: Primary care physicians: First stop for exercise advice? *Phys Sportsmed* 1983; 11:149–152.

40. Bassey EJ, Fentem PH, Skene PC: Health professionals view on exercise: A study. *J R Soc Health* 1984; 104:225–228.

41. American College of Sports Medicine: *Guidelines for Exercise Testing and Prescription*, ed 4. Lea & Febiger: Philadelphia, 1988.

42. Chisholm DM, et al.: Physical activity readiness. *Br Columbia Med J* 1975; 17:375–378.

43. Summary of the Second Report of the National Cholesterol Education Program (NCEP) Expert Panel on Detection, Evaluation, and Treatment of High Blood Cholesterol in Adults (Adult Treatment Panel II). *JAMA* 1993; 269:3015–3023.

44. Sox HC Jr, Garber AM, Littenberg B: The resting electrocardiogram as a screening test: A clinical analysis. *Ann Intern Med* 1989; 111:489–502.

45. Sox HC Jr, Littenberg B, Garber AM: The role of exercise testing in screening for coronary artery disease. *Ann Intern Med* 1989; 110:456–469.

46. Siscovick DS, et al.: The incidence of primary cardiac arrest during vigorous exercise. *N Engl J Med* 1984; 311:874–877.

47. Froelicher VF, et al.: The prognostic value of the exercise test. *Dis Mon* 1988; 34:677–735.

48. Cheitlin MD: Finding the high-risk patient with coronary artery disease. *JAMA* 1988; 259:2271–2277.

49. Gettman LR, Pollock ML: Circuit weight training: A critical review of its physiological benefits. *Phys Sportsmed* 1981; 9:44–60.

50. Goldberg L, Elliot DL, Kuehl KS: Assess-

ment of exercise intensity formulas by use of ventilatory threshold. *Chest* 1988; 94: 95–98.

51. Borg G, Linderholm H: Perceived exertion and pulse rate during graded exercise in various age groups. *Acta Med Scand* 1967; 472:194–206.

52. Borg GA: Psychophysical bases of perceived exertion. *Med Sci Sports Exerc* 1982; 14:377–381.

53. Waller BF, Roberts WC: Sudden death while running in conditioned runners aged 40 years or over. *Am J Cardiol* 1980; 45: 1292–1300.

54. Thompson PD, et al.: Incidence of death during jogging in Rhode Island from 1975 through 1980. *JAMA* 1982; 247:2535–2538.

55. Siscovick DS, et al.: Physical activity and primary cardiac arrest. *JAMA* 1982; 248: 3113–3117.

56. Koplan JP, et al.: An epidemiologic study of the benefits and risks of running. *JAMA* 1982; 248:3118–3121.

57. Richie DH, Kelso SF, Bellucci PA: Aerobic dance injuries: A retrospective study of instructors and participants. *Phys Sportsmed* 1985; 13:130–140.

58. Lane NE, et al.: Aging, long-distance running, and the development of musculoskeletal disability: A controlled study. *Am J Med* 1987; 82:772–780.

59. Panush RS, et al.: Is running associated with degenerative joint disease? *JAMA* 1986; 255:1152–1154.

60. Pollock ML, et al.: Effects of frequency and duration of training on attrition and incidence of injury. *Med Sci Sports Exerc* 1977; 9:31–36.

61. Kruse DL, McBeath AA: Bicycle accidents and injuries: A random survey of a college population. *Am J Sports Med* 1980; 8: 342–344.

62. Knochel JP: Heat stroke and related heat stress disorders. *Dis Mon* 1989; 35:301–377.

63. Hubbard RW, Armstrong LE: Hyperthermia: New thoughts on an old problem. *Phys Sportsmed* 1989; 17:97–113.

64. Coleman VR: Physician behavior and compliance. *J Hypertension* 1985; 3(suppl): 69–71.

65. Meichenbaum D, Turk DC: *Facilitating Treatment Adherence: A Practitioners' Handbook*. Plenum Press: New York, 1987.

66. Carter WB, et al.: Developing and testing a decision model for predicting influenza vaccination compliance. *Health Services Res* 1986; 20:897–932.

67. Becker MH, Maiman LA: Strategies for enhancing patient compliance. *J Community Health* 1980; 6:113–135.

68. Becker MH, Maiman LA: Sociobehavioral determinants of compliance with health and medical care recommendations. *Med Care* 1975; 13:10–25.

69. Gettman LR, et al: Physiologic effects on adult men of circuit strength training and jogging. *Arch Phys Med Rehabil* 1979; 60:115–120.

70. Oldridge NB: Compliance and exercise in primary and secondary prevention of coronary heart disease: A review. *Prev Med* 1982; 11:56–70.

71. Durbeck DC, et al.: The National Aeronautics and Space Administration-U.S. Public Health Service Health Evaluation and Enhancement Program: Summary of results. *Am J Cardiol* 1972; 30:784–790.

72. Dishman RK, Sallis JF, Orenstein DR: The determinants of physical activity and exercise. *Public Health Rep* 1985; 100:158–171.

PART II

Cardiovascular Disorders

CHAPTER 2

EXERCISE AS TREATMENT FOR ESSENTIAL HYPERTENSION

LINN GOLDBERG, MD, and DIANE L. ELIOTT, MD

Hypertension is a common health problem[1] and represents a significant risk for development of coronary heart disease, stroke, and congestive heart failure (CHF).[2-5] A systolic pressure above 150 mm Hg more than doubles a patient's risk of developing heart disease when compared to the normotensive state.[4] It is becoming clear that control of even mild blood pressure elevation (diastolic pressure of 90 to 104 mm Hg) has the potential to reduce the untoward consequences of hypertension.[6,7]

Since hypertension is primarily distributed among residents of industrialized nations and is uncommon in less technologic societies, its cause is likely to include lifestyle patterns (Table 2–1).[8-13]

Although significant adverse sequelae such as stroke and CHF can be

Table 2–1 **LIFESTYLE FACTORS INFLUENCING BLOOD PRESSURE**

High sodium intake
Low potassium consumption
Cigarette smoking
High dietary saturated fat
Alcohol ingestion
Obesity
Sedentary lifestyle

reduced by antihypertensive drug therapy, randomized treatment trials[14] have failed to demonstrate an improvement in rates of either fatal or nonfatal myocardial infarction. Paradoxically, large blood pressure reductions induced by pharmacologic agents can increase myocardial ischemia and mortality.[15-17] In addition, antihypertensive drug therapy can be expensive, and many medications have significant adverse effects. Some unfavorably alter other coronary risk factors.[18-22]

Nonpharmacologic measures have been recognized as primary therapeutic options for blood pressure control, and higher levels of physical fitness may reduce the risk of developing hypertension.[23,24] Both dietary modification and exercise are recommended for initial and long-term intervention.[1,25] Because hypertension is often associated with other cardiovascular risk factors,[26,27] and because physical training can favorably impact on those parameters[28-31] (also see Chapters 8, 9, and 10), a program of regular exercise provides an attractive therapeutic option.

This chapter focuses on (1) potential factors associated with the development of essential hypertension, (2) exercise hemodynamics among normotensive individuals and those with elevated blood pressure, (3) research investigating exercise as antihypertensive therapy, (4) the potential mechanism of action of physical activity as treatment for hypertension, (5) exercise–drug interactions, and (6) training guidelines for patients with high blood pressure.

Factors Associated with Essential Hypertension

Systemic blood pressure reflects the product of cardiac output (CO) and systemic vascular resistance (SVR).

$$BP \sim CO \times SVR$$

Hypertension can be due to factors that either increase CO, elevate SVR, or both.[15] Similarly, a favorable modification of either CO or SVR can reduce blood pressure. Understanding the treatment of elevated blood pressure requires insight into variables that affect its genesis.

AGE

Development of hypertension often begins early in life, with blood pressure levels rising from childhood to adulthood.[32] Higher baseline values are associated with elevated blood pressures over time.[33] Compared with normotensive subjects, those with borderline high blood pressure have at least twice the risk of developing hypertension.[3]

Exercise can both alter baseline blood pressure and retard its progression to hypertension. Cross-sectional research[34] has observed that children with higher fitness levels have lower blood pressures. When the blood pressure status and physical activity index of young adults were followed, pressures remained lower among the fittest and those who performed the greatest amount of regular exercise.[24]

In their initial presentation, younger individuals with elevated blood pressure often display a cardiogenic hypertension with heightened CO.[35] Likewise, borderline hypertensive subjects younger than age 30 have a higher cardiac index than similarly aged normotensive subjects.[36] As those with high blood pressure approach middle age, CO normalizes and elevated peripheral vascular resistance becomes a greater factor for sustained hypertension.[35] Finally, older hypertensive subjects exhibit increased total peripheral resistance as the predominant feature of their disease.[4,37] Among these older individuals, CO decreases in association with reduced beta-adrenoreceptor responsiveness, while renin and aldosterone levels fall.[37] These physiologic and hormonal profiles can influence treatment.

Young hypertensive patients' hyperdynamic circulation is often due to higher adrenergic activity, which can be countered by beta blockade.[38] With increasing age, catecholamines undergo alteration. Levels of norepinephrine tend to increase, and epinephrine concentrations decrease.[36-38] This age-dependent change in the norepinephrine-to-epinephrine ratio tends to shift the hemodynamic profile; high-cardiac-output hypertension evolves toward elevated-vascular-resistance hypertension.[37] In addition, elderly hypertensive individuals have decreased distensibility of arterial vessels and lowered plasma volume.[39]

OBESITY

Weight gain can contribute to the development of hypertension.[40] One's body mass index is associated with mean arterial pressure, plasma volume, and total exchangeable sodium.[41]

Obese hypertensive individuals have unique characteristics that may be explained in part by hormonal differences. Obese adolescents with elevated blood pressure have greater salt sensitivity, which correlates to fasting plasma insulin and aldosterone levels.[42] Insulin resistance could explain some of these changes, as both sodium retention and catecholamine levels are enhanced by higher insulin concentrations.[43,44] As expected, increased sympathetic activity, especially elevated norepinephrine levels, is present in young obese hypertensive individuals.[40] Other changes involve attenuated renal dopaminergic and natriuretic activity.[45]

Overall, these alterations appear to be expressed as volume expansion and increased sodium sensitivity. This physiologic state leads to elevated CO with either normal or slightly elevated peripheral resistance.[41]

Table 2-2 **PREDICTORS OF DEVELOPING HYPERTENSION**

Increased left ventricular mass index
High body mass index
Elevated 24-hour urine Na^+/K^+ excretion (mean, 3.6)
Race (African American)
Elevated blood pressure response to handgrip isometric exercise
Lower fitness level
Elevated blood pressure response to dynamic exercise
Family history of hypertension

PREDICTORS OF HYPERTENSION

Research has identified those individuals with a greater potential to develop sustained hypertension. As listed in Table 2-2, anthropometric data, race, exercise capacity, and blood pressure response to physical activity, as well as echocardiographic and urinary findings, can identify individuals at higher risk.[46-50] Institution of nonpharmacologic therapy to favorably influence one or more of these factors may delay or prevent future development of hypertension.

Exercise Hemodynamics

NORMOTENSIVE RESPONSE

Blood pressure and heart rate responses to physical activity differ with exercise modes. Hemodynamic sequelae of endurance (dynamic) exertion, in which large muscle groups are exercised in rhythmic contraction and relaxation at increasing work loads, can be compared with static (isometric) handgrip exertion at various work load levels or percentage of maximal contraction (Table 2-3).

During progressive dynamic exercise (walking, running, bicycling, and so on), systolic blood pressure and heart rate increase until a maximal level is achieved.[51] Vasodilatation occurs in the vascular beds of exercising muscle, reducing peripheral resistance and lowering diastolic blood pressure. Due to an elevated systolic and reduced diastolic blood pressure, mean arterial pressure is either unchanged or only slightly elevated during dynamic exertion. During static (isometric) small-muscle-group (i.e., handgrip) exertion, a pressor response occurs secondary to increased heart rate, with little change in peripheral resistance.[52] Systolic, diastolic, and mean arterial pressure and heart rate increase in proportion to (1) the percentage of maximal voluntary contraction (MVC) of the exercised muscle group, and (2) the duration of the activity.[53] At

Table 2-3 HEMODYNAMIC SEQUELAE OF ENDURANCE (DYNAMIC) EXERTION

	Exercise Mode	
Hemodynamic Parameters	Dynamic (e.g., Treadmill, Cycle)	Static (Isometric Handgrip)
Systolic blood pressure	↑ to ↑↑↑↑	↑ to ↑↑↑↑
Diastolic blood pressure	↔ to ↓	↑ to ↑↑
Heart rate	↑ to ↑↑↑↑	↑ to ↑↑
Mean arterial pressure	↔ to ↑	↑ to ↑↑↑
Systemic vascular resistance	0 to ↓	0 to ↑

Key: ↑ = mild increase; ↑↑ = moderate increase; ↑↑↑ = high increase; ↑↑↑↑ = very high increase;
↓ = mild decrease; ↔ = no significant change.
Modified from Blomquist CG, et al. Similarity of the hemodynamic responses to static and dynamic exercise of small muscle groups. *Circ Res* 1981; 48:87–92.

greater percentages of MVC, the intramuscular pressure may be so high that blood flow to the muscle is obstructed.

HYPERTENSIVE RESPONSE

Hypertension affects blood pressure regulation at rest and during physical activity. Although some patients with hypertension have an augmented blood pressure increase during exercise as compared to normal subjects of the same age, this is not a consistent finding.[54,55] In fact, most individuals with mild to moderate hypertension have blood pressure elevations during dynamic activity similar to those of normotensive individuals.[54,55] Higher ending levels merely reflect elevated resting systolic pressures. Similar blood pressure increases also occur among both groups during isometric exercise.[56,57] The duration of hypertension may affect the pressure response, however, because a correlation has been found between the degree of systolic blood pressure rise during exertion and left ventricular mass.[58]

In hypertensive individuals both systolic and diastolic pressures are reduced below resting values immediately following dynamic exercise.[59,60] Systolic blood pressure can be lowered for 60 to 90 minutes; diastolic blood pressure often returns to pre-exercise levels within 1 hour.[55,59] Hypertensive patients of various ages maintain a parallel, higher peripheral resistance during physical activity when compared to their normotensive counterparts.[54,60] This hemodynamic alteration may be responsible for the finding that diastolic blood pressure does not always decrease during dynamic exercise for those with sustained hypertension.[54]

Other cardiovascular changes can occur with elevated blood pressure and alter exercise hemodynamics and capacity. Patients with established hypertension have higher end-systolic volume as well as a lower ejection fraction, stroke volume, and maximal oxygen uptake (VO_{2max}).[61] These abnormalities can occur secondary to hypertension alone, without associated left ventricular hypertrophy or ischemic heart disease.[61] With increasing age, asymptomatic hypertensive patients have been observed to have higher exercise systolic blood pressure and lower VO_{2max}.[54] Likewise, CO becomes progressively reduced as hypertensive individuals become older.

Exercise as Antihypertensive Therapy

EPIDEMIOLOGIC EVIDENCE

Cross-sectional research considering adults and children has observed that greater physical fitness is associated with lower blood pressure. The Loma Linda Child/Adolescent blood pressure study[34] assessed exercise capacity and blood pressure among preadolescent and adolescent children. A significant relationship was found between fitness, as determined by treadmill exercise, and resting systolic blood pressure for preadolescent boys and adolescents of both sexes. Likewise, diastolic pressures were lower among children with above-average fitness as compared to those with average fitness in both pre-adolescent and adolescent boys and girls. These differences were present even when adjusted for height, weight, and age.

The development of hypertension can be altered by regular physical activity and by an individual's fitness level. Paffenbarger and colleagues[24] observed that adults performing greater amounts of weekly dynamic exercise had lower systemic blood pressure than less active adults. Also, individuals with higher aerobic fitness may lower their future risk of developing hypertension compared to individuals of low fitness. Blair and colleagues[23] observed 4,276 men for an average of 8.5 years after performing exercise tolerance tests. Blood pressure at rest and during exercise remained lower for the most aerobically fit. The physically inactive subjects had up to a 52% greater chance of developing hypertension, independent of other factors known to influence blood pressure.

In addition to a relationship between findings of blood pressure and dynamic exertion, cross-sectional study[62] demonstrated that those with greater job exposure to isometric-style exercise also had significantly lower blood pressure.

PROSPECTIVE TRAINING STUDIES

Fitness can delay the onset of hypertension, and also may be a useful treatment for those with established blood pressure elevation. A review[63] of 11 studies assessed exercise training's effectiveness in reducing blood pressure among subjects with essential hypertension. After training, systolic blood pressure was reduced by an average of 11 mm Hg; diastolic, by 8 mm Hg. However, some of these investigations lacked adequate control groups. A subsequent, larger review[64] of 25 exercise and hypertension studies used the technique of meta-analysis. Just as with various pharmacologic agents, exercise did not normalize or lower blood pressure in all subjects, but the overall effect was a significant decrement in both systolic and diastolic blood pressure.

Blood pressure reductions produced by physical activity do not appear to correlate with the intensity of training.[64] Improved aerobic fitness, as determined by increased VO_{2max}, may not be required for blood pressure reduction. Animal evidence suggests that lower training intensity (40% to 60% of VO_{2max}) can decrease blood pressure.[65] Likewise, blood pressure reduction has been unrelated to increases in VO_{2max} after conditioning among adolescents and adults with hypertension.[66] Hypertensive women had their blood pressures lowered to the same degree by 3 and 12 months of low-intensity training as by

12 months of high-intensity exertion.[67] Significant decrements in blood pressure have been found after regular exercise at or below the lactate threshold.[68,69] Similarly, circuit weight training, an exercise that has only a small effect on VO_{2max}, has resulted in lower blood pressure among those with diastolic hypertension.[70]

The amount of time required to lower resting blood pressure by physical activity has not been established. Diastolic blood pressure reduction, in part, seems to be related to the duration of the exercise program[64]; that is, the greater the length of the program, the more likely a hypotensive effect. Nevertheless, blood pressure reduction has occurred after just several weeks to 6 months of regular training.[70–72]

RESISTIVE EXERCISE AND BLOOD PRESSURE

Strength training (resistive exercise) also may lower blood pressure. Among normotensive individuals, diastolic blood pressure was reduced after just 9 to 10 weeks of circuit weight training.[70,73] A significant decrement in resting systolic blood pressure has been observed with 8 weeks of Olympic-style weight lifting.[74] Despite extreme blood pressure elevation (302/250 mm Hg) during maximal lifts by trained body builders,[75] resistive training studies have failed to observe untoward cardiovascular complications.[70,73,74,76]

Circuit weight training, when combined with traditional aerobic exercise, has been found to reduce blood pressure in hypertensive men.[77] Previously hypertensive adolescents who reduced their blood pressure by aerobic exercise were able to maintain blood pressure control by weight lifting, despite discontinuance of regular aerobic training.[78] Also, resistive exercise has resulted in beneficial effects on blood pressure among borderline hypertensive adults who were not previously engaged in aerobic activity.[70] Although cardiac adaptations to resistive exercise can involve increased left ventricular wall thickness, there appears to be no untoward effect on cardiac function.[79] Thus, weight training could offer another exercise mode to assist in the nonpharmacologic management of hypertension.

The use of isometric exercise to lower blood pressure has not been studied in hypertensive individuals. One investigation[80] found that intermittent hand-grip contractions reduced systolic and diastolic blood pressure by 13 and 15 mm Hg, respectively, but these subjects were healthy and did not have elevated blood pressure.

DURATION OF ACTION

Normalization of blood pressure after conditioning appears to act like a drug, in that the lower pressure is maintained only during periods of treatment. The previous elevated blood pressure levels return within weeks after resuming a sedentary lifestyle.[81]

EXERCISE COMBINED WITH DRUG THERAPY

Exercise may complement pharmacologic intervention and allow for the reduction of antihypertensive medication. Hypertensive sedentary men, performing a 10-week regimen of circuit weight training and aerobic conditioning, reduced average blood pressure from 145/97 mm Hg to 131/84 mm Hg, such that drug treatment (either diltiazem hydrochloride or propranolol) provided no additional benefit.[77] In another study,[82] men with mild hypertension were given either a placebo, the nonselective beta blocker propranolol, or the selective beta antagonist atenolol. Subjects were observed during a 10-week aerobic exercise program. After the subjects attained normotensive blood pressures with training, beta blockade therapy was withdrawn over a 2-week period as conditioning continued. Blood pressures remained reduced despite cessation of pharmacologic therapy.

Potential Mechanisms of Action

Several mechanisms responsible for the hypotensive effect of physical activity have been suggested. Differences in age, body composition, genetics, hypertensive physiology (cardiogenic versus peripheral resistance), and hormonal alterations in the hypertensive individual may play a role in the effectiveness of exercise. Animal models[83] suggest that a greater response to conditioning occurs among younger hypertensive individuals, and that there may be a genetic predisposition to blood pressure reduction by exercise. Human evidence has not confirmed age-related differences, because no adequate controlled trials have been performed among elderly individuals.

BODY COMPOSITION

Obesity is a risk factor for development of hypertension among children and young adults.[10,40] Obese hypertensive individuals are more likely to be salt sensitive and to have elevated catecholamine and insulin levels. Elevated insulin levels with relative insulin resistance may be at least partially responsible for hypertension in obese individuals.[84] Weight loss by diet and exercise has resulted in lower insulin levels and reduced blood pressure.[85,86]

Although exercise may lower blood pressure by reducing body fat, decreasing adiposity is not always necessary. Physical conditioning has been shown to result in decreased blood pressure among normotensive individuals and in those with mild hypertension, whether or not they are obese, and independent of body composition changes.[87,88] The magnitude of systolic and diastolic blood pressure reduction induced by exercise, in fact, may be unrelated to baseline body weight and may not require body composition changes.[64]

It is likely that exercise could exert some of its effect by changing body composition. This could increase insulin sensitivity due to body fat reduction alone or in conjunction with physical activity's synergistic effect on insulin action. The resulting lower insulin levels could result in lower salt sensitivity, lower catecholamine concentrations, and improved blood pressure control.

CATECHOLAMINES

Exercise training can influence the sympathetic nervous system,[88] as reflected by the observation that trained athletes have lower blood pressure, heart rate, and catecholamine responsiveness than sedentary controls.[89] Aerobically trained animal models[90,91] had their exercise blood pressure reduced by altering their sympathoadrenal response to exercise. Both indirect animal evidence[92] and direct assessments of catecholamines among humans[69,93] suggest a lowering in the "adrenergic state" after exercise conditioning. Thus, the hyperfunctional catecholamine levels often observed early in the course of hypertension[37,94] can be reduced with training.

Parallel reductions in resting blood pressure and sympathetic tone have been found after regular exercise among normotensive individuals and those with established hypertension.[69,93] After conditioning, a given submaximal work load can be performed with less sympathetic nervous system activity and lower circulating catecholamine levels.[69,95] Even among individuals with ischemic heart disease, 3 months of training improved maximal treadmill time while lowering plasma norepinephrine levels.[96]

Duncan and coworkers[88] evaluated 56 patients with mild hypertension before and after exercise conditioning. Subjects with mild diastolic hypertension (90 to 100 mm Hg) were classified as either normoadrenergic or hyperadrenergic, based on plasma catecholamine levels. After aerobic training, all exercisers improved fitness and lowered their systolic and diastolic blood pressures as compared to sedentary controls. These reductions were observed despite no change in body weight, dietary habits, or consumption of alcohol or caffeine. The greatest effect was found among the hyperadrenergic group, in whom reduced norepinephrine levels were correlated with the long-term hypotensive effect of regular exercise.

Although contrary data regarding the effects of exercise on blood pressure and catecholamines exist, these studies have been small and without adequate controls.[97] Most investigations support altered sympathetic function as one explanation for the antihypertensive effects of physical activity.

INSULIN LEVELS

Insulin has been shown to facilitate sodium reabsorption in the distal renal tubule, increase catecholamine levels, and act as a trophic factor for vascular hypertrophy.[43,44,98,99] Hypertensive subjects, even with average body weight and normal glucose tolerance, can be relatively insulin resistant.[86] Although hypertension, like obesity and type II diabetes, is associated with insulin resistance,[84,100] it is unclear whether (1) increased insulin levels result in hypertension, (2) the hypertensive state causes higher insulin concentrations, or (3) the association is noncausal.[101]

Insulin levels can be modified by exercise. Although increases occur with age, older, normotensive, fit individuals have the same low insulin concentrations as young, normotensive, fit subjects.[102] Likewise, blood pressure correlates directly with plasma insulin levels and inversely with physical fitness among normoglycemic, nonobese middle-aged men with a family history of type II diabetes.[84] Adolescents who lost weight by combining dietary restriction and exercise reduced both their blood pressure and plasma insulin levels.[85] Furthermore, prospective studies[103,104] have found that plasma insulin concentrations decrease with declining blood pressure during exercise training of obese subjects. Even among hemodialysis patients, 12 months of endurance training resulted in lower blood pressure, reduced requirements for antihypertensive medication, and increased glucose disappearance rates, with a 52% reduction in fasting insulin levels.[105]

Plasma insulin lowering is a potential link between blood pressure reduction and exercise training. This change has occurred for both nonobesity-related and obesity-related hypertension. Reduced insulin concentrations could promote greater natriuresis by decreasing renal reabsorption of sodium, by lowering catecholamine generation, or both, either of which could lower blood pressure.

VOLUME CHANGES

Plasma volume reduction represents another potential adaptation in blood pressure control after exercise conditioning. In normotensive individuals, plasma volume often expands after endurance training,[106] but volume changes after conditioning may differ in hypertensive individuals.[107] One explanation is the effect of exercise on specific plasma hormone levels. Exercise promotes atrial natriuretic factor (ANF) production in both normotensive and hypertensive individuals, with levels related to left ventricular mass, which often is greater in those with elevated blood pressure.[108,109] This peptide also suppresses plasma renin activity and aldosterone production.[110,111] In those with greater ventricular mass, an expected effect would be increased ANF secretion and the promotion of intravascular volume loss, leading to lower blood pressure after training. Also, since elevated insulin levels can result in sodium retention,[43] the reduced insulin concentrations that accompany physical conditioning[103,104] could decrease plasma volume.

Intravascular volume has been observed among hypertensive individuals engaged in an exercise program.[69] In those who exercised at the lactate threshold on a cycle ergometer for 10 weeks, both blood and plasma volume were lowered, and systolic and mean arterial pressure were reduced.[69] Although the results are preliminary, exercise training among hypertensive subjects could result in favorable blood pressure changes, in part due to plasma volume reduction.

Dynamic Exercise and Antihypertensive Drugs

Antihypertensive medications may influence blood pressure changes during submaximal and maximal exertion and may affect exercise capacity, the conditioning response to regular physical activity, and other coronary artery risk factors (Table 2–4). Understanding the various drug classes and their impact on exercise can assist in prescribing activities for those who require pharmacologic agents and can provide insight into therapeutic decisions for active hypertensive individuals.

CALCIUM CHANNEL ANTAGONISTS

Calcium channel antagonists inhibit transmembranous influx of calcium ions and reduce intracellular calcium concentration.[112] Despite varying electrophysiologic effects, these drugs all are vasodilating agents and decrease peripheral vascular resistance at rest and during physical activity.[113] Calcium channel antagonists have the potential to alter exercise tolerance, There is evidence that verapamil hydrochloride can impair left ventricular perform-

Table 2-4   **EXERCISE-RELATED EFFECTS OF ANTIHYPERTENSIVE DRUGS**

Drug Class	Submaximal Exercise Blood Pressure	Maximal Exercise Blood Pressure	VO_{2max}	Exercise Training Improvement	Effect on Other Risk Factors
Calcium channel antagonists	↓	↔ or ↓	↔	↔	↔
Beta blockers (selective and non-selective)	↓	↓	↓	↓*	Can increase LDL-C and TG, decrease HDL-C, and worsen glucose tolerance
Alpha and beta blockers	↓	↓	↔	↔	↔
Diuretics	↓	↔	↔	↔	Can increase LDL-C and TG, decrease HDL-C, and worsen glucose tolerance
ACE inhibitors	↓	↔	↔	↔	↔
Peripheral vasodilators**†	↓	↓	↔	↔	↔
Central alpha agonists**†	↓	↔	↔	↔	↔

*When beta blockade is withdrawn after conditioning, the training effect is observed.
†Probable effect (not well established).
Key: VO_{2max} = maximal oxygen uptake, ↓ = reduced levels, ↔ = no effect or no difference from pre-drug response, LDL-C = low-density lipoprotein cholesterol, TG = triglycerides, HDL-C = high-density lipoprotein cholesterol.

ance.[114] Using the technique of first-pass radionuclide angiography, however, no differences in exercise hemodynamics or left ventricular function were observed when verapamil was used at therapeutic doses in normal men.[115]

Calcium channel antagonists may affect heart rate and blood pressure during exercise. The two calcium channel blockers that slow cardiac conduction, verapamil and diltiazem hydrochloride, often cause a mild dose-dependent reduction in exercise heart rate.[116,117] Nifedipine, a member of the dihydropyridine subgroup, has greater peripheral vasoactivity without producing cardiac conduction changes. Nifedipine does not appear to alter the heart-rate response to physical activity.[118] Other vasoactive calcium channel antagonists, such as nicardipine, felodipine, and isradipine, probably act much like nifedipine with regard to exercise hemodynamics. During exercise, calcium channel antagonists have been observed to reduce systolic and diastolic pressure at submaximal work loads,[119] but higher systolic blood pressures achieved during maximal exercise without therapy were not lowered by either verapamil or nifedipine.[120-122] Verapamil has failed to reduce maximal exercise blood pressure even though it reduces SVR at rest and during peak exercise.[122]

When assessing exercise tolerance by maximal oxygen uptake (VO_{2max}), most studies suggest that calcium channel antagonists do not alter exercise capacity.[120,123,124] However, in one training study,[125] although nifedipine did not appear to block the conditioning response, VO_{2max} significantly increased after drug discontinuance.

BETA BLOCKERS

In the mid-1980s, beta-adrenergic blockers accounted for over one third of the total dollars spent by Americans on antihypertensive drug therapy.[126] Although they antagonize the cardiovascular effects of catecholamines, their antihypertensive effect is not clearly understood. Beta blockers can vary with regard to lipid solubility, intrinsic sympathomimetic activity, and cardioselectivity. The clinical significance of these differences in their ability to control blood pressure is small.

Following beta blockade, heart rate, blood pressure, maximal cardiac output and skeletal muscle blood flow are reduced during exercise (see Table 2−4).[127-129] These effects account for the observation that most selective and nonselective beta-adrenoreceptor antagonists adversely alter aerobic capacity.[129-131] The most negative effects of these drugs on exercise capacity have been found among healthy, highly conditioned subjects who have high aerobic capacities.[131] The reduction of maximal oxygen consumption by beta blockers is less pronounced in moderately or poorly conditioned individuals.[131] Studies reporting no changes in aerobic fitness levels have generally involved low doses of beta blockers or subjects with reduced exercise tolerance prior to drug treatment.[130] Although there have been reports that selective beta blockers may not reduce exercise capacity as much as nonselective agents, they all appear to lower VO_{2max} especially in fitter individuals.[129-131] The addition of calcium channel antagonists to beta blocker therapy does not appear to reduce VO_{2max} beyond the reduction in exercise capacity caused by beta blockade alone.[132]

Beta-adrenergic blocking drugs not only reduce established fitness levels, but also can attenuate the conditioning response to aerobic training.[133-136] Thirty hypertensive individuals were randomized to the nonselective beta blocker, propranolol, a beta-1 selective antagonist, metoprolol tartrate, or placebo along with a 10-week exercise program.[137] After training, systolic blood pressure was similarly lowered with exercise and placebo (146 to 135 mm Hg) when compared to beta blocker therapy (144 to 133 mm Hg). A 24% improvement in VO_{2max} was found in the placebo exercise group, an 8% increase occurred for those exercising while taking metoprolol, and no change was observed among those who trained and were treated with propranolol. When subjects discontinued beta blocker therapy, however, oxygen uptake increased so that no differences in VO_{2max} were present among the groups.

Another study[138] observed a blunting of the conditioning effect when sedentary hypertensive men were treated with atenolol along with 10 weeks of exercise. Although exercise capacity was not increased during drug therapy, the effect was not irreversibly inhibited by beta blockers, as improved VO_{2max} was observed just 3 to 5 days after discontinuing atenolol. Thus, although beta blockers are effective antihypertensives, they can reduce exercise capacity and conceal the aerobic conditioning effects of training while therapy is continued.

Beta-adrenoreceptor antagonists with additional alpha-blocking properties (e.g., labetalol) allow increased tissue blood flow and do not appear to alter VO_{2max} (see Table 2–4).[139,140] Also, labetalol has not been found to alter aerobic training as determined by maximal oxygen uptake.[140] The combination alpha- and beta-adrenoreceptor antagonist may be a preferred beta blocker among physically active individuals. However, labetalol should not be substituted as the sole agent used to treat myocardial ischemia in addition to elevated blood pressure.

DIURETICS

Diuretics have been first-line antihypertensive agents for many years.[141,142] Their hypotensive effect may result from reduced plasma volume, increased arteriolar dilatation, and lowered receptor sensitivity to various vasopressors.[143] Although other pharmacologic therapies have been shown to reduce hypertension-induced left ventricular hypertrophy, diuretics do not provide this effect.[144]

Few studies have observed the effect of diuretic therapy on exercise performance, and existing evidence reveals that peak blood pressures induced by physical activity may not always be controlled with diuretics.[145–147] Although the heart-rate response to dynamic exertion is not altered, SVR is lowered.[147]

ANGIOTENSIN CONVERTING ENZYME INHIBITORS

Angiotensin converting enzyme (ACE) inhibitors reduce blood pressure by lowering peripheral vascular resistance. This effect is achieved by inhibiting production of a vasoconstrictor, angiotensin II, from the relatively inert angiotensin I.[148] The contributing influence of tissue ACE inhibition or alterations in the kinin system by these drugs is, as yet, unclear.[149,150] ACE inhibitors reduce SVR without altering heart rate or CO in hypertensive individuals, and they do not alter the cardiovascular response to autonomic reflexes.[151]

The effects of ACE inhibition during physical activity have not been well studied. Despite effectively lowering blood pressure at rest, captopril did not reduce systolic blood pressure at maximal dynamic exertion,[152] but enalapril maleate, alone or in combination with a diuretic, did.[153] During isometric exercise, blood pressure and heart rate do not appear to be affected.[151,154] ACE inhibitors do not alter VO_{2max} (see Table 2–4).[153]

CASE: H.T., a 64-year-old white man, developed mild hypertension (diastolic blood pressure of 100 mm Hg) after 20 years of borderline blood pressure elevation. He had a strong family history of hypertension and had exercised for the previous 15 years by jogging each day. Initially, he was treated with a cardioselective beta blocker, atenolol. This resulted in complaints of impotence, generalized fatigue, and reduced running times. Because of these symptoms, therapy was changed to verapamil-SR, but abdominal discomfort secondary to constipation became a major complaint. As a result, he was treated with enalapril, an ACE inhibitor. Soon after therapy was begun and his dose was titrated to 10 mg each day, his energy level improved and he felt more as he had prior to pharmacologic therapy. His impotence resolved, and his general vigor returned to pre-drug levels, as did his "times" for 5-km and 10-km runs.

COMMENT: Enalapril is a competitive inhibitor of the angiotensin converting enzyme, an enzyme that also stimulates prostaglandin biosynthesis. ACE inhibitors have been shown to have a more favorable adverse-effect profile in hypertensive adults than other agents.[155] These drugs do not inhibit endurance exercise tolerance as do beta blockers.[134,153] Treatment efficacy and quality of life can be enhanced with use of ACE inhibitors or other drugs that do not impair VO_{2max} in the active hypertensive patient.

OTHER ANTIHYPERTENSIVES

The influence of centrally acting agents and peripheral vasodilating antihypertensives has been observed during exercise. Despite controlling blood pressure at rest and during light work, methyldopa and central alpha stimulants have not been effective at reducing systolic blood pressure during high-intensity exertion.[147,156] Few studies have observed the effect of the central alpha stimulant, clonidine hydrochloride, on exercise, but it does not appear to reduce endurance or interfere with aerobic training.[157] Likewise, prazosin hydrochloride, a postsympathetic alpha-adrenergic inhibitor, has been found to reduce blood pressure at rest and during both submaximal and maximal exercise without adversely altering exercise capacity.[158]

ISOMETRIC EXERCISE AND ANTIHYPERTENSIVE THERAPY

The hemodynamic effect of antihypertensives during isometric (static) exertion also has not been well studied. During isometric exercise, the increase in systolic blood pressure has been reduced by various nonselective and selective beta antagonists, and the alpha- and beta-adrenergic antagonist, labetalol.[159] Although these drugs reduced systolic blood pressure, no clear alteration of diastolic blood pressure was observed with static handgrip effort. Generally, ACE inhibitors have not been found to affect the blood pressure response to isometric exertion.[151]

ADVERSE EFFECTS OF ANTIHYPERTENSIVE DRUGS

Whereas exercise can improve blood pressure control and other cardiovascular risk factors, antihypertensive drugs can unfavorably alter cardiovascular risk (see Table 2–4). Diuretic treatment was associated with an increase in coronary artery disease mortality in hypertensive men with abnormal findings on the resting electrocardiogram in the Multiple Risk Factor Intervention Trial.[160] Other side effects of diuretics include hyperuricemia, hypokalemia, and a potential increase in cardiac arrhythmias during physical activity.[161,162] Also, insulin levels are increased with diuretics, and glucose intolerance may result.[20] Thiazides and loop diuretics can raise triglycerides, total cholesterol and low-density lipoprotein cholesterol levels, and in some cases, reduce high-density lipoprotein (HDL) cholesterol concentrations.[18,19,163] The lipid and hormonal alterations may be large enough to negate the benefits of blood pressure reduction in coronary heart disease prevention.[164,165]

Other antihypertensives also have side effects that alter exercise capacity or change cardiovascular risk. Beta-adrenergic blockers can result in bronchospasm and hypertriglyceridemia, lower HDL cholesterol, and exacerbate glucose intolerance and peripheral vascular disease.[21,22,166,167] Although ACE inhibitors have a low side-effect profile, they can cause reversible renal deterioration, hyperkalemia, cough, hypotension, and angioedema.[151,168,169] Calcium antagonists, such as verapamil or diltiazem, may cause constipation, whereas nifedipine, nicardipine, isradipine, and felodipine can result in tachycardia and peripheral edema. Several calcium channel antagonists have the potential to cause headache (nifedipine, nicardipine, isradipine, and felodipine), and some can precipitate cardiac conduction abnormalities (verapamil and diltiazem).

> **CASE:** F.H. is a 45-year-old man. When first seen at age 40, he had a 10-year history of hypertension, treated by various agents including diuretics, vasodilators, and beta blockers. He has a family history of coronary artery disease. Leg cramps occurred during diuretic therapy, mild headaches were reported with therapy with various peripheral vasodilators, and fatigue and depression developed during beta blocker treatment. His blood pressure was controlled with hydralazine and the combination diuretic Dyazide (triamterene and hydrochlorothiazide), but he "did not feel well" on these agents. After encouragement, he began training at the Oregon Health Sciences University exercise clinic. Because of his age and coronary risk profile, a treadmill test was performed prior to physical conditioning and exercise guidelines were established.
>
> After 12 weeks of training, he discontinued drug therapy on his own. No weight loss occurred, and he reported no dietary changes. With exercise (stationary cycling, aerobic dance, and jogging) 3 to 5 days a week, his resting blood pressure remained normal (124/82 mm Hg) even after stopping antihypertensive agents. Five years later, F.H. has remained normotensive and continues to exercise regularly.

> **CASE:** T.M., a 29-year-old man, developed borderline hypertension (140/90 mm Hg) and wished to begin a regular exercise program. Results of his physical examination, aside from his blood pressure, were normal. T.M. began jogging for 30 minutes three to four times each week and played racquetball once each week. His follow-up blood pressure after 16 weeks of exercise was 128/82 mm Hg. Follow-up at 6 months revealed similar normotensive levels.
>
> At 1-year follow-up, T.M.'s blood pressure was 148/98 mm Hg. He related that because of work and the winter season, he had been unable to exercise regularly and doubted he could return to an active lifestyle in the near future. Therapy with verapamil 180 SR was initiated, and T.M.'s blood pressure was controlled (122/80 mm Hg at 3 months of follow-up). After 6 months of pharmacologic therapy, T.M. began another exercise program, similar to his previous regimen. After 2 months, drug treatment was stopped. At follow-up, T.M.'s blood pressure remained controlled (126/84 mm Hg) as exercise conditioning continued.

> **COMMENT:** Exercise can be complementary to pharmacologic agents, and in some individuals, regular physical activity can replace antihypertensive drugs. As long as exercise is continued, blood pressure can be controlled in patients responsive to this intervention. However, as in T.M.'s case, blood pressure often will return to its previous elevated level if training is discontinued.[87]

Exercise Training Guidelines

Physical activity, as outlined in Chapter 1 or as recommended by the American College of Sports Medicine,[170] can treat those with asymptomatic hypertension. A pre-exercise evaluation should be used to identify other risk factors and detect concurrent disease and end-organ damage. The type, intensity, duration, and frequency of training, as well as progression, should be assessed regularly. We believe that if two or more cardiovascular risk factors (male gender, diabetes, dyslipidemia, family history of early coronary artery disease, and smoking) are present in an asymptomatic, hypertensive, sedentary individual, a symptom-limited exercise test should be performed with continuous electrocardiographic monitoring. In addition to assessing exercise capacity, an exercise test will evaluate submaximal and maximal blood pressure responses. Those with an exaggerated systolic blood pressure response (over 250 mm Hg) or failure to reduce diastolic pressure (below 90 mm Hg) should have drug therapy initiated before an exercise program proceeds.

Training intensity need not be high. Intensity can be prescribed based on maximum heart rate, using a calculated formula (220 − age) or measured during a maximal exercise test. Lower levels (65% to 70% of maximum heart rate) may be just as effective as higher intensities (70% to 85%). After an initial conditioning period (12 to 16 weeks), antihypertensive medication can be slowly reduced in an attempt to prevent rebound hypertension or unmask previously treated myocardial ischemia. Biweekly follow-ups should be implemented during and immediately after the tapering of medication, to determine the chronic effect of training on blood pressure. However, no reduction in medication should be attempted until blood pressure is adequately controlled.

Summary

A lifestyle that includes regular exercise has the potential to decrease blood pressure and, at the same time, favorably alter other cardiovascular risk factors. This nonpharmacologic approach may be effective alone or when used concurrently with antihypertensive drug therapy. Exercise should be promoted as an initial intervention strategy for treatment of hypertension.

REFERENCES

1. The fifth report of the Joint National Committee on Detection, Evaluation, and Treatment of High Blood Pressure (JNC V). *Arch Intern Med* 1993; 153: 154–183.
2. Kannel WB, Sorlie P: Hypertension in Framingham. In Paul O, ed: *Epidemiology in Controlled Hypertension.* Symposia Specialist: Miami, 1975, pp 553–592.
3. Kannel WB, et al.: Components of blood pressure and risk of atherothrombotic brain infarction: The Framingham Study. *Stroke* 1976; 7:327–331.
4. Kannel WB, et al.: Role of blood pressure in the development of congestive heart failure: The Framingham Study. *N Engl J Med* 1972; 287:781–787.
5. Cornoni-Huntley J, LaCroix AZ, Havlik RJ: Race and sex differentials in the impact of hypertension in the United States: The National Health and Nutrition Examination Survey I Epidemiologic Follow-up Study. *Arch Intern Med* 1989; 149: 780–788.
6. Medical Research Council Working Party: MRC trial of treatment of mild hypertension: Principal results [letter]. *BMJ* 1985; 291:97–104.
7. Hypertension Detection and Follow-up Program Cooperative Group: Five-year

findings of the hypertension detection and follow-up program, I: Reduction in mortality of persons with high blood pressure, including mild hypertension. *JAMA* 1979; 242:2562–2571.

8. *The Lipid Research Clinics Population Studies Data Book, Vol I. The Prevalence Study.* Bethesda, MD: U.S. Dept. of Health and Human Services publication. NIH 80-1527. July 1980:86–89.

9. Sparrow D, et al.: Factors in predicting blood pressure change. *Circulation* 1982; 65:789–794.

10. Aristimuño GG, et al.: Influence of persistent obesity in children on cardiovascular risk factors: The Bogalusa Heart Study. *Circulation* 1984; 69:895–904.

11. Stamler RJ, et al.: Relationship of multiple variables to blood pressure: Findings from our Chicago epidemiological studies. In Paul O, ed: *Epidemiology and Control of Hypertension.* Symposia Specialist: Miami, 1975, pp 307–356.

12. Krishna GG, Miller E, Kapoor S: Increased blood pressure during potassium depletion in normotensive men. *N Engl J Med* 1989; 320:1177–1182.

13. Ullian ME, Linas SL: Hemodynamic effects of potassium. *Semin Nephrol* 1987; 7: 239–252.

14. MacMahon SW, et al.: The effects of drug treatment for hypertension on morbidity and mortality from cardiovascular disease: A review of randomized controlled trials. *Prog Cardiovasc Dis* 1986; 29(suppl 1): 99–118.

15. Cruickshank JM, Thorp JM, Zacharias FJ: Benefits and potential harm of lowering high blood pressure. *Lancet* 1987; 1: 581–584.

16. Cooper SP, et al.: The relation between degree of blood pressure reduction and mortality among hypertensives in the Hypertension Detection and Follow-up Program. *Am J Epidemiol* 1988; 127:387–403.

17. Farnett L, et al.: The J-curve phenomenon and the treatment of hypertension: Is there a point beyond which pressure reduction is dangerous? *JAMA* 1991; 265: 489–495.

18. Bloomgarden ZT, et al.: Elevated hemoglobin A1c and low-density lipoprotein cholesterol levels in thiazide-treated diabetic patients. *Am J Med* 1984; 77: 823–827.

19. Ames RP, Hill P: Increase in serum lipids during treatment of hypertension with chlorthalidone. *Lancet* 1976; 1:721–723.

20. Breckenridge A, et al.: Glucose tolerance in hypertensive patients on long-term diuretic therapy. *Lancet* 1967; 1:61–64.

21. Leon AS, et al.: Blood lipid effects of antihypertensive therapy: A double-blind comparison of the effects of methyldopa and propranolol. *J Clin Pharmacol* 1984; 24:209–217.

22. Bielmann P, Leduc G: Effects of metoprolol and propranolol on lipid metabolism. *Int J Clin Pharmacol Biopharm* 1979; 17: 378–382.

23. Blair SN, et al.: Physical fitness and incidence of hypertension in healthy normotensive men and women. *JAMA* 1984; 252:487–490.

24. Paffenbarger RS Jr, et al.: Physical activity and incidence of hypertension in college alumni. *Am J Epidemiol* 1983; 117: 245–257.

25. Briazgunov IP: The role of physical activity in the prevention and treatment of noncommunicable diseases. *World Health Stat Q* 1988; 41:242–250.

26. Kaplan NM: Importance of coronary heart disease risk factors in the management of hypertension: An overview. *Am J Med* 1989; 86(suppl 1B):1–4.

27. National Education Programs Working Group report on the management of patients with hypertension and high blood cholesterol. *Ann Intern Med* 1991; 114: 224–237.

28. Goldberg L, Elliot DL: The effect of exercise on lipid metabolism in men and women. *Sports Med* 1987; 4:307–321.

29. Hurley BF, et al.: Resistive training can reduce coronary risk factors without altering VO_{2max} or percent body fat. *Med Sci Sports Exerc* 1988; 20:150–154.

30. Butler RM, Goldberg L: Exercise and prevention of coronary heart disease. *Primary Care* 1989; 16:99–114.

31. Cooper KH, et al.: Physical fitness levels vs selected coronary risk factors: A cross-sectional study. *JAMA* 1976; 236:166–169.

32. Hagberg JM, et al.: Relation between casual blood pressure readings in youth and age 40: A retrospective study. *J Chron Dis* 1964; 17:397–404.

33. Paffenbarger RS Jr, Thorne MC, Wing AL: Chronic disease in former college students: VIII. Characteristics in youths predisposing to hypertension in later years. *Am J Epidemiol* 1968; 88:25–32.

34. Fraser GE, Phillips RL, Harris R: Physical fitness and blood pressure in school children. *Circulation* 1983; 67:405–412.

35. Widimsky J, Fejfarova MH, Fejfar Z: Changes in cardiac output in hypertensive disease. *Cardiologia* 1957; 31: 381–389.

36. Messerli FH, et al.: Borderline hypertension: Relationship between age, hemodynamics and circulating catecholamines. *Circulation* 1981; 64:760–764.

37. Messerli FH, et al.: Essential hypertension in the elderly: Hemodynamics, intravascular volume, plasma renin activity, and circulating catecholamine levels. *Lancet* 1983; 2:983–986.

38. Ulrych ME, et al.: Cardiac output and distribution of blood volume in central and peripheral circulations in hypertensive

and normotensive man. *Br Heart J* 1969; 31:570–574.

39. Applegate WB: Hypertension in elderly patients. *Ann Intern Med* 1989; 110: 901–915.

40. Kannel WB, et al.: The relation of adiposity to blood pressure and development of hypertension: The Framingham Study. *Ann Intern Med* 1967; 67:48–59.

41. Messerli FH, et al.: Disparate cardiovascular effects of obesity and arterial hypertension. *Am J Med* 1983; 74:808–812.

42. Rocchini AP, et al.: The effect of weight loss on the sensitivity of blood pressure to sodium in obese adolescents. *N Engl J Med* 1989; 321:580–585.

43. DeFronzo RA: Insulin and renal sodium handling: Clinical implications. *Int J Obesity* 1981; 5(suppl 1):93–104.

44. Reaven GM, Hoffman BB: A role for insulin in the aetiology and course of hypertension? *Lancet* 1987; 2:435–437.

45. Kikuchi K, et al.: The pathophysiological role of water-sodium balance and renal dopaminergic activity in overweight patients with essential hypertension. *J Clin Hypertens* 1987; 3:3–11.

46. de Simone G, et al.: Echocardiographic left ventricular mass and electrolyte intake predict arterial hypertension. *Ann Intern Med* 1991; 114:202–209.

47. Parker FC, et al.: The association between cardiovascular response tasks and future blood pressure levels in children: Bogalusa Heart Study. *Am Heart J* 1987; 113: 1174–1179.

48. Chaney RH, Arndt S: Predictability of blood pressure response to isometric stress. *Am J Cardiol* 1983; 51:787–790.

49. Chaney RH, Eyman RK: Predicting the development of hypertension from blood pressure measurements during isometric exercise. *Cardiol Board Rev* 1990; 7: 131–138.

50. Thomas CB: The heritage of hypertension. *Am J Med Sci* 1952; 224:367–376.

51. Longhurst JC, Mitchell HH: Does endurance training benefit the cardiovascular system? *J Cardiovasc Med* 1983; 8: 227–236.

52. Bezucha GR, et al.: Comparison of hemodynamic responses to static and dynamic exercise. *J Appl Physiol* 1982; 53: 1589–1593.

53. Asmussen E: Similarities and dissimilarities between static and dynamic exercise. *Circulation Res* 1981; 48(part 2):I3–I10.

54. Amery A, et al.: Influence of hypertension on the hemodynamic response to exercise. *Circulation* 1967; 36:231–237.

55. Sannerstedt R: Hemodynamic response to exercise in patients with arterial hypertension. *Acta Med Scand-Suppl* 1966; 458:1–83.

56. Sannerstedt R, Julius S: Systemic hemodynamics in borderline arterial hypertension: Responses to static exercise before and under the influence of propranolol. *Cardiovasc Res* 1972; 6:398–403.

57. Hoel BL, Lorentsen E, Lund-Larsen PG: Hemodynamic responses to sustained hand-grip in patients with hypertension. *Acta Med Scand* 1970; 188:491–495.

58. Gottdeiner JS, et al.: Left ventricular hypertrophy in men with normal blood pressure: Relation to exaggerated blood pressure response to exercise. *Ann Intern Med* 1990; 112:161–166.

59. Bennett T, Wilcox RG, MacDonald IA: Post-exercise reduction of blood pressure in hypertensive men is not due to acute impairment of baroreflex function. *Clin Sci* 1984; 67:97–103.

60. Kaufman FL, Hughson OL, Schaman JP: Effect of exercise on recovery blood pressure in normotensive and hypertensive subjects. *Med Sci Sports Exerc* 1987; 19:17–20.

61. Miller DD, et al.: Effects of systemic hypertension on exercise ejection fraction. *Hypertens Vascular Dis* 1987; 4:21–39.

62. Buck C, Donner AP: Isometric occupational exercise and the incidence of hypertension. *J Occup Med* 1985; 27: 370–372.

63. Hagberg JM, Seals DR: Exercise training and hypertension. *Acta Med Scand-Suppl* 1986; 711:131–136.

64. Hagberg JM: Exercise, fitness and hypertension. In Bouchard C, et al., eds: *Exercise, Fitness and Health: A Consensus of Current Knowledge.* Human Kinetics Books: Champaign, Ill. 1990.

65. Tipton CM, et al.: Influences of exercise intensity, age, and medication on resting systolic blood pressure of SHR populations. *J Appl Physiol* 1983; 55:1305–1310.

66. Hagberg JM, et al.: Effect of exercise training on the blood pressure and hemodynamic features of hypertensive adolescents. *Am J Cardiol* 1983; 52: 763–768.

67. Roman O, et al.: Physical training program in arterial hypertension: A long term prospective follow-up. *Cardiol* 1981; 67: 230–243.

68. Kiyonaga A, et al.: Blood pressure and hormonal responses to aerobic exercise. *Hypertens* 1985; 7:125–131.

69. Urata H, et al.: Antihypertensive and volume-depleting effects of mild exercise on essential hypertension. *Hypertens* 1987; 9:245–252.

70. Harris KA, Holly RG: Physiological response to circuit weight training in borderline hypertensive subjects. *Med Sci Sports Exerc* 1987; 19:246–252.

71. Choquette G, Ferguson RJ: Blood pressure reduction in "borderline" hypertensives following physical training. *Can Med Assoc J* 1973; 108:699–703.

72. Boyer JL, Kasch FW: Exercise therapy in hypertensive men. *JAMA* 1970; 211: 1668–1671.

73. Wilmore JH, et al.: Strength, endurance, BMR and body composition changes during circuit weight training. Med Sci Sports Exerc 1976; 8:59–60.

74. Stone MH, et al.: Cardiovascular responses to short-term Olympic style weight training in young men. Can J Appl Sport Sci 1983; 8:134–139.

75. MacDougall JD, et al.: Arterial blood pressure response to heavy resistance exercise. J Appl Physiol 1985; 58:785–790.

76. Goldberg L, et al.: Changes in lipid and lipoprotein levels after weight training. JAMA 1984; 252:504–506.

77. Kelemen MH, et al.: Exercise training combined with antihypertensive drug therapy: Effects on lipids, blood pressure, and left ventricular mass. JAMA 1990; 263:2766–2771.

78. Hagberg JM, et al.: Effect of weight training on blood pressure and hemodynamics in hypertensive adolescents. J Pediatr 1984; 104:147–151.

79. Effron MB: Effects of resistive training on left ventricular function. Med Sci Sports Exerc 1989; 21:694–697.

80. Wiley RL, et al.: Isometric exercise training lowers resting blood pressure. Med Sci Sports Exerc 1992; 24:749–754.

81. Cade R, et al.: Effect of aerobic exercise training on patients with systemic arterial hypertension. Am J Med 1984; 77:785–790.

82. Madden DJ, Blumenthal JA, Ekelund LG: Effects of beta-blockade and exercise on cardiovascular and cognitive functioning. Hypertens 1988; 11:470–476.

83. Squire JM, Myers MM, Fried R: Cardiovascular responses to exercise and stress in the borderline hypertensive rat. Med Sci Sports Exerc 1987; 19:11–16.

84. Ferrannini E, et al.: Insulin resistance in essential hypertension. N Engl J Med 1987; 317:350–357.

85. Rocchini AP, et al.: Insulin and blood pressure during weight loss in obese adolescents. Hypertens 1987; 10:267–273.

86. Reisin E, et al.: Cardiovascular changes after weight reduction in obesity hypertension. Ann Intern Med 1983; 98:315–319.

87. Bjorntorp P: Hypertension and exercise. Hypertens 1982; 4(suppl 3):56–59.

88. Duncan JJ, et al.: The effects of aerobic exercise on plasma catecholamines and blood pressure in patients with mild essential hypertension. JAMA 1985; 254:2609–2613.

89. Winder W, et al.: Training-induced changes in hormonal and metabolic responses to submaximal exercise. J Appl Physiol 1979; 46:766–771.

90. Cox RH, et al.: Cardiovascular and sympathoadrenal responses to stress in swim-trained rats. J Appl Physiol 1985; 58:1207–1214.

91. Galbo H, et al.: Diminished hormonal responses to exercise in trained rats. J Appl Physiol 1977; 43:953–958.

92. Askew EW, et al.: Response of rat tissue lipases to physical training and exercise. Proc Soc Exp Biol Med 1972; 141:123–129.

93. Jennings GL, et al.: Effects of changes in physical activity on blood pressure and sympathetic tone. J Hypertens-Suppl 1984; 2:S139–S141.

94. Klein AA, et al.: Sympathetic nervous system and exercise tolerance response in normotensive and hypertensive adolescents. J Am Coll Cardiol 1984; 3:381–386.

95. Hartley LH, et al.: Multiple hormonal responses to graded exercise in relation to physical training. J Appl Physiol 1972; 33:602–606.

96. Cooksey JD, et al.: Exercise training and plasma catecholamines in patients with ischemic heart disease. Am J Cardiol 1978; 42:372–376.

97. Cleroux J, Peronnet F, de Champlain J: Effects of exercise training on plasma catecholamines and blood pressure in labile hypertensive subjects. Eur J Appl Physiol Occup Physiol 1987; 56:550–554.

98. Baum M: Insulin stimulates volume absorption in the rabbit proximal convoluted tubule. J Clin Invest 1987; 79:1104–1109.

99. Lever AF: Slow pressor mechanisms in hypertension: A role for hypertrophy of resistance vessels? J Hypertens 1986; 4:515–524.

100. Foster DW: Insulin resistance: A secret killer? [editorial] N Engl J Med 1989; 320:733–734.

101. Donahue RP, et al.: Hyperinsulinemia and elevated blood pressure: Cause, confounder, or coincidence? Am J Epidemiol 1990; 132:827–836.

102. Seals DR, et al.: Glucose tolerance in young and older athletes and sedentary men. J Appl Physiol 1984; 56:1521–1525.

103. Krotkiewski M, et al.: Effects of long-term physical training on body fat, metabolism, and blood pressure in obesity. Metabolism 1979; 28:650–658.

104. Bjorntorp P, et al.: The effect of physical training on insulin production in obesity. Metabolism 1970; 19:631–638.

105. Goldberg AP, et al.: Exercise training reduces coronary risk and effectively rehabilitates hemodialysis patients. Nephron 1986; 42:311–316.

106. Holmgren A, et al.: Effect of training on work capacity, total hemoglobin, blood volumes, heart volume and pulse rate in recumbent and upright positions. Acta Physiol Scand 1960; 50:70–83.

107. Beretta-Piccoli C, et al.: Relation of arterial pressure with exchangeable and total body sodium and with plasma exchangeable and total body potassium in essential hypertension. Clin Sci 1981; 61(Suppl 7):81s–84s.

108. Papademetriou V, et al.: Exercise blood

pressure response and left ventricular hypertrophy. *Am J Hypertens* 1989; 2: 114–116.

109. Mannix ET, et al.: Atrial natriuretic peptide and the renin-aldosterone axis during exercise in man. *Med Sci Sports Exerc* 1990; 22:785–789.
110. Shenker Y, et al.: Plasma levels of immunoreactive atrial natriuretic factor in healthy subjects and in patients with edema. *J Clin Invest* 1985; 76:1684–1687.
111. Richards AM, et al.: Plasma atrial natriuretic peptide concentrations during exercise in sodium replete and deplete normal man. *Clin Sci* 1987; 72:159–164.
112. Fleckenstein A: *Calcium Antagonism in Heart and Smooth Muscle: Experimental Facts, Therapeutic Prospects.* John Wiley & Sons: New York, 1983.
113. Henry PD: Comparative pharmacology of calcium antagonists: Nifedipine, verapamil and diltiazem. *Am J Cardiol* 1980; 46: 1047–1058.
114. Newman RK, et al.: Effect of verapamil on left ventricular performance in conscious dogs. *J Pharmacol Exp Ther* 1977; 201: 723–730.
115. D'Agostino HJ Jr, et al.: Effect of verapamil on left ventricular function at rest and during exercise in normal men. *J Cardiovasc Pharmacol* 1983; 5:812–817.
116. Klein W, et al.: Role of calcium antagonists in the treatment of essential hypertension. *Circ Res* 1983; 52(suppl): I174–I181.
117. Stein DT, et al.: Effects of nifedipine and verapamil on isometric and dynamic exercise in normal subjects. *Am J Cardiol* 1984; 54:386–389.
118. Chick TW, et al.: The effect of nifedipine on cardiopulmonary responses during exercise in normal subjects. *Chest* 1986; 89:641–646.
119. Szlachcic J, et al.: Diltiazem versus propranolol in essential hypertension: Responses of rest and exercise blood pressure and effects on exercise capacity. *Am J Cardiol* 1987; 59:393–399.
120. Goldberg L, Elliot DL: Comparison of labetalol and verapamil at rest and during maximal exercise among hypertensives. *Med Sci Sports Exerc* 1989; 21:S87.
121. Stein DT, et al.: Effects of nifedipine and verapamil on isometric and dynamic exercise in normal subjects. *Am J Cardiol* 1984; 54:386–389.
122. Cody RJ, et al.: Exercise hemodynamics and oxygen delivery in human hypertension: Response to verapamil. *Hypertension* 1986; 8:3–10.
123. Raffestin B, et al.: Effects of nifedipine on responses to exercise in normal subjects. *J Appl Physiol* 1985; 58:702–709.
124. Yamakado T, et al.: Effects of diltiazem on cardiovascular responses during exercise in systemic hypertension and comparison

to propranolol. *Am J Cardiol* 1983; 52: 1023–1027.

125. Duffey DJ, Horwitz LD, Brammell HL: Nifedipine and the conditioning response. *Am J Cardiol* 1984; 53:908–911.
126. *Drug Utilization in the U.S.—1984.* Washington D.C.: U.S. Department of Health and Human Services; March 1986. Report No FDA\CDB-86\112.
127. Nordenfelt I: Blood flow of working muscles during autonomic blockade of the heart. *Cardiovasc Res* 1974; 8:263–267.
128. Trap-Jensen J, et al.: The effects of beta-adrenoceptor blockers on cardiac output, liver blood flow and skeletal muscle blood flow in hypertensive patients,. *Acta Physiol Scand* 1976; 440(Suppl):30.
129. McSorley PD, Warren DJ: Effects of propranolol and metroprolol on the peripheral circulation. *BMJ* 1978; 2:1598–1600.
130. Tesch PA: Exercise performance and beta-blockade. *Sports Med* 1985; 2:389–412.
131. Joyner MJ, et al.: Effects of beta-blockade on exercise capacity of trained and untrained men: A hemodynamic comparison. *J Appl Physiol* 1986; 60(4):1429–1434.
132. Gordon NF, et al.: Effect of dual beta-blockade and calcium antagonism on endurance performance. *Med Sci Sports Exerc* 1987; 19:1–6.
133. Sable DL, et al.: Attenuation of exercise conditioning by beta-adrenergic blockade. *Circulation* 1982; 65:679–684.
134. Willmore JH, et al.: Beta-blockade and response to exercise: Influence of training. *Phys Sportsmed* 1985; 13:60–69.
135. Wolfel EE, et al.: Effects of selective and nonselective beta-adrenergic blockade on mechanisms of exercise conditioning. *Circulation* 1986; 74:664–674.
136. Marsh RC, et al.: Attenuation of exercise conditioning by low dose beta-adrenergic blockade. *J Am Coll Cardiol* 1983; 2: 551–556.
137. Ades PA, et al.: Hypertension, exercise and beta-adrenergic blockade. *Ann Intern Med* 1988; 109:629–634.
138. Morrow TA, et al.: Aerobic training and hypertensives: Does atenolol inhibit or conceal the conditioning effect? *Med Sci Sports Exerc* 1990; 22:S26.
139. Fagard R, et al.: Response of the systemic and pulmonary circulation to alpha- and beta-receptor blockade (labetalol) at rest and during exercise in hypertensive patients. *Circulation* 1979; 60:1214–1217.
140. Goldberg L, et al.: A comparison of labetalol v atenolol on exercise training of sedentary hypertensives. *Med Sci Sports Exerc* 1990; 22:S26.
141. Gifford RW Jr: Role of diuretics in treatment of essential hypertension. *Am J Cardiol* 1986; 58:15A–17A.
142. *The 1984 Report of the Joint National Committee on Detection, Evaluation, and Treat-*

ment of High Blood Pressure. Bethesda, MD: Dept. of Health and Human Services publication NIH 84-1088, 1984.

143. McMahon FG: *Management of Essential Hypertension: The Once-A-Day Era.* Futura Publication Co: New York, 1978.

144. Messerli FH, et al.: Hypertension and sudden death: Disparate effects of calcium entry blocker and diuretic therapy on cardiac dysrhythmias. *Arch Intern Med* 1989; 149:1263–1267.

145. Lund-Johansen P: Hemodynamic changes in long-term diuretic therapy of essential hypertension: A comparative study of chlorthalidone, polythiazide and hydrochlorothiazide. *Acta Med Scand* 1970; 187:509–518.

146. Lee WR, Fox LM, Slotkoff LM: Effects of antihypertensive therapy on cardiovascular response to exercise. *Am J Cardiol* 1979; 44:325–328.

147. Rosendorff C, Goodman C, Coull A: Effect of antihypertensive therapy on left ventricular function and myocardial perfusion at rest and during exercise. *J Hypertens* 1984; 2(Suppl 2):63–68.

148. Lever AF: Angiotensin II, angiotensin-converting enzyme inhibitors, and blood vessel structure. *Am J Med* 1992; 92(Suppl 4B):35S–38S.

149. Doyle AE: ACE inhibition: Benefits beyond blood pressure control. *Am J Med* 1992; 92(Suppl 4B):1S–2S.

150. Dzau VJ: Short- and long-term determinants of cardiovascular function and therapy: Contributions of circulation and tissue renin-angiotensin systems. *J Cardiovasc Pharmacol* 1989; 14(Suppl 4):S1–S5

151. Williams GH: Converting-enzyme inhibitors in the treatment of hypertension. *N Engl J Med* 1988; 319:1517–1525.

152. Pickering TG, et al.: Comparison of antihypertensive and hormonal effects of captopril and propranolol at rest and during exercise. *Am J Cardiol* 1982; 49:1566–1568.

153. Leon AS, et al.: Enalapril alone and in combination with hydrochlorothiazide in the treatment of hypertension: Effect on treadmill exercise performance. *J Cardiopulmon Rehabil* 1986; 6:251–256.

154. Reid JL, Millar JA, Campbell BC: Enalapril and autonomic reflexes and exercise performance. *J Hypertens* 1983; 1(suppl): 129–134.

155. Williams GH: Quality of life and its impact on hypertensive patients. *Am J Med* 1987; 82:98–105.

156. Lund-Johansen P: Hemodynamic changes at rest and during exercise in long-term clonidine therapy of essential hypertension. *Acta Med Scand* 1974; 1-2:111–115.

157. Davies SF, et al.: Comparative effects of transdermal clonidine and oral atenolol on acute exercise performance and response to aerobic conditioning in subjects with hypertension. *Arch Intern Med* 1989; 149:1551–1556.

158. Lund-Johansen P: Hemodynamic changes at rest and during exercise in long-term prazosin therapy for essential hypertension. *Postgrad Med* Nov 1975: 45–52.

159. Pandhi T, Sharma PL: Comparative effects of beta-, alpha- and combined beta- plus alpha-adrenoceptor blocking agents in stress-induced increase in arterial blood pressure. *Int J Pharmacol Ther Toxicol* 1987; 25:297–300.

160. Multiple Risk Factor Intervention Trial Research Group: Multiple Risk Factor Intervention Trial: Risk factor changes and mortality results. *JAMA* 1982; 248:1465–1477.

161. Lake CR, Ziegler MG, Coleman MD: Hydrochlorothiazide-induced sympathetic hyperactivity in hypertensive patients. *Clin Pharmacol Ther* 1979; 26:428–432.

162. Medical Research Council Working Party on Mild to Moderate Hypertension: Ventricular extrasystoles during thiazide treatment: Substudy of MRC mild hypertension trial. *BMJ* 1983; 287:1249–1253.

163. Ames RP: Metabolic disturbances increasing the risk of coronary heart disease during diuretic-based antihypertensive therapy: Lipid alterations and glucose intolerance. *Am Heart J* 1983; 106:1207–1214.

164. Samuelsson O, et al.: Cardiovascular morbidity in relation to change in blood pressure and serum cholesterol levels in treated hypertension: Results from the primary prevention trial in Göteburg, Sweden. *JAMA* 1987; 258:1768–1776.

165. Heyden S, Schneider KA, Fodor GJ: Failure to reduce cholesterol as explanation for the limited efficacy of antihypertensive treatment in the reduction of CHD: Examination of the evidence from six hypertension intervention trials. *Klin Wochenschr* 1987; 65:828–832.

166. Johnson BF, et al.: Comparative effects of propranolol and prazosin upon serum lipids in thiazide-treated hypertensive patients. *Am J Med* 1984; 76:109–112.

167. Lehtonen A, Marniemi J: Effect of atenolol on plasma HDL cholesterol subfractions. *Atherosclerosis* 1984; 51:335–338.

168. Bender W, La France N, Walker WG: Mechanism of deterioration in renal function in patients with renovascular hypertension treated with enalapril. *Hypertens* 1984; 6:I193–I197.

169. Jenkins AC, et al.: Captopril in hypertension: Seven years later. *J Cardiovasc Pharmacol* 1985; 7(suppl 1):S96–S101.

170. *The Recommended Quantity and Quality of Exercise for Developing and Maintaining Cardiorespiratory and Muscular Fitness in Healthy Adults.* American College of Sports Medicine Position Stand, 1990.

CHAPTER 3

CARDIAC REHABILITATION

TERENCE KAVANAGH, MD

The emergence of cardiac rehabilitation is due to a combination of circumstances. First was the ascendance of ischemic heart disease and its major manifestation, acute myocardial infarction (MI), as a leading cause of death and disability. Then, in the 1950s, Levine and Lown[1] introduced early mobilization after a heart attack, an approach conferring psychologic and physiologic benefits, without increasing the incidence of cardiac rupture, sudden death, or left ventricular aneurysm formation. Early movement resulted in a more rapid recovery, whereas prolonged bed rest was associated with muscle wasting, bone loss, poor cardiovascular performance, and thromboembolic episodes.[2] Furthermore, evidence suggests that a sedentary lifestyle is a major risk factor for ischemic heart disease; conversely, regular exercise exerts a protective effect, both in primary prevention and in rehabilitation following a cardiac event.

In this chapter, I review the mechanisms of the beneficial effects of exercise for those with atherosclerotic cardiac disease, valvular abnormalities, and conduction defects, and following cardiac transplantation. Specific recommendations for a cardiac rehabilitation program are provided.

The Benefits of Exercise

PRIMARY PREVENTION OF ISCHEMIC HEART DISEASE

Regular physical activity may delay the onset of ischemic heart disease or protect against the disease. An inverse relationship exists between physical activity and cardiac disease, and the reported benefit is a twofold to threefold reduction in risk. A study from the Centers for Disease Control[3] subjected 43 published studies to careful epidemiologic and statistical analysis and concluded that physical activity was inversely related to the incidence of coronary heart disease, with the risk of inactivity similar in magnitude to that of hypertension, hypercholesterolemia, and smoking. Because a higher proportion of U.S. adults lead a sedentary lifestyle (60%) than suffer from hypertension (10%) or hypercholesterolemia (10%), or smoke a pack or more of cigarettes a day (18%), increasing the general population's physical activity may have a greater effect on reducing the incidence of ischemic heart disease than modification of the other three risk factors.[3]

MECHANISMS

Physical training could exert a favorable influence on the atherosclerotic or thrombotic processes by several possible mechanisms. Evidence from animal models indicates that chronic exercise can increase coronary artery diameter, the extent of myocardial capillarization,[4,5] and coronary collateral growth.[6-8] Heightened resistance of the ischemic heart to ventricular fibrillation also has been demonstrated in treadmill-trained animals.[9,10] Nontrained macaque monkeys, fed an atherosclerotic diet, developed severe coronary atherosclerosis and fatal MI, whereas their treadmill-trained counterparts who were fed the same diet had large-caliber coronary arteries free from atherosclerosis.[11]

Among healthy humans, exercise training has effects on both cardiac dimensions and performance. Prolonged vigorous activity, particularly when started in adolescence, increases ventricular volume and wall thickness, with these changes correlating closely with increased maximal oxygen uptake (VO_{2max}).[12-15] Unlike the hypertrophy due to disease, changes in the athlete's heart are accompanied by a proportionate increase in coronary artery vasculature.[16] However, there is little evidence that similar dimensional changes occur in middle-aged subjects, particularly in the presence of ischemic heart disease. The aging myocardium may be incapable of such adaptation, especially when poorly perfused. An alternative explanation for lack of such changes is that the training stimulus was inadequate. The latter possibility is supported by reports[17,18] of increased left ventricular mass in post–MI patients when they undertook 8 to 12 months of high-intensity jogging.

Regular physical exercise results in a reduction in heart rate, both at rest and during a fixed submaximal work load. This reduction has been attributed to increased resting vagal tone and reduced sympathetic drive during exercise. There is still debate as to whether this originates in the heart or the periphery.

In an effort to solve the problem, some investigators have trained the upper or the lower limbs, and then carried out exercise testing on the "trained" and "untrained" limbs to measure the cardiovascular responses to training. Arm training did not result in this "training effect" when individuals were evaluated with leg exercise,[18a-20] supporting the contention that peripheral stimuli predominate. A number of studies, however, have demonstrated that some 50% of the training effects developed by leg exercise can be evoked by subsequent arm testing.[21-24] In the final analysis, the differing results may be a reflection of variations among subjects, as well as the mode, intensity, and duration of the training.

Our experience at the Toronto Rehabilitation Centre with cardiac transplantation patients supports both peripheral and central effects of physical conditioning. Resting and submaximal bradycardia were observed in the denervated hearts of transplantation recipients, but only in those who achieved an exercise quantity of 32 km or more per week of walking-jogging over a 2-year period.[25] We reasoned that this reflected reduced catecholamine levels, down-regulation, or both in either sensitivity or density of myocardial adrenoreceptors. Conversely, for some heterotopic transplant recipients (in which the donor's heart augments the native heart), compliance to the exercise program was not high, and thus no training effect was seen in the denervated donor heart.[26] However, the innervated native heart did develop a training bradycardia. These findings infer that central and peripheral mechanisms coexist and are induced by differing types and levels of training stimuli.

In addition to resting bradycardia, the product of systolic blood pressure and heart rate ("double product") during similar work loads is reduced after training. The lower double product reflects reduced myocardial oxygen consumption at a given external exercise level.[27] Also, the lower heart rate at a given work load signifies an increase in the period of diastole. Since coronary blood flow occurs during this phase of the cardiac cycle, its prolongation can reduce myocardial ischemia. Both a reduction in double product and an increased diastole are likely explanations for the reduction in anginal symptoms at a given work load reported following endurance training.[28-30]

Although maximum heart rate is unchanged by training, stroke volume and maximum cardiac output are increased, which can be explained by peripheral circulatory changes. Total peripheral resistance is reduced because of the increased vascularity and vasodilatation of the trained skeletal muscles.[31] Among healthy individuals, higher stroke volumes are partly due to improved myocardial contractility,[32,33] but stroke volume was not increased among a group of 12 post–MI patients who participated in a 3-month training program.[34] Thus, the improvement in maximal oxygen uptake in these patients was ascribed entirely to an increase in peripheral oxygen extraction. On the other hand, a randomized study[35] carried out on 79 post–MI patients attending the Toronto Rehabilitation Centre demonstrated a 10% increase in stroke volume. Interestingly, this change was apparent only after 12 months of training. Prior to this, fitness gains were due to increased peripheral oxygen extraction.

Peripheral mechanisms can result in increased exercise capacity and increased VO_{2max} for patients with coronary disease who have reduced ventricular function. Regular exercise increases capillarization of skeletal muscle, raises myoglobin levels, increases the number and size of mitochondria, and enhances oxidative enzyme activity.[31,36] The net result is a more efficient oxygen transport system and greater arteriovenous oxygen difference after training, resulting in more external work accomplished with less cardiac work.

Finally, a number of other changes accompanying regular exercise impact on coronary artery disease, including increase in plasma high-density lipoprotein cholesterol,[37-39] reduction in plasma catecholamine levels,[40,41] improved insulin sensitivity,[42,43] and enhanced fibrinolytic activity with reduction in platelet aggregation.[44,45]

Exercise Rehabilitation

BENEFITS FROM EXERCISE AFTER MYOCARDIAL INFARCTION

For the patient recovering from an acute MI, exercise training offers benefits in addition to a possible reduction in subsequent cardiac events. The stricken individual, previously in apparent good health, is abruptly confronted with the fact of his or her mortality; an immediate fear of death may give way to depression and a loss of self-confidence. A strategy of early mobilization and exercise training is effective in alleviating depression, restoring self-confidence, and reducing anxiety.[46,47]

By means of a training program, individuals can increase exercise capacity and the stimulus required to induce angina. This adaptation is due primarily to a reduction in the double product and a prolongation of diastole. It has also been suggested that exercise may increase pain tolerance[48] and coronary arteriovenous oxygen difference.[49] Debate continues as to whether exercise, particularly in the presence of coronary stenosis, can enhance development of coronary collaterals. Confirmation in man has proven difficult, possibly because these vessels are small, located intramurally, and undetectable by routine coronary angiography. There is circumstantial evidence for the development of collaterals, however, from studies showing that vigorous training results in higher double products for equivalent levels of myocardial ischemia (as measured by onset of angina or amount of ST-segment depression).[50-53] Exercise scintigraphy has detected training-induced collateral circulation after regular exercise.[54-56] Finally, there is increasing evidence that combining a low-fat diet and intensive exercise training can improve myocardial perfusion by regression of coronary atherosclerosis.[57,58]

Thus, it appears that exercise can enhance the patient's quality of life, improve functional capacity, counteract risk factors, and encourage a return to work. For these reasons, post–MI exercise therapy is firmly advocated by the World Health Organization,[59] as well as by many international and national organizations involved in the public health aspects of atherosclerotic heart disease.

In the final analysis, it is still unclear whether exercise training improves prognosis. A number of prospective randomized controlled trials have addressed this problem. Some investigations show a statistically significant beneficial effect, while others fail to do so. The reasons for the inconsistency are not peculiar to exercise therapy, but rather to the disease process being investigated. Given that coronary atherosclerosis takes years to develop, it follows that combative techniques will require equal time to establish statistical and clinical validity. For many, the disease may have progressed so far that a relatively brief therapeutic intervention is inadequate to alter its course. Equally important is the relatively low number of subjects studied. As an example of the large subject number required, the Lipid Research Clinic's Coronary Primary Prevention Trial[60] followed approximately 10,000 hypercholesterolemic men for an average of 7 years and failed to find any difference in the incidence of fatal MI between treated and untreated groups. Only by accounting for nonfatal MIs and extrapolating this to the population as a whole could the results be used to justify the present public health strategy of reducing serum cholesterol levels to 5.2 mmol/L or less.

Given the problems of inadequate patient numbers and short-term follow-up, meta-analysis has been used to pool results and analyze them as a single group. Although no trial studying exercise showed a significant reduction in mortality, all but one had a positive trend favoring physical training.[61] By combining results, a significant (19%) reduction in total mortality was found among the exercisers. The use of meta-analysis was particularly appropriate, since pooled studies closely resemble each other in format, time from acute event to entry, and freedom from pharmacologic factors. When 10 other randomized prospective trials were subjected to meta-analysis,[62] a highly significant reduction of 25% in recurrent fatal MI was noted in the exercising group. This is "as beneficial an effect as has been reported for beta-blockade therapy after acute myocardial infarction, a form of intervention now widely accepted. . . ."[63] The most recent review[64] analyzed 22 published trials, involving a total of 4,554 patients who were followed for an average of 3 years, and obtained similar results; the exercisers experienced 20% to 25% less mortality from heart attack than the nonexercisers.

PATIENT SELECTION

Historically, cardiac rehabilitation has involved the MI survivor, and these patients still constitute the majority of referrals. However, cardiac rehabilitation has been extended to individuals following bypass surgery and coronary angioplasty, pacemaker placement, and cardiac transplantation and, in recent years, to those with stable, chronic heart failure.

Variant Angina

For those with Prinzmetal's, or variant, angina, there is less evidence for the beneficial effect of training. Classically, these patients suffer from unprovoked nocturnal angina, which awakens them or occurs shortly after rising. However, at least 50% of affected individuals experience chest pain in relation to excitement or exertion. With the advent of calcium channel blockers and their potential for relieving coronary artery spasm, these patients are candidates for cardiac rehabilitation.

Coronary Artery Bypass Grafting

Coronary artery bypass graft (CABG) surgery has increased dramatically since it was first introduced in the mid-1960s. Many cardiac rehabilitation programs include patients recovering from CABG, who may experience a psychologic boost associated with rapid mobilization after surgery. It is hoped that the rehabilitation approach, by reducing risk factors, may favorably influence the reported 5% annual angina recurrence rate due to graft closure, native coronary disease progression, or both.[65,66] Post–CABG patients can be mobilized 24 hours after surgery and progress more rapidly during the in-hospital phase. They can commence an endurance training regimen 5 to 6 weeks after surgery.[67,68]

The training program for post–CABG patients requires little modification, apart from awareness that chest wall pain and, in the case of a venous graft, leg discomfort may slow the patient's progress. Upper-limb exercises may be a valuable component in preventing adhesions, muscle weakness, and resultant poor posture.[67,68]

With the increasing interest in cost-effectiveness, CABG surgery should be evaluated for its ability to improve the quality and extent of life in terms of returning patients to employment. Surgical patients are less likely to return to employment than medically treated post–MI patients.[69–73] However, the CABG patient may have more disease and thus be more disabled. Also, return-to-work status may reflect many personal and socioeconomic variables, as well as surgical outcome.[73,74] An uncontrolled study[75] noted that 1 year after bypass surgery, 350 patients participating in exercise rehabilitation reported significant increases in time spent on physical activities such as walking, hiking, bicycling, bowling, and golf, but these findings are of less impact because there was no control group.

Percutaneous Transluminal Coronary Angioplasty

Many patients who undergo percutaneous transluminal coronary angioplasty (PTCA) underestimate the chronic nature of their coronary artery disease and perceive the procedure as a "quick fix," not recognizing the necessity for rehabilitation. PTCA patients can start training 2 to 4 weeks after the procedure. The incidence of post-operative stenosis within the first 12 months has been estimated at between 25% and 30%.[76] Whether a vigorously pursued rehabilitation regimen can favorably affect this outcome remains a subject for further research. However, the close observation, serial exercise testing, and telemetry associated with exercise training affords an excellent opportunity for early detection of restenosis.

Valve Surgery

Patients recovering from cardiac valve surgery, despite an excellent hemodynamic result, may be disabled by years of presurgical restricted activity and deconditioning; they also are candidates for exercise rehabilitation.[77,78] Patients with mechanical prosthetic valves, however, receive anticoagulant therapy and may not tolerate vigorous, weightbearing activities. Also, mechanical prostheses have fixed orifices, which place some limitation, at least theoretically, on cardiac performance during maximal effort.

Pacemaker Patients

Exercise regimens can be of value for individuals with permanent transvenous pacemakers.[79–81] Since heart rate is limited to the programmed level, those with fixed-rate ventricular synchronous devices will require monitoring by blood pressure and perceived exertion scales, with close attention to symptoms of cerebral ischemia. Direct measurement of oxygen uptake during an exercise test is recommended because it ensures the accurate prescription of a safe and effective training intensity. In general, patients who perform satisfactorily on an exercise test can safely follow the customary modes of endurance training, although vigorous upper-body activities may not be advisable.

Chronic Heart Failure

It had been believed that patients with severe left ventricular dysfunction (i.e., ejection fraction less than 30%) should avoid exercise. In these patients, effort is limited by inadequate stroke volume and cardiac output, with resultant poor skeletal muscle perfusion and marked limitation in aerobic capacity.[82-85] The combination of pulmonary venous congestion and low cardiac output can result in frank congestive heart failure (CHF). However, neither resting nor exercise ejection fraction is an adequate measure of exercise tolerance, as patients with the same ejection fractions vary widely in exercise capacity. Exercise testing, particularly with metabolic measurements, can provide an assessment of exercise capacity by determining VO_{2max} and ventilatory threshold. These measures of physical capacity can be used to stratify patients more accurately than the subjective indices of fatigue and dyspnea.[86-90]

Despite potential adverse effects, exercise training has benefited individuals with impaired ventricular function. Eight post–MI patients with an ejection fraction of less than 45% exercised for 2 months.[91] The authors reported no adverse effects, but the subjects showed no change in ejection fraction or any other measure of ventricular function. Nevertheless, all patients were symptomatically improved and increased their exercise capacity by 17%, with a concomitant 13% fall in heart rate and a 7% blood pressure reduction.

In another study,[92] 18 patients with ejection fractions less than 40% trained for 12 to 42 months. Resting heart rate decreased, exercise performance improved, and there was no change in ventricular function. Others[93,94] have confirmed that patients with CHF placed on an exercise program achieve a training effect and enhanced well-being without evidence of improved cardiac function. Twelve patients with CHF trained for 16 to 24 weeks, using a combination of stationary cycling, stair climbing, walking, and jogging.[95] They demonstrated a 52% increase in work capacity, 23% higher maximal oxygen uptake, and 20% improvement in the oxygen uptake level at the ventilatory threshold.

The first controlled, randomized crossover comparison of physical training and restriction of physical activity was reported in 1990, and involved 11 patients with stable heart failure and a mean ejection fraction of 19%.[96] Eight weeks of home-based cycle ergometer training resulted in an 18% increase in maximal oxygen uptake, an 18% decrease in submaximal rate-pressure production, an 8% reduction in resting heart rate, and improved scores for breathlessness, fatigue, general well-being, and ease of normal daily activities.

Thus, although it might be premature to advocate widespread admission of CHF patients to exercise programs, there is increasing evidence that physical training will benefit a number of these patients.

Following Myocardial Infarction

The majority of individuals in cardiac rehabilitation will have had a recent MI. Clinical observation and symptom-limited exercise testing 3 to 4 weeks following the infarct identifies patients with high, moderate, and low risks.[97-99] Lower-risk patients are those individuals who can perform more than 5-6 METs (metabolic equivalents) of exercise (oxygen uptake of 17.5-21 mL/kg/min) without ischemia. Those patients who can exercise to eight or more METs (oxygen uptake of 28 mL/kg/min or more) can perform most physical activities. For the latter subset of low-risk patients, rehabilitation may be considered for psychologic reasons or patient preferences but is not needed to enhance exercise capacity.

Individuals considered at higher risk develop ischemia at a heart rate of less than 130 bpm or five METs. Other high-risk patients include those with reduced ventricular function (ejection fraction less than 30%), complex ventricular arrhythmias, angina or ST depression at low-level exercise, and sudden-death survivors. The high-risk patients are generally referred for angiography and further intervention. Although ideally all high-risk and many moderate-risk patients will be identified before referral to rehabilitation programs, in practice some will only be recognized at the time of an admission exercise test, or even later, during training sessions.

Typically, one half of post-MI patients are in the low-risk category. They will be referred to a rehabilitation program on the basis of their needs, as perceived by themselves and their physicians. Some will require assistance to return to heavy labor or to vigorous recreational activity. For others, restoration of self-confidence by demonstrating the ability to participate in a training program may be necessary to attain full recovery. All low-risk patients should be assessed for rehabilitation, as even those who consider themselves fit may be exercising at an inappropriately high intensity. This group will not require close monitoring or prolonged supervision and can often continue on their own after attending classes for a few weeks to several months.

A significant proportion of the moderate- to high-risk patients will undergo revascularization; the remainder will likely constitute less than 30% of MI survivors, including the inoperable and those declining surgery. For some, exercise training will be absolutely contraindicated (Table 3-1). The others

Table 3-1 **CONTRAINDICATIONS TO AN EXERCISE TRAINING REGIMEN**

Unstable angina
Severe aortic outflow obstruction
Acute myocarditis or pericarditis
Uncontrolled complex arrhythmias
Active congestive heart failure
Recent pulmonary embolism or thrombophlebitis
Untreated third-degree heart block
Severe systemic hypertension that is not
   responding to medication
Uncontrolled diabetes
Acute infections

will need varying degrees of close observation, including telemetry, ambulatory monitoring, and one-on-one supervision.

Once candidates are chosen for exercise rehabilitation, the question of how soon to start after the acute event must be addressed. Although mobilization with low-level activities occurs just days after uncomplicated MI or CABG surgery, evidence suggests that exercise conditioning programs that begin within 8 weeks after the MI may be associated with a higher incidence of recurrent MI.[62]

PROGRAM COMPONENTS

It has been customary to categorize cardiac rehabilitation programs into phase I, II, and III, according to whether they take place before hospital discharge, during a 3- to 6-month outpatient period, or thereafter as maintenance therapy. For most patients, the period of hospitalization is 7 to 10 days. Routine care usually includes early mobilization, health education, and referral to an outpatient exercise program. Since the mortality rates following an acute MI fall off steeply after the first year, this period is a time for intensive rehabilitation, with its attendant counseling, testing, and monitoring.

EFFECTS OF MEDICATION

Many patients entering a cardiac rehabilitation program are taking agents that affect their response to physical exertion. Awareness of drug effects allows appropriate interpretation of exercise testing and advice on training parameters (see also Chapter 2).

Beta-blocking agents are used for the treatment of angina and hypertension. There also is evidence that the administration of a beta blocker to post– MI patients can reduce mortality from recurrent infarctions by as much as 25%.[62] These drugs block cardiac adrenoreceptors, resulting in reduced heart rate and blood pressure at rest and during exercise. As a result, the double product is decreased, lowering myocardial oxygen demand. This will enable the patient with angina to achieve a higher exercise work load without symptoms. However, angina (or ST-segment depression) will recur at the previous product of heart rate times systolic blood pressure. Although VO_{2max} can be reduced, oxygen consumption during submaximal work largely is unaffected by beta-blockade.[100-102] Similarly, there appears to be little effect on ratings of perceived exertion.[103]

Drug-induced exercise bradycardia invalidates the use of age-related heart rate tables for establishing maximal or target rates, although the linear relationship of heart rate to oxygen uptake remains unaltered.[104,105] Therefore, exercise intensity still can be related to the customary percentage of the maximal heart rate achieved on beta-blockade. Since blood levels and the drug's chronotropic effect will vary with the time of ingestion, training sessions and repeat appointments for exercise testing should be arranged to maintain a constant time between activity and medication dosing.

Evidence shows that cardiac patients receiving beta blockers can achieve a training effect.[103-110] The beta blockers can reduce utilization of fatty acids,[111] and possibly glycogen,[112] by skeletal muscle, however. This, together with the reduced cardiac output and peripheral vasoconstriction, may be the cause of fatigue experienced by some patients.

Calcium channel blockers act by slowing calcium passage into smooth-muscle cells of the myocardium and blood vessel walls, resulting in vasodilatation of coronary and peripheral vasculature. They are prescribed for the treatment of angina, hypertension, and some (verapamil hydrochloride and diltiazem hydrochloride), for supraventricular arrhythmias. The use of calcium channel blockers for angina and hypertension is increasing, and may ultimately equal that of the beta blockers. Several are currently available in North America: verapamil, diltiazem, nifedipine, nicardipine, isradipine, and felodipine. These drugs do not affect exercise capacity in the absence of angina. Nifedipine, isradipine, felodipine, and nicardipine can result in tachycardia; diltiazem, a mild bradycardia; and verapamil, either no effect on heart rate or a slight bradycardia. Cardiac conduction is not altered by nifedipine, nicardipine, felodipine, or isradipine, whereas both verapamil and diltiazem can produce varying degrees of atrioventricular block.

Digitalis, or digoxin, enhances cardiac contractility and is used in the treatment of CHF. It also is prescribed for atrial fibrillation, to reduce ventricular rate. Although not frequently indicated among cardiac rehabilitation patients, it has a bradycardic effect and can cause nonischemic ST-segment depression at rest and during exertion. This can potentially overstate the ischemic response during exercise testing.

Nitrates relieve angina by dilating coronary and peripheral vessels. The types of nitrates prescribed include the short-acting sublingual nitroglycerin tablet, long-acting isosorbide dinitrate, and nitroglycerin in a dermal patch or ointment and oral spray. All forms of nitrates reduce preload, increase heart rate, and lower blood pressure, enabling the patient to exercise without angina. Thus, they may be used prior to an exercise session to offset ischemia. However, they also can give rise to complaints of headache or hypotension, with the potential for syncope.

EXERCISE TESTING

Exercise testing and prescription for healthy subjects were addressed in Chapter 1. For cardiac patients, the most important prescription parameter is exercise intensity, which should be sufficient to achieve a training effect without inducing myocardial ischemia. Hence the need for an exercise test before beginning a program.

Whether the test is carried out on a treadmill or a cycle ergometer, the purpose is the same; that is, to study the cardiorespiratory responses to increasing physical effort. The noninvasive parameters usually monitored are symptoms, heart rate, blood pressure, exercise electrocardiogram (ECG), and a rating of perceived exertion. A further refinement is the collection and analysis of expired air to measure ventilation, oxygen consumption and carbon dioxide production, and the ventilatory threshold. In some laboratories, blood gases or oxygen saturation, pH, and lactate levels also can be measured.

During a symptom-limited maximal test, the work load is increased at regular prearranged intervals or continuously (ramping protocol) until the patient is exhausted or untoward symptoms or signs develop. Proof of true maximal effort is provided by failure of the heart rate or oxygen uptake to increase, despite a rise in workload. The maximum heart rates, which decrease with age, can be estimated from age-related tables, or by subtracting the patient's age from 220, if drugs that alter the chronotropic response to exercise (i.e., beta blockers) are not used.[113] A submaximal test is one carried out to a predetermined submaximal target heart rate.

Testing Protocols

In general, treadmills are used more commonly in clinical cardiology, and cycle ergometers tend to be used by those involved in respiratory physiology. The advantages of the cycle ergometer are:

1. Pedaling action is simple and does not arouse anxiety
2. Mechanical efficiency and work load are largely independent of body mass
3. The upper body remains stable, making it easier to obtain accurate metabolic and circulatory measurements.

A possible disadvantage is early quadriceps fatigue, particularly among those unaccustomed to cycling. The treadmill, on the other hand, employs the more customary and natural walking motion, but the use of the railings for support can reduce the energy cost of a given speed and slope, so the work load attained during the test is overestimated, in the absence of metabolic measurements. However, if this balance aid is proscribed during treadmill testing, it may produce fear in older or more disabled patients.

In the typical cycle ergometer test, the power output is increased by a constant value, usually 100 kpm·min⁻¹ (17 watts), every minute or two until the maximal or target heart rate is reached.[113] Protocols differ only in the time it takes for the subject to reach either of these goals. The Balke and Naughton treadmill protocols are the best suited for the early post–MI patient (Table 3–2). The Bruce (probably the most popular) and the Ellestad protocols begin with higher work loads and have greater incremental increases, and thus are less time-consuming (Table 3–3).[113a]

Occasionally patients are referred for a program that will involve arm training. These patients include paraplegics, lower-limb amputees, and anyone suffering from severe musculoskeletal or circulatory leg problems. Arm ergometry elicits different responses than treadmill walking or cycle ergometry, mainly because of differing amounts of muscle mass and prior conditioning. At equivalent levels of submaximal effort, the heart rate, systolic and diastolic blood pressure, minute ventilation, and oxygen uptake are higher and the stroke volume is lower during arm work than during leg work.[114-116] The maximal oxygen uptake achieved during arm ergometry generally is reported as 60% to 80% of that for the treadmill or cycle ergometer, or even less if contributions from the trunk muscles are prevented by use of a shoulder support and harness.[117] However, even if one calculates oxygen uptake on the basis of limb volume, the values are slightly higher during arm work as opposed to leg work.[118,119] Maximum values for cardiac output are lower, while values for heart rate and systolic blood pressure are similar.[120]

Often candidates for arm ergometry are in poor physical condition and will only be able to tolerate small increments in power output, such as 50 kpm·min⁻¹ (8 watts per minute). The test is usually discontinuous in type, with

Table 3-2 **PROTOCOLS FOR TREADMILL EXERCISE TEST: BALKE AND NAUGHTON**

	Balke		
Stage	Speed 3.3 mph	Grade (%)	Duration (min)
1	Constant	2	2
2	Constant	6	4
3	Constant	10	6
4	Constant	14	8
5	Constant	18	10
6	Constant	22	12

	Naughton*			
Stage	2.0 mph Grade (%)	3.0 mph Grade (%)	3.4 mph Grade (%)	Duration (min)
1	—	—	—	2
2	0.0	—	—	2
3	3.5	0.0	—	2
4	7.0	2.5	2.0	2
5	10.5	5.0	4.0	2
6	14.0	7.5	6.0	2
7	17.5	10.0	8.0	2
8	—	12.5	10.0	2
9	—	15.0	12.0	2
10	—	17.5	14.0	2
11	—	20.0	16.0	2
12	—	22.5	18.0	2
13	—	25.0	20.0	2
14	—	27.5	22.0	2
15	—	30.0	24.0	2
16	—	32.5	26.0	2

*Lower speeds suitable for cardiac patients and those with low tolerance.

work stages of 2 minutes and rests of 1 minute between stages. This pause allows time for a blood pressure reading and an ECG tracing that is free from muscle artifact. Usually, the maximal power output achieved is quite low but sufficient to demonstrate ischemic ST-segment changes.[121]

Responses to Testing

Exercise heart rate, whatever testing mode, is determined from the ECG, and increases linearly with work load and oxygen consumption. An attenuated response to increasing effort, or less commonly, failure of the heart rate to rise (termed "chronotropic incompetence" by Ellestad[122]) may be a feature of ischemic heart disease. There also can be reductions in resting and exercise heart rates as a result of treatment with beta-blocking agents or some of the calcium channel antagonists. Maximal heart rate (HR_{max}) is reached a minute or so before Vo_{2max}; this asymptote leads to the discrepancy when comparable levels are expressed as percentages, e.g., 50% Vo_{2max} = 65% HR_{max}.

Systolic pressure also increases as work load is augmented. An inadequate systolic blood pressure response, so-called "inotropic incompetence," suggests left ventricular dysfunction (usually a manifestation of severe coronary artery

Table 3–3 **PROTOCOLS FOR TREADMILL EXERCISE TEST: BRUCE AND ELLESTAD**

	Bruce		
Stage	Speed (mph)	Grade (%)	Duration (min)
1	1.7	10	3
2	2.5	12	3
3	3.4	14	3
4	4.2	16	3
5	5.0	18	3
6	5.5	20	3
7	6.0	22	3
	Ellestad		
Stage	Speed (mph)	Grade (%)	Duration (min)
1	1.7	10	3
2	3.0	10	2
3	4.0	10	2
4	5.0	10	3
5	5.0	15	2
6	6.0	15	3

disease) or aortic outflow obstruction.[123] The double product (heart rate $\times$ systolic blood pressure) correlates well with myocardial oxygen consumption during exercise and can be used to identify a threshold for angina from test to test. Diastolic pressure remains unchanged from rest, or can decrease slightly during dynamic exercise.[124]

CASE: G.D., a 46-year-old man, was evaluated for exercise rehabilitation 11 weeks after an acute anterior MI; the initial submaximal exercise test is shown in Table 3–4. He was not taking any medications.

Following this symptom-free test, in which the heart rate and blood pressure responded appropriately and the ECG was within normal limits, G.D. began an exercise program and returned to his work as a traveling salesman. Although his exercise regimen progressed satisfactorily, after 3 months he began to complain of extreme fatigue. He was advised to stop exercising, and a second exercise test (Table 3–5) was performed.

Table 3–4 **INITIAL POST–MI SUBMAXIMAL EXERCISE TEST**

Power Output (kpm/min)	Heart Rate (bpm)	Blood Pressure (mm Hg)	ECG	Symptoms
Rest	82	120/70	Normal	None
100	113	134/80	Normal	None
200	120	146/90	Normal	None
300	132	156/90	Normal	None
400	144	162/90	Normal	None
500	153	174/90	Normal	None
600	162	188/90	ST −0.6 mm	None
		Recovery		
4 min	111	110/70	Normal	None

Table 3–5 **FOLLOW-UP EXERCISE TEST**

Power Output (kpm/min)	Heart Rate (bpm)	Blood Pressure (mm Hg)	ECG	Symptoms
Rest	68	90/60	Normal	None
100	94	100/70	Normal	None
200	110	116/70	Normal	None
300	132	130/70	Normal	None
400	148	122/70	Normal	None
500	156	120/70	Normal	None
600	164	116/70	ST −1.7 mm	Breathless
Recovery				
1 min.	80	106/70	Normal	None
7 min	78	90/60	Normal	None

As a result of this test, in which there was a marked difference in the systolic blood pressure response, further investigations were planned. Unfortunately, before these could be performed, the patient died suddenly. An autopsy revealed a slightly enlarged heart and extensive coronary atherosclerosis, with scarring of the anterior, anteroseptal and anterolateral left ventricular walls. There was no evidence of recent infarction.

COMMENT: Failure of the systolic blood pressure to rise, or a fall in blood pressure in response to increasing effort, is an ominous sign. The most commonly sought exercise-induced ECG abnormality is ST-segment depression. This is observed most readily in the bipolar CM_5 lead, in which the positive electrode is placed at the V_5 position and the negative electrode on the manubrium.[125] The addition of two other leads (e.g., V_1 and III) increases the sensitivity and allows easier analysis of ectopic beats.

Horizontal or downward sloping ST-segment depression of 1 mm or more (measured 80 milliseconds from the "J" point) in any lead generally indicates myocardial ischemia. However, it can occur in a number of nonischemic conditions such as hypokalemia, left ventricular hypertrophy, bundle-branch block, Wolff-Parkinson-White syndrome, and the use of various pharmaceutical agents (e.g., digitalis). Elevation of the ST segment of $\geq$ 1 mm, although infrequent, may be more specific for ischemia and may be associated with areas of ventricular dyskinesia or akinesia.

Exercise-induced ventricular ectopic beats can occur in healthy individuals, but are more commonly seen in patients with coronary disease. Uniform, isolated ventricular extrasystoles have no particular significance. However, when multiform or frequent (more than 3 in 10 beats, couplets, or ventricular tachycardia), occurring in the presence of ST-segment depression or poor ventricular function and at low levels of exercise, they are associated with a poorer prognosis.[126,127] Likewise, the appearance of complex ectopy during any exercise stage is an indication for stopping the test.

The appearance of complex ventricular arrhythmias in the first few minutes of recovery also can be a cause for concern. It often is due to the rapid increase in plasma catecholamine levels and accompanying abrupt fall in blood pressure.[128] This may be offset by having the patient warm-down in the recovery period, such as stepping in place or cycling at zero load.

Changes in the amplitude of the QRS complex during exercise are considered by some to be a predictor of coronary artery disease.[129] Normally the R wave decreases in size with increasing heart rate. Some investigators believe that an increase in R-wave amplitude, even in the absence of ST-segment depression, indicates three-vessel disease and poor ventricular function. However, this has not been fully substantiated, and more evidence is required before it can be accepted. Rarely, inverted U waves are seen during exercise or in the recovery phase. This appears to be a reliable indicator of coronary artery disease.[130]

Many laboratories include pulmonary and metabolic measurements to determine exercise intensity. A further guide to intensity is the rating of perceived exertion (RPE).[131] To define RPE, the patient is asked to indicate a number on the exertion scale at each test stage. The scale shown in Table 3–6 or a 10-point scale such as Table 1–6 can be used.

Contraindications to exercise testing are the same as those that preclude a patient from entering a training program. Reasons for terminating the exercise test are shown in Table 3–7.

An exercise test cannot replicate all of the adverse components that may be associated with heavy physical effort, particularly such psychologic stresses as fear, extreme apprehension, or intense competition. In such cases, it may be necessary to monitor the subject under actual or simulated exercise conditions.

CASE: L.C., a 59-year-old firefighter, complained of chest pain while attending a fire and was subsequently referred by his family physician for assessment. He achieved a power output of 1,000 kpm.min^{-1} (170 watts) on the cycle ergometer, with a heart rate of 145 bpm and a systolic blood pressure of 220 mm Hg before stopping because of leg fatigue. The exercise ECG showed an occasional isolated multiform ventricular ectopic beat, and 1.2 mm of upsloping ST-segment depression during the final 1 minute of effort. The patient was asymptomatic throughout. Analysis of expired air revealed a peak oxygen uptake of 29 mL/kg/min (normal for a sedentary 59-year-old is 36 mL/kg/min) without evidence of a plateau (i.e., the test was not a maximal one).

Table 3–6 **RATING OF PERCEIVED EXERTION**

6	
7	Very, very light
8	
9	Very light
10	
11	Fairly light
12	
13	Somewhat hard
14	
15	Hard
16	
17	Very hard
18	
19	Very, very hard
20	

From Borg G[141]

Table 3–7   **REASONS FOR TERMINATING EXERCISE TESTS**

Failure of heart rate or systolic blood pressure to rise, or a fall, with increasing effort
Systolic blood pressure exceeding 260 mm Hg, or diastolic blood pressure exceeding 120 mm Hg
Frequent (3 in 10 or more) complex ventricular premature beats, ventricular tachycardia
Sustained supraventricular tachycardia or atrial fibrillation
Development of second- or third-degree heart block
ST-segment depression in excess of 2 mm (horizontal or down-sloping)
Increasing anginal symptoms
Any adverse change in the patient's apperance or attitude, e.g., pallor, excessive sweating, confusion
Failure of monitoring equipment

To complete the evaluation, telemetry was carried out at the Fire Hall while the subject performed a search and rescue drill in the "maze." This involved crawling through 16 meters of smoke-filled, cramped (1 meter by 1 meter), interconnected passages, while encumbered with 30 kg of protective clothing and breathing apparatus. The temperature was maintained at 22.2°C (72°F), and there was an upper time limit of 20 minutes to complete the circuit. During this procedure his heart rate increased to 160 bpm, systolic blood pressure to 250 mm Hg, and the ECG showed bigeminy and trigeminy, with couplets, and 2.3 mm of ST-segment depression at the highest heart rates. He complained of heaviness in the chest, which resolved within 2 minutes of completing the drill.

As a result of these findings, he came under the care of a cardiologist, who elected to treat him medically. The fire department appointed him to supervisory duties, without loss of rank, and he was enrolled in the exercise rehabilitation program.

COMMENT: On occasion, the exercise test fails to mimic all aspects of work-related effort.

Test Interpretation

How accurate is the exercise ECG, and in particular ST-segment depression, in identifying coronary artery disease? The answer requires familiarity with the concept of probability. The probability that the test will be positive in the presence of disease is referred to as *sensitivity*. The probability that the test will be negative in the absence of disease is its *specificity*. Both values are expressed as percentages and are obtained from the following formulas:

$$\text{sensitivity} = \frac{TP}{TP + FN} \times 100 \qquad \text{specificity} = \frac{TN}{TN + FP} \times 100$$

where TP = true positives, FN = false negatives, TN = true negatives, and FP = false positives.

Stated another way, sensitivity reflects those with *disease* who have a positive test, and specificity reflects those *without disease* who have a negative test.

Comparison between coronary angiography and exercise testing, using 0.1 mV of horizontal or downsloping ST-segment depression as the criterion for a positive test, reveals a sensitivity of approximately 70% (70% of those with angiographic evidence of disease are correctly identified), and a specificity of approximately 90% (90% of those without angiographic disease have a normal test). Altering the test criterion for abnormality (i.e., increasing the level of ST-segment depression considered positive) will alter the sensitivity and specificity in a reciprocal manner. For example, using 0.2 mV of ST-segment depression as the criterion increases the specificity but decreases sensitivity.

A perfect diagnostic test would be 100% sensitive and 100% specific, and therefore, its results would be totally conclusive. Exercise ECG testing falls short of perfection, and results must be interpreted in terms of probability, or likelihood. Bayes' theorem relates the probable outcome of a test to our knowledge of prior outcomes.[132] The predictive value of a test is the clinical significance of a positive test, or the likelihood that a positive test is true. For an abnormal test, it is determined by the equation:

$$\text{positive predictive value} = \frac{TP}{TP + FP} \times 100$$

In order to calculate the predictive value, one needs to know the test's sensitivity and specificity, and the prevalence of coronary artery disease in the population being tested, which is sometimes referred to as the prior probability of disease. For example, given a 70% sensitivity and a 90% specificity, in a population of 10,000 patients with a disease prevalence of 5% (500 patients with disease), the total number of true positive tests will be 350 (70% sensitivity × 500), with 950 results being false positives (10% [90% specificity] × 9,500). The predictive value is therefore 27% (350 ÷ [350 + 950]). That is, in this low-prevalence population, only 27% of positive tests indicate disease, and most positives are false positives.

As a second example, when the prevalence or prior probability is increased to 50%, the number of true positives will be 3,500, false positives 500, and the predictive value of a positive test would be 88%.

Applying Bayes' theorem requires knowledge of the pre-test likelihood of coronary disease. This is usually estimated from the presence or absence of risk factors and anginal pain, together with its character, position, radiation, and duration, and aggravating or relieving factors. The pre-test probability of coronary heart disease will be altered by the exercise ECG to provide a post-test probability of significant coronary atherosclerosis. The pre-test odds for coronary disease, as determined by age, sex, and other clinical variables, and the post-test probability of disease have been available in published tables[133,134] over the past two decades. For example, a history of classic effort angina in a middle-aged man indicates a 90% or 9:1 pre-test probability of coronary stenosis. Applying Bayes' theorem, if the individual had a positive exercise test, post-test odds are 98% (positive predictive value). However, if the exercise test was negative, its predictive value of no heart disease is only 34% (among those with a pre-test likelihood of 90%). That is, of those with negative ECG exercise tests, only 34% will not have disease if they have a 90% risk of having coronary artery disease prior to testing. Thus, among this high-risk population, a positive test only increases the chances of disease from 90% to 98%, whereas a negative test still leaves a 66% possibility of disease.

Alternatively, an atypical history of angina in a middle-aged man would result in a pre-test odds for disease of 50:50 (a 50% prevalence). The post-test odds of a positive test are then 88%, while 75% of those with a negative test have no disease. The exercise test has the greatest clinical use among those with an intermediate pre-test risk for coronary disease. For those with higher risks, a negative test will not exclude disease. For those with low risk (e.g., asymptomatic younger individuals and those without coronary risk factors), most positive tests will be false-positive results.

Exercise Training Protocols

A training session should include a warm-up and a cool-down, with flexibility routines to reduce injuries. Patients should be instructed in pulse-taking, recognition and interpretation of symptoms, the effect of various medications, the ability to cope with climatic conditions, and the choice of suitable footwear and clothing.[135,136] Guidelines for supervised cardiac rehabilitation have been published by the American Heart Association[137] and American College of Sports Medicine,[138] which recommend that exercise sessions be attended by a physician or nurse with resuscitation equipment.

INTENSITY

The training intensity should be between 50% and 70% of peak oxygen uptake.[139] This is approximately the level of the ventilatory threshold and should not be exceeded during exercise.[140] On the original 20-point Borg scale, this threshold lies between 12 and 14 (see Table 3–6), or at level 5 to 6 of the 10-point scale (Table 1–6), when work is rated "somewhat strong."[141] If heart rate alone is used, the effort should result in a heart rate between 65% and 80% of maximum. The heart rate reserve formula, also referred to as the Karvonen formula, uses the percentage of the difference between resting and maximal heart rate (the chronotropic reserve) and the resting value (65% to 80%).

$$(HR_{max} - HR_{resting}) + HR_{resting} = HR_{training}^{142}$$

However, higher heart rates (77% and above) as determined by the Karvonen formula may be too intense; the training heart rate among lower-conditioned individuals is often above their ventilatory threshold.

> **CASE:** J.A., a 48-year-old man, was referred for exercise rehabilitation 12 weeks after an uncomplicated CABG procedure. An incremental exercise test on the cycle ergometer was performed to establish an initial exercise prescription. A maximal test was achieved, as evidenced by an oxygen uptake plateau in the final minutes of effort. The ventilatory-anaerobic threshold occurred at a work load of 500 $kpm \cdot min^{-1}$ and an oxygen uptake of 15.7 $mL \cdot kg^{-1} \cdot mm^{-1}$ (58% of peak oxygen uptake). This corresponded to 13 on the 20-point Borg scale, and a heart rate of 126 bpm (70% of maximum heart rate). All of these measurements conformed to a level of effort appropriate for achieving a training effect and did not cause adverse symptoms or signs.
>
> The oxygen uptake at the ventilatory threshold was equated to a walking speed of approximately 17 min/mile. A trial walk at this pace proved comfortable, pulse rate varied between 20 and 21 beats for a 10-second count, and there were no adverse symptoms. Within 4 weeks, the distance was increased to 3 miles at the same pace, and further progress was excellent.

COMMENT: The ventilatory threshold (which closely reflects the onset of the anaerobic threshold), peak oxygen uptake, maximal heart rate, and the RPE all can be used to identify an effective and safe training level.

When the test has been stopped prior to maximal levels because of signs or symptoms of ischemia, a percentage (usually 70% to 85%) of the heart rate or oxygen uptake measurement at the conclusion of the test ($HR_{max, symptom-limited}$, $VO_{2max, symptom-limited}$) is used for prescription purposes. Training intensity should never be greater than that attained during the exercise test.

SYMPTOMS DURING EXERCISE

In my practice, patients who experience angina during exercise are taught to reduce their pace or, if necessary, stop exercising for a few minutes until the symptoms disappear. Following this, they can restart exercise at reduced intensity. Only if symptoms do not respond to these measures is medication indicated. If this approach proves impractical, then an interval-type training program is used (i.e., walk-run or brisk walking alternating with slow walking).[30]

TELEMETRY

Because routine telemetry or Holter monitoring for all cardiac patients is prohibitively expensive and has not been shown to be a consistently effective safety measure, it cannot be advocated. On the other hand, telemetry does provide a valuable safety net for patients identified as having severe ST-segment changes or frequent complex arrhythmias. It may also be helpful for those who, after starting the program, report effort-induced bouts of pulse irregularity or symptoms consistent with cerebral ischemia, such as light-headedness.

TRAINING MODE

The training activity generally should involve repetitive movement of large muscle groups. Typical modes are brisk walking, slow jogging (the pace not to exceed 7.5 min/km or 12 min/mile), low-intensity swimming, bicycling, cross-country skiing, and circuit weight training. Walking and jogging have been used in the program at the Toronto Rehabilitation Centre for more than 25 years.[135,139,143] A starting level is based on 50% to 70% of the patient's peak oxygen uptake measurement, and progression takes place through a series of levels depending on the individual's training responses.[139] As conditioning improves, patients can participate in other more vigorous forms of physical recreation. A general guide to one's cardiovascular fitness level necessary to engage in these activities is listed on Table 3–8.

Some individuals require upper-limb strengthening to satisfy job needs or allow participation in physical activities that involve vigorous arm use. Arm training can be combined with leg work, using an arm-leg ergometer (e.g., Schwinn Airdyne), or exercises designed for the arms only, such as light weights (2–4 kg), arm ergometry, or wall pulleys. Since arm work results in higher heart rates and blood pressures than leg work at similar relative inten-

Table 3-8 **FITNESS FOR SPORTS***

You need to be fit to take part in recreational physical games and sports. How fit? That depends not only on the sport itself, but also on your individual skill. However, a good guide to your cardiovascular ability to participate is the level of your performance on the training tables.

To Participate In: Sport	You Need To Be Able To Walk-Jog 3 Miles (4.8 km) In: Time (minutes)
Archery	60-57
Badminton—social	39
—more vigorously	30-24
Basketball—recreational	39
—game	30-24
Bicycling— 8 mph	60
—10 mph	45
—12 mph	36
—15 mph	30
Bowling	54
Canoeing—leisurely	60-54
—vigorously	45-36
Gardening—raking	72
—mowing	42
—digging	36
Golf—using power cart	60
—pulling a club cart	48
—carrying clubs	42
Handball—easy	36
—more vigorously	30
Field hockey	30
Horseback riding—walking	60
—trotting	42
—galloping	33
Ice skating—leisurely	45
—quickly	36-30
Skiing—cross-country (very leisurely)	42-36
—cross-country (4 mph)	33
—cross-country (5 mph)	30
—cross-country (8 mph)	21
—downhill (easily)	42-36
—downhill (vigorously)	36-30
Snowshoeing	30-24
Soccer (depending on position and level of play)	54-36
Squash	25-18
Swimming (assuming a reasonably proficient swimmer, and optimal water temperature of 82°-86°F [28°-30°C]).	
—breast stroke	30-27
—crawl stroke	33-30
—back stroke	33-30
—side stroke	36-33
—treading water	60-54
Tennis—doubles	48
—singles	33

*Values are based on a 150-lb (70-kg) person.
From Kavanagh[139]

sity, however, the training work load should be appropriately reduced. According to Schwade and colleagues,[120] similar heart rate and blood pressure responses are obtained with arm work loads one half that of leg work loads. Upper-extremity training for cardiac patients has been shown to be safe, and can result in improvements in arm ergometry values for peak power output and oxygen uptake.[144,145]

DURATION AND FREQUENCY

If training intensity has been chosen appropriately, a workout at a constant pace for at least 20 to 30 minutes will not cause excessive fatigue or symptoms. As fitness improves, this can be extended to 45 minutes, provided that the intensity does not lead to excessive breathlessness or discomfort. A minimum of three training sessions a week is needed to gain a benefit. The Toronto program advocates five sessions weekly. One session is carried out at the Centre under supervision; the remaining four are nonsupervised and away from the Centre.[135,146] With this approach, patients can be taught to exercise safely and effectively on their own. It appears that more is gained from weekly attendance at a formal class for 18 months than from attending three times weekly for 6 months. The Toronto program has obtained excellent compliance and significant improvement in physical fitness without compromising safety.

STRENGTH TRAINING

Traditionally, resistance training or weight lifting has been excluded from the cardiac patient's program, for what have appeared to be sound physiologic reasons.[147] Although weight training is not an isometric (static) exercise, it is similar during maximal lifts. A static muscle contraction that involves 70% or more of maximum effort results in a disproportionate increase in heart rate and blood pressure product for the absolute level of oxygen uptake,[143] and this has previously been felt to be harmful for the ischemic heart. In recent years, however, there has been interest in this form of training, using innovative types of weight training equipment. It appears that some of the cardiovascular dangers associated with this type of exercise may have been exaggerated.[148-150] Cardiac patients have undertaken supervised and prescribed weight training programs without ill effects.[151-154] Upper-limb strengthening is especially useful in preparation for return to an occupation that involves arm work or for participation in throwing or racquet sports.

OTHER PROGRAM COMPONENTS

Post-coronary health counseling and education programs appear most effective in changing lifestyle when combined with exercise training.[155-157] When the patient is attending exercise classes, there is an opportunity to offer educational lectures and discussions, and to work with the individual to identify specific risk factors. Advice can be offered regarding smoking cessation and dietary modification. General discussions are encouraged, with question-and-answer sessions in an atmosphere of club-like friendliness, rather than that of a hospital or other medical setting.

SAFETY

Given that patients with ischemic heart disease, latent or overt, are more likely to suffer a fatal MI or cardiac arrest than their healthy counterparts, it is reassuring to know that medically supervised cardiac exercise programs are safe. Haskell,[158] analyzing 30 centers, found one fatal cardiovascular event for every 116,402 patient hours of exercise and one nonfatal event for every 34,673 patient hours. More recently, Van Camp and Peterson,[159] evaluating 157 cardiac programs, reported one cardiac arrest per 111,996 patient hours of exercise, one nonfatal MI per 293,990 patient hours, and one fatality per 783,972 patient hours of exercise. The Toronto Rehabilitation Centre's record for the years 1968 to 1991 is one fatal and one nonfatal cardiovascular event for every 347,579 and 405,509 patient hours of exercise, respectively.

A number of routine precautionary measures can minimize the risk of a fatality. The training staff should caution patients to adhere to the following exercise rules:

1. Always warm up and warm down.[128,160,161]
2. Avoid extremes of heat and cold.[162,163]
3. Train regularly, avoiding excessive peaks of activity.
4. Avoid intensive competition.
5. Adhere to the prescribed limits.
6. Reduce the exercise load when either ischemic symptoms or anxiety develops.
7. Report all symptoms, particularly light-headedness, chest pain, or syncope, no matter how brief.

Cardiac Transplantation Patients*

Cardiac transplantation is an accepted treatment for end-stage cardiac disease, with actuarial survival rates of 81% for the first year[164] and 69% for the first 5 years after operation.[165] Since many patients have endured months of restricted activity prior to surgery, exercise rehabilitation should be a component of postoperative care.

With the advent of cyclosporine, more judicious tissue matching, and improved surgical techniques, the transplant patient frequently leaves the intensive care unit 48 hours after surgery. The average stay in hospital has gradually shortened, until it is now approximately 18 days. An exercise cycle may be used for rehabilitation beginning on the fourth postoperative day. The usual follow-up routine includes frequent return visits for blood tests, ECGs, radiographs, endomyocardial biopsy, exercise testing, echocardiography, and coronary angiography. If the exercise rehabilitation program is directed by the transplant unit, there is an opportunity to assess the patient's progress and adherence to the training program.

---

*The information contained in this section is based on experience gained from a pilot project between the Toronto Rehabilitation Centre and the Cardiac Transplant Unit, Harefield Hospital, Middlesex, England.

EXERCISE TESTING

The denervated transplanted heart has a high resting heart rate. Because there is no autonomic control and vagal tone is absent, the heart beats at the intrinsic rate of the sinoatrial node. The latter is a function of age, and ranges from an average of 110 bpm at age 30 to 80 bpm at age 50. Since donor hearts are usually obtained from young accident victims, the intrinsic rate of the transplanted heart often is in excess of 100 bpm.[166,167]

During the exercise test, because of the absence of direct sympathetic stimulation of myocardial beta-adrenoreceptors, the transplanted heart initially accelerates more slowly than normal. During the early phase of exercise, increase in cardiac output is achieved by a rise in stroke volume, due to augmented venous return and the Frank-Starling mechanism. As exercise becomes more vigorous, the heart rate increases more rapidly because of the chronotropic action of circulating catecholamines. After exercise, when the normal innervated heart decelerates rapidly (because of increased vagal tone), the transplanted heart rate may plateau for the first few minutes of recovery or even continue to rise, presumably because catecholamine levels are still high and increasing. Thereafter, the rate decreases gradually and may take as long as 20 minutes to return to resting levels.[168] Figure 3–1 shows a typical transplant patient's heart-rate responses to increasing effort.

After cardiac transplantation, resting blood pressure is moderately raised, and peak exercise blood pressure is reduced. Both cardiac and peripheral

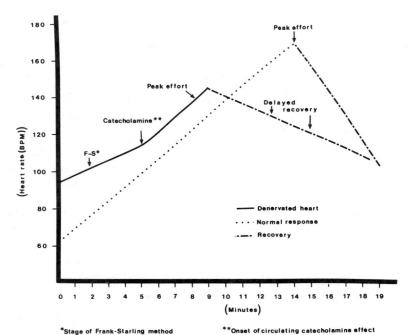

*Stage of Frank-Starling method   **Onset of circulating catecholamine effect

Figure 3–1 Typical transplanted denervated heart rate response to an incremental exercise test on the cycle ergometer, compared with the response of a healthy subject matched for donor age. Note the high resting rate, the delayed acceleration and deceleration in rate during effort and recovery, and the tendency for the rate to continue to rise after the termination of exercise.

vascular changes probably contribute to these observations. Resting hypertension may reflect preoperative CHF and the resultant chronic plasma norepinephrine elevation.[169] Loss of sympathetic stimulation and resultant impairment of myocardial contractility may account for the low peak exercise systolic blood pressure. Chronically elevated serum catecholamine levels also may induce down-regulation of the peripheral arterial alpha receptors.[170]

The post-transplant patient often experiences muscle wasting due to physical inactivity. Because of this limitation, with low peak heart rate and blood pressure, the maximum power output or work load achieved is reduced to two thirds that of a normal age-matched population.

Ischemia of the denervated heart can be detected by the appearance of ST-segment depression and dysrhythmias, although angina symptoms will not occur. Because the transplanted heart is healthy, except during bouts of rejection, exercise ECG abnormalities are rare. Late development of an accelerated form of coronary atherosclerosis in the donor heart is not uncommon, however, and ischemia may eventually be seen in long-standing transplant recipients.[171]

TRAINING REGIMEN

The training prescribed following cardiac transplantation is similar to that for post–MI and post–CABG patients. Intensity is based on 50% to 70% of peak oxygen uptake, taking into account the ventilatory threshold and a perception of effort of 14 on the 15-point Borg scale. The training most commonly advocated by the author is walking-jogging. The initial prescription is 1 mile (1.6 km), 5 days each week, with the average pace varying between 18 and 23 minutes per mile (11-14 min/km). The distance is increased by 1 mile per session every 2 weeks, maintaining the same pace until the patient is walking 3 miles, five times weekly. At 6 weeks, the pace is then quickened by 1 minute per mile until the 3 miles are accomplished in 45 minutes (typically within 4 months after starting the program). Thereafter, 45-second bouts of slow jogging paced at 12 min/mile (7.5 min/km) are introduced every 0.5 mile (800 m), 0.25 mile (400 m), 0.125 mile (200 m), and so on until ultimately the entire 3 miles is completed in 36 minutes.

Because of the atypical heart-rate response and lack of angina as a symptom of myocardial ischemia, accurate pacing must be emphasized, as well as the concept of perceived exertion and recognition of untoward symptoms such as excessive dyspnea, unusual fatigue, light-headedness, and extrasystoles.

In our experience, compliance to the exercise program is good. Few workouts are missed because of injuries or other medical setbacks. Many patients have progressed to walking-jogging approximately 15 miles (24 km) per week at an average pace of 13.5 min/mile (8.5 min/km).

TRAINING BENEFITS

Physiologic changes include an increase in lean body mass, improved exercise performance with elevated peak oxygen uptake, and often a reduction in resting systolic and diastolic blood pressure. At comparable pretraining levels of submaximal effort, blood pressure and perceived exertion are lower, but submaximal heart rate is reduced only in those who attain the greatest conditioning.[31] The reduction in submaximal heart rate may be due to lowering of effort-induced norepinephrine levels, down-regulation in the sensitivity of cardiac beta-adrenoreceptors, or both. Both of these changes have been shown to occur in animals and humans exposed to vigorous training.[32]

Psychologic assessments show that the training effect is accompanied by an increased sense of vigor and a lessening of depression, anxiety, and fatigue.[172] We could find no correlation between the length of time from surgery and subsequent psychologic changes, and thus assume that they are associated with progressive training rather than spontaneous recovery.

> **CASE:** B.P., a 44-year-old male steelworker, developed congestive cardiomyopathy. Over the next 4 years, his condition deteriorated. He had cardiac transplantation and 16 weeks later, enrolled in the exercise rehabilitation program.
>
> The initial exercise test was carried out on the cycle ergometer. The test was uneventful, and B.P. was given an exercise prescription requiring him to walk 2 miles in 32 minutes, five times each week, aiming for a perceived exertion of 12 to 13 on the Borg scale, and a heart rate of 120 to 130 bpm. His progress was excellent, and 6 months later, he was averaging 20 miles/wk at a walk-jog pace of 13.5 min/mile. He expressed the desire to enter a marathon, and it was agreed that, provided no adverse medical circumstances arose, we would help him to train for the Boston Marathon.
>
> Throughout the subsequent winter, he trained assiduously, so that by the following spring, he was walk-jogging an average of 45 to 50 miles/wk. Throughout this time, results of regular blood tests and ECGs were normal, routine serial endomyocardial biopsies were negative for rejection, and results of cardiac catheterization studies were unremarkable.
>
> A final exercise test was carried out prior to the marathon. When compared with the results of the initial exercise study, it showed a reduction in resting and submaximal heart rates and an increase in peak oxygen uptake and power output (Figure 3-2). There was a reduction in body weight and estimated percentage of body fat (21.5% to 19.8%). Subjectively, the patient reported an enhanced sense of well-being.
>
> He entered the Boston Marathon, and became the first cardiac transplantation patient to complete such an event (April 16, 1985). Monitoring during the race showed a maximum heart rate of 142 beats·min[1], without ECG abnormalities. At no time did he experience adverse symptoms. Postrace ECGs were normal. He continues to feel well, jogs 15 to 20 miles/week, and participates in other recreational activities. Results of subsequent exercise tests, endomyocardial biopsies, and angiograms have been normal.
>
> **COMMENT:** Although marathoning is not recommended as a routine goal for cardiac transplant patients, this patient's feat has been a great source of inspiration for others preparing for or emerging from cardiac transplantation surgery.[173]

Summary

Evidence suggests that exercise rehabilitation affords psychologic and physiologic benefit to patients with ischemic heart disease, and in particular to post-MI patients. Although there has been conflicting opinion as to whether or

Figure 3–2 Increase in maximal measured oxygen consumption (VO_{2max}) in a cardiac transplantation patient from initial (Δ) to final ($\bullet$) cycle ergometer test, and an increase in ventilatory anaerobic threshold, expressed in terms of oxygen consumption (L/min). (AT, anaerobic threshold.)

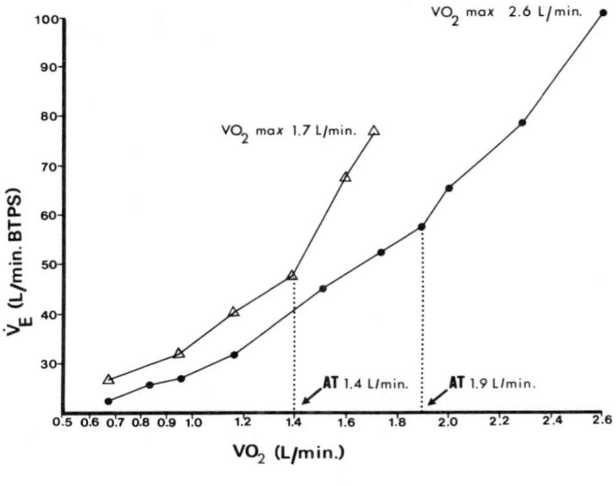

not prognosis is improved,[174] analysis of pooled data from randomized clinical trials is encouraging in this regard, showing a reduction in fatal recurrences in the order of 25%.[64] The training activity customarily employed is endurance or aerobic, with an appropriate intensity based on the results of an exercise test. In addition, more recent exercise programs have safely added weight lifting to enhance physical capacity. Implemented in this manner, cardiac rehabilitation can be safely conducted.

REFERENCES

1. Levine SA, Lown B: "Armchair" treatment of acute coronary thrombosis. *JAMA* 1952; 148:1365–1369.
2. Saltin B, et al.: Response to exercise after bed rest and after training. *Circulation* 1968; 38(5 Suppl):VII1–VII78.
3. Powell KE, et al.: Physical activity and the incidence of coronary heart disease. *Ann Rev Public Health* 1987; 8:253–287.
4. Leon AS, Bloor CM: The effect of complete and partial deconditioning on exercise-induced cardiovascular changes in the rat. In Manninen V, Holene PI, eds: *Physical Activity and Coronary Artery Disease: Advances in Cardiology.* S Karger: Basel, 1976.
5. Ljungqvist A, Unge G: The proliferative activity of the myocardial tissue in various forms of experimental cardiac hypertrophy. *Acta Pathol Microb Scand* 1973; 81(A):233–240.
6. Eckstein RW: Effect of exercise and coronary artery narrowing on coronary collateral circulation. *Circulation Res* 1957; 5:230–235.
7. Cohen MV, Yipintsoi, Scheuer J: Coronary collateral stimulation by exercise in dogs with stenotic coronary arteries. *J Appl Physiol* 1982; 52:664–671.
8. Heaton WH, et al.: Beneficial effect of physical training on blood flow to myocardium perfused by chronic collaterals in the exercising dog. *Circulation* 1978; 57:575–581.
9. Noakes TD, Higginson L, Opie LH: Physical training increases ventricular fibrillation thresholds of isolated rat hearts during normoxia, hypoxia, and regional ischemia. *Circulation* 1983; 67:24–30.
10. Billman GE, Schwartz PJ, Stone HL: The effects of daily exercise on susceptibility to sudden cardiac death. *Circulation* 1984; 69:1182–1189.
11. Kramsch DM, et al.: Reduction of coronary atherosclerosis by moderate conditioning exercise in monkeys on an atherogenic diet. *N Engl J Med* 1981; 305:1483–1489.
12. Morgenroth J, et al.: Comparative left ventricular dimensions in trained athletes. *Ann Intern Med* 1975; 82:521–524.
13. Raskoff WJ, Goldman S, Cohn K: The "athletic heart:" Prevalence and physiological significance of left ventricular enlargement on distance runners. *JAMA* 1976; 236:158–162.
14. Reindell H, Roskamm H, Steim H: Heiz und kerslang bei trainiesten. *Med Welt* 1960; 31:1557–1563.
15. Milliken MC, et al.: Left ventricular mass

as determined by magnetic resonance imaging in male endurance athletes. *Am J Cardiol* 1988;62:301–305.

16. Mellerowicz H: The effects of training on the heart and circulation. In Grupe O, Kurz D, Teipel JM, eds: *The Scientific View of Sport.* Springer-Verlag: Berlin, 1972.

17. Hindman MC, Wallace AG: Radionuclide exercise studies. In Cohen LS, Mock MB, Ringgvist I, eds: *Physical Conditioning and Cardiovascular Rehabilitation.* John Wiley & Sons: New York, 1981.

18. Ehsani AA, et al. Cardiac effects of prolonged and intense exercise training in patients with coronary artery disease. *Am J Cardiol* 1982; 50:246–254.

18a. Clausen JP, Trap-Jensen J, Lassen NA: The effects of training on the heart rate during arm and leg exercise. *Scand J Clin Lab Invest* 1970; 26:295–301.

19. Davies CTM, Sargeant AJ: Effects of training on the physiological responses to one- and two-leg work. *J Appl Physiol* 1975; 38:377–381.

20. Saltin B, et al.: The nature of the training response: Peripheral and central adaptations to one-legged exercise. *Acta Physiol Scand* 1976; 96:289–305.

21. Clausen JP, et al.: Central and peripheral circulatory changes after training of the arms or legs. *Am J Physiol* 1973; 225: 675–682.

22. Clausen JP: Effect of physical training on cardiovascular adjustments to exercise in man. *Physiol Rev* 1977; 57:779–815.

23. Lewis S, et al.: Transfer effects of endurance training to exercise with untrained limbs. *Eur J Appl Physiol Occup Physiol* 1980; 44:25–34.

24. Thompson PD, et al.: Effect of exercise training on the untrained limb exercise performance of men with angina pectoris. *Am J Cardiol* 1981; 48:844–850.

25. Kavanagh T, et al.: Cardiorespiratory responses to exercise training after orthotopic cardiac transplantation. *Circulation* 1988; 77(1):162–171.

26. Kavanagh T, et al.: Exercise rehabilitation after heterotopic cardiac transplantation. *J Cardiopulmonary Rehabil* 1989; 9:303–310.

27. Nelson RR, Gobel FL, Jorgensen CR: Hemodynamic predictors of myocardial oxygen consumption during static and dynamic exercise. *Circulation* 1974; 50: 1179–1189.

28. Council on Scientific Affairs: Physician-supervised exercise programs in rehabilitation of patients with coronary heart disease. *JAMA* 1981; 245:1463–1466.

29. Frick MH, Katila: Haemodynamic consequences of physical training after myocardial infarction. *Circulation* 1968; 37: 192–202.

30. Kavanagh T, Shephard RJ: Conditioning of postcoronary patients: Comparison of continuous and interval training. *Arch Phys Med Rehabil* 1975; 56:72–76.

31. Scheur J, Tipton CM: Cardiovascular adaptations to physical training. *Ann Rev Physiol* 1977; 39:221–251.

32. DeMaria AN, et al.: Alterations in ventricular mass and performance induced by exercise training in man evaluated by echocardiography. *Circulation* 1978; 57: 237–244.

33. Parker BM, et al.: The noninvasive cardiac evaluation of long-distance runners. *Chest* 1978; 73:376–381.

34. Detry JM, et al.: Increased arteriovenous oxygen difference after physical training in coronary heart disease. *Circulation* 1971; 44:109–118.

35. Paterson DH, et al.: Effects of physical training on cardiovascular function following myocardial infarction. *J Appl Physiol* 1979; 47:482–489.

36. Holloszy JO: Biochemical adaptations in muscle: Effects of exercise on mitochondrial oxygen uptake and respiratory enzyme activity in skeletal muscle. *J Biol Chem* 1967; 242:2278–2282.

37. Heath GW, et al.: Exercise training improves lipoprotein lipid profiles in patients with coronary artery disease. *Am Heart J* 1984; 105:889–895.

38. Kavanagh T, et al.: Influence of exercise and life-style variables upon high-density lipoprotein cholesterol after myocardial infarction. *Arteriosclerosis* 1983; 3: 249–259.

39. Hartung GH, Squires WG, Gotto Am Jr: Effects of exercise training on plasma high-density lipoprotein cholesterol in coronary disease patients. *Am Heart J* 1981; 101:181–184.

40. McCrimmon DR, et al.: Effect of training on plasma catecholamines in post myocardial infarction patients. *Med Sci Sports Exerc* 1976; 8:152–156.

41. Hartley LH, et al.: Multiple hormonal responses to graded exercise in relation to physical training. *J Appl Physiol* 1972; 33:602–606.

42. Ruderman NB, Ganda OB, Johansen KL: The effect of physical training on glucose tolerance and plasma lipids in maturity-onset diabetes. *Diabetes* 1979; 28(suppl 1):89–92.

43. Petersen O, Beck-Nielson H, Heading L: Increased insulin receptors after exercise in patients with insulin dependent diabetes mellitus. *N Engl J Med* 1980; 302: 886–892.

44. Williams RS, Eden S, Anderson J: Reduced epinephrine-induced platelet aggregation following cardiac rehabilitation. *J Cardiac Rehabil* 1981; 1:127–132.

45. Williams RS, et al.: Physical conditioning augments fibrinolytic response to venous occlusion in healthy adults. *N Engl J Med* 1980; 302:987–991.

46. Kavanagh T, Shephard RJ, Tuck JA: De-

pression after myocardial infarction. *Can Med Assoc J* 1975; 113:23–27.

47. Kavanagh T, et al.: Depression following myocardial infarction: The effects of distance running. *Ann NY Acad Sci* 1978; 301:1029–1038.

48. Bergman H, Varnauskas E: Placebo effect in physical training of coronary heart disease. In Larsen OA, Malmborg RO, eds: *Coronary Heart Disease and Physical Fitness.* Ejnar Munksgaards Forlag: Cophenhagen, 1971.

49. Varnauskas E, Holmberg S: Myocardial blood flow during exercise in patients with coronary heart disease: Comments on training effects. In Larson OA, Malmborg RO, eds: *Coronary Heart Disease and Physical Fitness.* University Park Press: Baltimore, 1971, pp 102–104.

50. Redwood DR, Rosing DR, Epstein SE: Circulatory and symptomatic effects of physical training in patients with coronary-artery disease and angina pectoris. *N Engl J Med* 1972; 286:959–965.

51. Raffo JA, et al.: Effects of physical training on myocardial ischemia in patients with coronary artery disease. *Br Heart J* 1980; 43:262–269.

52. Laslett LJ, Paumer L, Amsterdam EA: Increase in myocardial oxygen consumption indexes by exercise training at onset of ischemia in patients with coronary artery disease. *Circulation* 1985; 71: 958–962.

53. Ehsani AA, et al.: Effects of 12 months of intense exercise training on ischemic ST-segment depression in patients with coronary artery disease. *Circulation* 1981; 64: 1116–1124.

54. Froelicher V, et al.: Cardiac rehabilitation: Evidence for improvement in myocardial perfusion and function. *Arch Phys Med Rehabil* 1980; 61:517–522.

55. Schuler G, et al.: Low-fat diet and regular, supervised physical exercise in patients with symptomatic coronary artery disease: Reduction of stress-induced myocardial ischemia. *Circulation* 1988; 77: 172–181.

56. Todd IC, et al.: Effects of daily high-intensity exercise on myocardial perfusion in angina pectoris. *Am J Cardiol* 1991; 68:1593–1599.

57. Ornish D, et al.: Can lifestyle changes reverse coronary heart disease? The Lifestyle Heart Trial. *Lancet* 1990; 336: 129–133.

58. Schuler G, et al.: Myocardial perfusion and regression of coronary heart disease in patients on a regimen of intensive physical exercise and low fat diet. *J Am Coll Cardiol* 1992; 19:34–42.

59. Report of a WHO Committee: *Prevention of Coronary Heart Disease.* Technical Report Series 678. Geneva: World Health Organization, 1982.

60. The Lipid Research Clinics Coronary Primary Prevention Trial results: I. Reduction in incidence of coronary heart disease. *JAMA* 1984; 251:351–364.

61. May GS, et al.: Secondary prevention after myocardial infarction: A review of long-term trials. *Prog Cardiovasc Dis* 1982; 24:331–352.

62. Oldridge NB, et al.: Cardiac rehabilitation after myocardial infarction: Combined experience of randomized clinical trials. *JAMA* 1988; 260:945–950.

63. Yusof S, et al.: Beta blockade during and after myocardial infarction: An overview of the randomized trials. *Prog Cardiovasc Dis* 1985; 27:335–371.

64. O'Connor GT, et al.: An overview of randomized trials of rehabilitation with exercise after myocardial infarction. *Circulation* 1989; 80:234–244.

65. Leaman DM, Brower RW, Meester GT: Coronary artery bypass surgery: A stimulus to modify existing risk factors? *Chest* 1982; 81:16–19.

66. Campeau L, et al.: The relation of risk factors to the development of atherosclerosis in saphenous-vein bypass grafts and the progression of disease in the native circulation: A study 10 years after aortocoronary bypass surgery. *N Engl J Med* 1984; 311:1329–1332.

67. Dion WF, et al.: Medical problems and physiologic responses during supervised inpatient cardiac rehabilitation: The patient after coronary artery bypass grafting. *Heart Lung* 1982; 11:248–255.

68. Exercise rehabilitation after heart transplantation. In Kapoor AS, et al., eds: *Cardiomyopathies and Heart-Lung Transplantation.* McGraw-Hill: New York, 1991, pp 359–368.

69. Oberman A, et al.: Employment status after coronary artery bypass surgery. *Circulation* 1982; 65(Suppl 2):115–119.

70. Varnauskas E: Survival, myocardial infarction, and employment status in a prospective randomized study of coronary bypass surgery. *Circulation* 1985; 72 (Suppl V):V90–V101.

71. Wenger NK: Rehabilitation of the coronary patient: Status 86. *Prog Cardiovasc Dis* 1986; 29:181–204.

72. Naughton J: Vocational and avocational rehabilitation for coronary patients. In Wenger NK, Hellerstein HK, eds. *Rehabilitation of the Coronary Patient.* Wiley Medical: New York, 1984, pp 484–492.

73. Kavanagh T, Matosevic V: Assessment of work capacity in patients with ischemic heart disease: Methods and practices. *Eur Heart J* 1988; 9(Suppl L):67–73.

74. Naughton J: Role of physical activity as a secondary intervention for healed myocardial infarction. *Am J Cardiol* 1985; 55:21D–26D.

75. Barboriak JJ, Anderson AJ, Rimm AA: Changes in avocational activities follow-

ing coronary artery bypass surgery. *J Cardiac Rehabil* 1983; 3:214–216.

76. Vandormael MG, et al.: Multilesion coronary angioplasty: Clinical and angiographic follow-up. *J Am Coll Cardiol* 1987; 10:246–252.

77. Newell J, et al.: Physical training after heart valve replacement. *Br Heart J* 1980; 44:638–649.

78. Carstens V, Behrenbeck DW, Hilger HH: Exercise capacity before and after cardiac valve surgery. *Cardiol* 1983; 70: 41–49.

79. Superko H: Effects of cardiac rehabilitation in permanently paced patients with third-degree heart block. *J Cardiac Rehabil* 1983; 3:561–568.

80. Obina R, Keritzinsky G, Anderson R: Exercise for pacemaker patients. *Phys Sportsmed* 1984; 12:127–130.

81. American College of Sports Medicine: *Guidelines for Exercise Testing and Prescription,* ed 3. Lea & Febiger: Philadelphia, 1986, pp 65–68.

82. Harris P: Evolution and the cardiac patient. *Cardiovasc Res* 1983; 17:313–319, 373–437.

83. Wilson JR, et al.: Evaluation of energy metabolism in skeletal muscle of patients with heart failure with gated phosphorus-31 nuclear magnetic resonance. *Circulation* 1985; 71:57–62.

84. Weber KT, Janicki JS: Lactate production during maximal and submaximal exercise in patients with chronic heart failure. *J Am Coll Cardiol* 1985; 6:717–724.

85. Weber KT, et al.: Oxygen utilization and ventilation during exercise in patients with chronic cardiac failure. *Circulation* 1982; 65:1213–1223.

86. Franciosa JA, Ziesche S, Wilen M: Functional capacity of patients with chronic left ventricular failure: Relationship of bicycle exercise performance to clinical and hemodynamic characterization. *Am J Med* 1979; 67:460.

87. Weber KT, Janicki JS: Cardiopulmonary exercise testing for evaluation of chronic cardiac failure. *Am J Cardiol* 1985; 55:22A–31A.

88. Lipkin DP: The role of exercise testing in chronic heart failure. *Br Heart J* 1987; 58:559–566.

89. Wilson JR, et al.: Use of maximal bicycle exercise testing with respiratory gas analysis to assess exercise performance in patients with congestive heart failure secondary to coronary artery disease or to idiopathic dilated cardiomyopathy. *Am J Cardiol* 1986; 58:601–606.

90. Szlachcic J, et al.: Correlates and prognostic implication of exercise capacity in chronic congestive heart failure. *Am J Cardiol* 1985; 55:1037–1042.

91. Letac B, Cribier A, Desplanches JF: A study of left ventricular function in coronary patients before and after physical training. *Circulation* 1977; 56:375–378.

92. Lee AP, et al.: Long-term effects of physical training on coronary patients with impaired ventricular function. *Circulation* 1982; 60:1519.

93. Cobb FR, et al.: Effects of exercise training on ventricular function in patients with recent myocardial infarction. *Circulation* 1982; 66:100–108.

94. Conn EH, Williams RS, Wallace AG: Exercise responses before and after physical conditioning in patients with severely depressed left ventricular function. *Am J Cardiol* 1982; 49:296–300.

95. Sullivan MJ, Higginbotham MB, Cobb FR: Exercise training in patients with chronic heart failure delays ventilatory anaerobic threshold and improves submaximal exercise performance. *Circulation* 1989; 79:324–329.

96. Coats AJ, et al.: Effects of physical training in chronic heart failure. *Lancet* 1990; 335:63–66.

97. DeBusk RF, et al.: Identification and treatment of low-risk patients after acute myocardial infarction and coronary-artery bypass graft surgery. *N Engl J Med* 1986; 314:161–166.

98. American College of Physicians: Evaluation of patients after recent acute myocardial infarction. *Ann Intern Med* 1989; 110:485–488.

99. Moss AJ, Benhorin J: Prognosis and management after a first myocardial infarction. *N Engl J Med* 1990; 322:743–753.

100. Van Baak MA, et al.: Long-term antihypertensive therapy with beta-blockers: Submaximal exercise capacity and metabolic effects during exercise. *Int J Sports Med* 1987; 8:342–347.

101. Van Baak MA, et al.: Metabolic effects of verapamil and propranolol during submaximal endurance exercise in patients with essential hypertension. *Int J Sports Med* 1987; 8:270–274.

102. Wilcox RG, et al.: The effects of acute or chronic ingestion of propranolol or metoprolol on the physiological responses to prolonged, submaximal exercise in hypertensive men. *Br J Clin Pharmac* 1984; 17:273–281.

103. Van Herwaarden CLA, et al.: Effects of propranolol and metoprolol on hemodynamic and respiratory indices and on perceived exertion during exercise in hypertensive patients. *Br Heart J* 1979; 41: 99–105.

104. Van Baak MA, Jennen W, Verstappen FTJ: Maximal aerobic power and blood pressure in normotensive subjects after acute and chronic administration of metoprolol. *Eur J Clin Pharmac* 1985; 28: 143–148.

105. Hossack KF, Bruce RA, Clarke LJ: Influence of propranolol on exercise prescrip-

tion of training heart rates. *Cardiol* 1980; 65:47–58.

106. Fletcher GF: Exercise training during chronic beta blockade in cardiovascular disease. *Am J Cardiol* 1985; 55:110D–113D.

107. Froelicher V, et al.: Can patients with coronary artery disease receiving beta blockers obtain a training effect? *Am J Cardiol* 1985; 55:155D–161D.

108. Pratt CM, et al.: Demonstration of training effect during chronic beta-adrenergic blockade in patients with coronary artery disease. *Circulation* 1981; 64:1125–1129.

109. Horgan JH, Teo KK: Training response in patients with coronary artery disease receiving beta-adrenergic blocking drugs with or without partial agonist activity. *J Cardiovasc Pharm* 1983; 5:1019–1024.

110. Ehsani AA: Altered adaptive responses to training by nonselective beta-adrenergic blockade in coronary artery disease. *Am J Cardiol* 1986; 58:220–224.

111. Frisk-Holmberg M, Jorfeldt L, Juhlin-Dannfelt A: Metabolic effects in muscle during antihypertensive therapy with $beta_1$ and $beta_1/beta_2$-adrenoreceptor blockers. *Clin Pharmacol Ther* 1981; 30:611–618.

112. Hossack KF, Bruce RA, Kusumi F: Altered exercise ventilatory responses by apparent propranolol-diminished glucose metabolism: Implications concerning impaired physical training benefit in coronary patients. *Am Heart J* 1981; 102:378–382.

113. Jones NL, et al.: *Clinical Exercise Testing.* WB Saunders: Philadelphia, 1988.

113a. Pollock ML, Wilmore JH, Fox SM: *Exercise in Health and Disease Evaluation and Prescription for Prevention and Rehabilitation.* WB Saunders: Philadelphia, 1984.

114. Astrand P-O, et al.: Intra-arterial blood pressure during exercise with different muscle groups. *J Appl Physiol* 1965; 20:253–256.

115. Bevegard S, Freyschuss U, Strandell T: Circulatory adaptation to arm and leg exercise in supine and sitting position. *J Appl Physiol* 1966; 21:37–46.

116. Stenberg J, et al.: Hemodynamic response to work with different muscle groups, sitting and supine. *J Appl Physiol* 1967; 22:61–70.

117. Davies CT, Sargeant AJ: Physiological responses to standardized arm work. *Ergonomics* 1974; 17:41–49.

118. Fardy PS, Webb D, Hellerstein HK: Benefits of arm exercise in cardiac rehabilitation. *Phys Sportsmed* 1977; 5:30–41.

119. Shaw DJ, et al.: Arm-crank ergometry: A new method for the evaluation of coronary artery disease. *Am J Cardiol* 1974; 33:801–805.

120. Schwade J, Blomqvist CH, Shapiro W: A comparison of the response to arm and leg work in patients with ischemic heart disease. *Am Heart J* 1977; 94:203–208.

121. Acker J Jr, Martin D: Angina and ST-segment depression during treadmill and arm ergometer testing in patients with coronary artery disease. *Phys Ther* 1988; 68:195–198.

122. Ellestad MH: *Stress Testing, Principles and Practice*, ed 3. FA Davis: Philadelphia, 1986.

123. Bruce RA, DeRoven TA, Hossack KF: Value of maximal exercise tests in risk assessment of primary coronary heart disease events in healthy men: Five years' experience of the Seattle Heart Watch Study. *Am J Cardiol* 1980; 46:371–378.

124. Lang-Anderson K, et al.: *Fundamentals of Exercise Testing.* Geneva: World Health Organization, 1971.

125. Blackburn H: The exercise electrocardiogram: Technological, procedural and conceptual developments. In *Measurement in Exercise Electrocardiography.* Charles C Thomas: Springfield, Ill., 1969.

126. Sandberg L: The significance of ventricular premature beats or runs of ventricular tachycardia developing during exercise tests. *Acta Med Scand* 1961; 169:1.

127. Udall JA, Ellestad MH: Predictive implications of ventricular premature contractions associated with treadmill stress testing: A follow-up of 6,500 patients after maximum treadmill stress testing. *Circulation* 1977; 56:985–989.

128. Dimsdale JE, et al.: Postexercise peril: Plasma catecholamines and exercise. *JAMA* 1984; 251:630–632.

129. Bonoris PE, et al.: Evaluation of R wave changes vs. ST segment depression in stress testing. *Circulation* 1978; 57:904.

130. Lepeschkin E: Physiological basis of the U wave. In Schlant RC, Hurst JW, eds: *Advances in Electrocardiography*, vol. 2. Grune & Stratton: New York, 1977.

131. Borg G, Holmgren A, Lindblad I: Quantitative evaluation of chest pain. *Acta Med Scand* 1981; 644:43–45.

132. Rifkin RD, Hood WB: Bayesian analysis and elctrocardiographic exercise stress testing. *N Engl J Med* 1977; 297:681–686.

133. American Heart Association: *Coronary Risk Handbook.* American Heart Association: New York, 1973.

134. Froelicher VF: *Exercise Testing and Training.* LeJacq: New York, 1983, p 83.

135. Kavanagh T: Distance running and cardiac rehabilitation: Physiologic and psychosocial considerations. In Franklin BA, ed: *Clinics in Sports Medicine: Symposium on Cardiac Rehabilitation.* W.B. Saunders Company: Philadelphia, 1984, pp 513–526.

136. Kavanagh T: Consideration and guidelines for cardiac patients exercising out-

doors in cold weather. *J Cardiol Rehabil* 1983; 3:70–73.

137. American Heart Association: *Exercise Standards: A Statement for Health Professionals.* American Heart Association: Dallas, 1991.

138. American College of Sports Medicine: *Guidelines for Graded Exercise Testing and Exercise Testing and Exercise Prescription,* ed 3. Lea & Febiger: Philadelphia, 1986.

139. Kavanagh T: *Take Heart.* Key Porter Books: Toronto, 1992.

140. Davis JA, Vodak P, Wilmore JH: Anaerobic threshold and maximal aerobic power for three modes of exercise. *J Appl Physiol* 1976; 41:544–550.

141. Borg G: *Physical Performance and Perceived Exertion.* Gleerup: Lund, Sweden, 1962, pp 1–63.

142. Karvonen M, Kentala K, Mustala O: The effects of training on heart rate: A longitudinal study. *Ann Med Exp Biol Ferm* 1957; 35:307–315.

143. Shephard RJ: *Endurance Fitness,* ed 2. University of Toronto Press: Toronto, 1977.

144. Magell JR, et al.: Metabolic and cardiovascular adjustment to arm training. *J Appl Physiol* 1978; 45:75–79.

145. Wrisley D, et al.: Effects of exercise training on arm and leg aerobic capacity in cardiac patients. (Abst) *Med Sci Sports Exerc* 1983; 15:92.

146. Kavanagh T: The Toronto Rehabilitation Centre's Cardiac Exercise Program. *J Cardiac Rehab* 1982; 2:496–502.

147. Lind AR, McNichol GW: Muscular factors which determine the cardiovascular responses to sustained and rhythmic exercise. In Proceedings of the International Symposium on Physical Activity and Cardiovascular Health. *Can Med Assoc J* 1967; 96:706–712.

148. DeBusk RF, et al.: Comparison of cardiovascular responses to static-dynamic and dynamic effort alone in patients with ischemic heart disease. *Circulation* 1979; 59:977–984.

149. Fardy PS: Isometric exercise and the cardiovascular system. *Phys Sportsmed* 1981; 9:43–56.

150. Ferguson RJ, et al.: Coronary blood flow during isometric and dynamic exercise in angina pectoris patients. *J Cardiac Rehabil* 1981; 1:21–27.

151. Saldivar M, et al.: Safety of a low-weight, low-repetition strength training program in patients with heart disease (abst). *Med Sci Sports Exerc* 1983; 15:119.

152. Vander LB, et al.: Acute cardiovascular responses to Nautilus exercise in cardiac patients: Implications for exercise training. *Ann Sports Med* 1986; 2:165–169.

153. Kelemen MH, et al.: Circuit weight training in cardiac patients. *J Am Coll Cardiol* 1986; 7:38–42.

154. Butler RM, Beierwaltes WH, Rogers FJ: The cardiovascular response to circuit weight training in patients with cardiac disease. *J Cardiopulmonary Rehabil* 1987; 7:402–409.

155. Pozen MW, et al.: A nurse rehabilitator's impact on patients with myocardial infarction. *Med Care* 1977; 15:830–837.

156. Rahe RH, Ward HW, Hayes V: Brief group therapy in myocardial infarction rehabilitation: Three- to four-year follow-up of a controlled trial. *Psychosom Med* 1979; 41:229–242.

157. Burgess AW, et al.: A randomized control trial of cardiac rehabilitation. *Soc Sci Med* 1987; 24:359–370.

158. Haskell WL: Safety of out-patient cardiac exercise programs: Issues regarding medical supervision. In Franklin BA, Rubenfire M, eds: *Cardiac Rehabilitation (Clinics in Sports Medicine).* WB Saunders: Philadelphia, 1984, p 471.

159. Van Camp SP, Peterson RA: Cardiovascular complications of outpatient cardiac rehabilitation programs. *JAMA* 1986; 256:1160–1163.

160. Barnard RJ, et al.: Ischemic response to sudden strenuous exercise in healthy men. *Circulation* 1973; 48:936–942.

161. Foster C, et al.: Left ventricular function during sudden strenuous exercise. *Circulation* 1981; 63:592–596.

162. Kavanagh T, Shephard RJ: Fluid and mineral needs of post-coronary distance runners. In Landry F, Orban WR, eds: *Sports Medicine.* Symposia Specialists: Miami, 1978.

163. Kavanagh T: Guidelines for cold weather exercise. *J Cardiac Rehab* 1983; 3:70–73.

164. Buxton M, et al.: Costs of the Heart Transplant Programmes at Harefield and Papworth Hospitals. Her Majesty's Stationery Office: London, 1985.

165. Kriett JM, Kaye MP: The registry of the international society for heart transplant programmes at Harefield and Papworth Hospitals. Her Majesty's Stationery Office: London, 1985.

166. Jose A, Collision D: The normal range and determinants of the intrinsic heart rate in man. *Cardiovasc Res* 1970; 4:160.

167. de Marneffe M, et al.: Variations of normal sinus node function in relation to age: Role of autonomic influence. *Eur Heart J* 1986; 7:662–672.

168. Savin WM, et al.: Cardiorespiratory responses of cardiac transplant patients to graded, symptom-limited exercise. *Circulation* 1980; 62:55.

169. Borow KM, et al.: Left ventricular contractility and contractile reserve in humans after cardiac transplantation.

170. Borow KM, et al.: Clinical evidence for differential sensitivity of alpha and beta adrenergic receptors after cardiac transplantation. *Circulation* 1985; 72(III):III.

171. Nitkin RS, Schroeder JS: Accelerated cor-

onary artery disease risk in heart transplanted patients. *J Am Coll Cardiol* 1985; 5:535A.

172. Kavanagh T, Yacoub M, Tuck J: Receptiveness and compliance of cardiac transplant patients to an exercise rehabilitation program. *Circulation* 1987; 74(4) Suppl 2: II–10 (abstract).

173. Kavanagh T, et al.: Marathan running after cardiac transplantation: A case history. *J Cardiopul Rehabil* 1986; 6: 16–20.

174. Greenland P, Chu JS: Efficacy of cardiac rehabilitation services: With emphasis on patients after myocardial infarction. *Ann Intern Med* 1988; 109:650–663.

PART III

Musculoskeletal Disorders

CHAPTER 4

THE USE OF EXERCISE TO TREAT RHEUMATIC DISEASE

SHARON R. CLARK, PhD, FNP,
CAROL S. BURCKHARDT, RN, PhD,
and ROBERT M. BENNETT, MD

Musculoskeletal disorders are second to circulatory diseases in restricting activity, and are the number-two cause of work disability.[1] For many years, the most common exercise prescribed for rheumatic disorders was rest, range-of-motion (ROM) exercises, and more rest.[2-5] More recently, recommendations have changed from complete bed rest to local rest of the acutely involved joints. During the 1970s, investigators began to question these recommendations, which may have played a role in deconditioning and increased disability among patients with rheumatic diseases. Evidence[6] disputes the long-held belief that regular exercise results in further joint destruction in patients with rheumatic disease.

This chapter will discuss the current state of knowledge about the use of exercise as a treatment modality for rheumatoid arthritis, the most common form of inflammatory arthritis; anklyosing spondylitis, the most common inflammatory spondyloarthropathy; and fibrositis or fibromyalgia, the most common chronic soft-tissue disorder. Diagnostic criteria, clinical features, and specific recommendations for exercise prescription are provided.

83

Rheumatoid Arthritis

Rheumatoid arthritis (RA) is a chronic, systemic, inflammatory disease of unknown etiology, characterized by synovial inflammation.[7] The severity of the synovitis is directly related to the degree of joint damage.[8,9]

DIAGNOSTIC CRITERIA

The diagnostic criteria for RA were revised in 1987, and the previously used classification system was eliminated.[7] Of particular interest and use for purposes of evaluating exercise are functional class criteria. The Steinbrocker[10] functional categories were adopted as the official classification by the American College of Rheumatology. The Arthritis Impact Measurement Scales (AIMS) was published by Meenan and colleagues.[11] That original document included 7 demographic and 55 health-status items arranged into 9 scale groups. The American College of Rheumatology categories and a modification of AIMS can be found in Table 4–1. Classifying patients' functional abilities from these scales can be of particular use in monitoring the effects of exercise for patients with RA.

COURSE OF DISEASE

Although unrelenting progressive disease may be seen, RA typically has a pattern of remissions and exacerbations with a tendency toward incremental deterioration and progressive decline in a patient's functional capacity.[12-15] Even when disease activity has decreased, the level of disability continues to increase,[16] especially early in the disease.[17]

One proposed explanation for the increase in disability observed in RA patients is progressive muscle weakness. Muscle biopsy and electromyography findings are consistent with type II (fast twitch) muscle atrophy.[18] Herbison and associates[19] report that muscle atrophy is a hallmark of RA and that, while mild RA has been shown to be associated with type II muscle atrophy, severe RA has a decrease in both type II and type I (slow twitch) muscle fibers. Atrophy of both types of muscle fiber will result in decreased strength and endurance, common complaints of patients with RA.

EXERCISE CAPACITY OF PATIENTS WITH RA

Despite the wide recognition of weakness and fatigue in patients with RA, it was not until the 1970s that investigators in Sweden began to evaluate their physical performance. A group led by Ekblom[20] studied 31 female patients with RA to determine their exercise capacity, assessing walk time, muscle strength, and maximal oxygen uptake (VO_{2max}). The variables of this study laid the foundation for future studies. A summary of these studies is found in Table 4–2. Patients with RA were found to have reduced capacity on all exercise variables when compared to normal controls.

In the 1980s other investigators reported findings regarding the physical conditioning of rheumatic patients. Measures of fitness that are available to all clinicians were evaluated by Burckhardt and colleagues,[21] who tested 70 women, aged 24 to 59 years, with either RA, fibrositis, or systemic lupus

Table 4–1 **FUNCTIONAL CLASSIFICATION SYSTEMS FOR RHEUMATOID ARTHRITIS: STEINBROCKER FUNCTIONAL CLASSIFICATION**

Class	Functional Ability
I	Able to perform normal activities
II	Moderate restriction: Adequate for normal activities
III	Marked restriction: Inability to perform most duties of usual occupation or self-care
IV	Incapacitation or confinement to bed or wheelchair

Modified Arthritis Impact Measurement Scale (AIMS)†
Mobility and Physical Activity Scales‡
(Circle one number that best applies.)

1. When you travel around your community, does someone have to assist you because of your health?
   - Yes, all of the time 5
   - Yes, most of the time 4
   - Yes, some of the time 3
   - Yes, a little of the time 2
   - No, none of the time 1
2. Are you able to use public transportation?
   - No, because of my health 3
   - No, for some other reason 2
   - Yes, able to use public transportation 1
3. Do you have to stay indoors most or all of the day because of your health?
   - Yes 2
   - No 1
4. Are you in bed or in a chair for most or all of the day because of your health?
   - Yes 2
   - No 1
5. Does your health limit the kind of vigorous activities you can do, such as running, lifting heavy objects, or participation in strenuous sports?
   - Can't do this at all 5
   - Yes, a great deal 4
   - Yes, somewhat 3
   - Yes, a little 2
   - No, not at all 1
6. Do you have any trouble either walking several blocks or climbing a few flights of stairs because of your health?
   - Can't do this at all 5
   - Yes, a great deal of trouble 4
   - Yes, a fair amount of trouble 3
   - Yes, a little trouble 2
   - No trouble 1
7. Do you have trouble bending, lifting, or stooping because of your health?
   - Can't do this at all 5
   - Yes, a great deal of trouble 4
   - Yes, a fair amount of trouble 3
   - Yes, a little trouble 2
   - No trouble 1
8. Do you have any trouble either walking one block or climbing one flight of stairs because of your health?
   - Can't do this at all 5
   - Yes, a great deal of trouble 4
   - Yes, a fair amount of trouble 3
   - Yes, a little trouble 2
   - No trouble 1

Continued

Table 4–1 **FUNCTIONAL CLASSIFICATION SYSTEMS FOR RHEUMATOID ARTHRITIS: STEINBROCKER FUNCTIONAL CLASSIFICATION**—*Continued*

9. Are you unable to walk unless you are assisted by another person or by a cane, crutches, artificial limbs, or braces?
   Yes 2
   No 1
10. Can you easily write with a pen or pencil?
    No 2
    Yes 1
11. Can you button articles of clothing?
    No, not at all 5
    Yes, with much difficulty 4
    Yes, with some difficulty 3
    Yes, with little difficulty 2
    Yes, easily 1
12. Can you turn a key in a lock?
    No, not at all 5
    Yes, with much difficulty 4
    Yes, with some difficulty 3
    Yes, with little difficulty 2
    Yes, easily 1
13. Can you tie a pair of shoes?
    No, not at all 5
    Yes, with much difficulty 4
    Yes, with some difficulty 3
    Yes, with little difficulty 2
    Yes, easily 1
14. Can you open a new jar of food?
    No, not at all 5
    Yes, with much difficulty 4
    Yes, with some difficulty 3
    Yes, with little difficulty 2
    Yes, easily 1
15. If you had the necessary transportation, could you go shopping for groceries or clothes?
    I am completely unable to do any shopping 4
    With quite a bit of help (help with most trips) 3
    With a little bit of help (help with some trips) 2
    Without help (take care of all shopping needs yourself) 1
16. If you had a kitchen, could you prepare your own meals?
    I am completely unable to prepare any meals 4
    With quite a bit of help (help with most things) 3
    With a little bit of help (help with some things) 2
    Without help (plan and cook full meals yourself) 1
17. If you had household tools and appliances (vacuum, mops, and so on), could you do your own housework?
    I am completely unable to do any housework 4
    With quite a bit of help (help with most things) 3
    With a little help (can do light housework, but need help with some things) 2
    Without help (can clean floors, windows, refrigerators, and so on) 1

*Adapted from Schumacher.[7]
†Adapted from Meenan, Gertman, and Mason.[11]
‡Higher score = greater disability.

Table 4–2 **SUMMARY OF STUDIES EVALUATING PHYSICAL CONDITION OF PATIENTS WITH RHEUMATOID ARTHRITIS**

Author	Subject Characteristics	Fitness Variables	Methods	Findings
Ekblom 1974[20]	31 F with mild RA of at least 3 years' duration	Cardiorespiratory fitness	850-m timed walk test Oxygen uptake	41.8% < normal values 30% < normal values
		Lower-extremity muscle strength	Up and down flight of 12 steps	60.9% < normal values
		Upper-extremity muscle strength	Strain gauge	33%–52% < normals
Beals 1985[26]	20 F, RA and OA compared functional class II	Cardiorespiratory fitness	50-feet timed walk test Oxygen uptake	No difference between age groups RA < OA < normals
		Lower-extremity muscle strength	Cybex II, knee	RA < OA < normals
Harkcom 1985[33]	20 F with RA functional class II	Cardiorespiratory fitness	Oxygen uptake	Improved oxygen uptake and RA symptoms Greater reported functional status 15- & 25-minute training > 35-minute training
Hsieh 1987[25]	16 subjects, RA functional class I or II	Quadricep/hamstring ratio	Cybex II	RA < controls
		Lower limb endurance	Cybex II	No difference
Minor 1988[23]	120 subjects, OA or RA	Cardiorespiratory fitness	Oxygen uptake	RA < OA < predicted values
Burckhardt 1988[21]	70 F; 28 RA, 13 SLE, 29 fibrositis	Cardiorespiratory fitness	Timed walk test 6 minute, 12 minute	78% poor fitness compared to normals. RA < fibrositis or SLE
		Lower-extremity muscle strength	Up and down flight of stairs	< Normal values, no difference between patient groups

Continued

Table 4-2 **SUMMARY OF STUDIES EVALUATING PHYSICAL CONDITION OF PATIENTS WITH RHEUMATOID ARTHRITIS**—*Continued*

Author	Subject Characteristics	Fitness Variables	Methods	Findings
		Upper-extremity muscle strength	Soft weights (10 lb or <) lifted overhead	No difference between groups
		Flexibility	Sit and reach box	No difference

Key: F = female, OA = osteoarthritis, RA = rheumatoid arthritis, SLE = systemic lupus erythematosus.

erythematosus. An age-matched group of women without rheumatic or other chronic illnesses served as controls. Cardiorespiratory fitness was assessed by having the subject walk as far as she could in 12 minutes. Those with rheumatic disease had lower fitness values when compared to either sedentary controls or published normal levels. No subject had experienced any adverse effects from the vigorous walking when contacted 1 week later. They found the distance walked in 6 minutes and 12 minutes to be highly correlated ($r = 0.95$). This study first identified the 6-minute walk test as a useful clinical tool for evaluating cardiorespiratory work capacity among those with chronic rheumatic disease. Endurance fitness values may be estimated from Table 4-3.

Another shorter-duration, timed walk test[22] correlated a 5-minute period of walking with expired gas analysis measurement of VO_{2max} among those with osteoarthritis (OA) and RA. Although all subjects had lower-extremity disease involvement, none experienced adverse effects from this exercise testing. Although these short-duration walk tests are not recommended to screen for coronary artery disease, they are a convenient method for evaluating and monitoring functional exercise capacity in many rheumatic patients.

Minor and associates[23] studied the largest number of subjects to determine the physical fitness of patients with either OA or RA. They used a standardized treadmill protocol and measured oxygen consumption in 120 subjects (OA n = 80, RA n = 40) with documented involvement of at least one weightbearing joint. The women with RA achieved 62% of expected VO_{2max}, while the men with RA achieved 81% of their predicted values.

Although the combined sample size of these studies is relatively small, with a collective total of 265 subjects, they confirm the clinical observation that patients with RA have reduced exercise tolerance. This appears due to decreases in both muscular strength and cardiorespiratory endurance, which can lead to further deconditioning and functional disability.*

Despite reduced exercise capacity and concerns of arthritic complication during maximal exertion, none of the subjects in these studies reported a flare in joint activity after high-intensity work.†

---

*References 6, 20, 21, 23-25.
†References 20, 22, 23, 25, 26.

Table 4-3 **6-MINUTE WALK NORMS FOR WOMEN (DISTANCE IN YARDS)**

Fitness Category	Under 30	Age in Years		
		30-39	40-49	50-59
Very poor	<660	<621	<587	<557
Poor	660-720	621-681	587-647	557-609
Fair	721-782	682-754	648-720	610-674
Good	783-880	755-845	721-812	675-754
Excellent	≥881	≥846	≥813	≥755

Adapted from Cooper M, Cooper KH: *Aerobics for Women*. Evans, New York: 1972, p. 74.

TRAINING STUDIES

It has been assumed that rest is the single most important factor in the treatment of active arthritis, but longitudinal studies to confirm its efficacy have not been performed.[27] In 1978 Smith and Polley[4] recommended that the ideal program for treatment of RA is a loading dose of complete bed rest followed by sufficient rest to prevent fatigue. Shortly thereafter, Lightfoot[28] suggested from empirical evidence that systemic rest can ameliorate an acute exacerbation of rheumatoid disease and stated, "any patient who wishes to institute a vigorous program of jogging, bicycling, or calisthenics in a misguided attempt to improve his joint function should be admonished to desist." However, since that time, he has modified this view to conclude that "using a stationary exercise cycle is of great value once control of synovitis in knees and hips has been achieved."[3]

Many investigations have demonstrated that vigorous exercise is not detrimental to the patient with RA. While methodologies have varied, all have included patients, primarily women, with definite or classic RA. Subjects have tended to be older, have a longer duration of disease, and be in functional class II or III. Some studies required no active disease at time of training, while others permitted mild to moderate disease activity.

Although patients with RA had lower than expected levels of physical fitness, even with mild disease present, the use of supervised strength and aerobic conditioning programs did not exacerbate symptoms. Some[6] contend that exercises that cause any pain at all exacerbate joint destruction. However, no one has observed that a supervised program results in further joint destruction. Interestingly, fewer joint symptoms and less destruction have been found after training.

In 1975, Ekblom and colleagues[29,30] evaluated 34 patients in a nonacute stage of RA, who had the disease for a minimum of 3 years. Twenty-three subjects were assigned to a special training group and 11 subjects served as controls. All participated in a physical therapy program consisting of muscle strengthening and ROM exercises. In addition, the training group exercised on a cycle ergometer for two to five training intervals of 3 to 5 minutes per interval, with equivalent rest time between intervals. Training was performed at an intensity of 50% to 70% of their maximum pretraining work load, five times per week, for 6 weeks. During periods of increased disease activity, the training recommendation was to ride a cycle ergometer without resistance, to minimize exercise-related pain. At the end of the study, the training group showed a significant improvement in a walk test and improved oxygen uptake. There was no change in joint status as evaluated by pain and swelling. A follow-up evaluation 6 months after the training revealed that 18 of the 23 had continued to exercise two or more times per week; those who had continued to exercise reported improved performance in various activities such as walking and stair climbing. Only one subject ceased training activity due to a flare of symptoms.

Subjects were reevaluated several years later. At the end of 8 years, those in the treatment group were three times more physically active, had less stiffness, and used less sick leave with fewer hospitalized days than the control group. Also, the exercise group had fewer intra-articular injections and radiologic changes, consistent with a decrease in their disease progression.[31] Thus, the exercise group was not only more physically active, but also had fewer indications of active disease and its complications.

Another group of 10 subjects with RA underwent a similar physical training program,[32] with muscle biopsies obtained before and after training. Exercise capacity improved and type II muscle fiber atrophy was reduced after training. No subject had an increase in joint disease activity due to training. Harkcom and coworkers[33] assigned 20 women with functional class II RA and low fitness to endurance exercise for 15, 25, or 35 minutes, three times weekly over a 12-week training period. These women were able to achieve improved oxygen uptake with as little as 15 minutes of endurance exercise. Also, exercise subjects had fewer actively involved joints, less morning stiffness, and an improved self-reported sleep pattern at the end of the training. Those who exercised either 15 or 25 minutes per session reported improvement in general mood, less fatigue, and an improved ability to do household and social activities when compared to controls or to the group who exercised for 35 minutes per session. This latter finding may illustrate the need to recommend that at first, deconditioned patients with RA train for a shorter duration until initial conditioning has occurred.

Investigators from Denmark[24] prescribed individual incremental exercise programs to subjects who were initially functional class II or III, without acute RA activity. Exercises were performed to avoid extreme joint positions, with reduction of intensity if there was a complaint of excessive fatigue, pain, or a joint effusion. The training consisted of three 5-minute bicycling periods at 50% to 70% maximum heart rate, two times per week, in addition to lower-body dynamic strength exercises. Of 20 subjects, 13 experienced a decrease in the number of swollen joints during the training program; only 2 had an increase in joint swelling, which required temporary cessation of strength training but allowed the continuation of aerobic conditioning. The authors concluded that RA patients in a phase of moderate disease activity can tolerate controlled strength and aerobic training.

TREATMENT: CONDITIONING PARAMETERS

When prescribing exercise as a component of a treatment program, the clinician needs to be cognizant of specific modifiers based on the patient's characteristics. The RA activity will influence the recommendations for exercise. Potential systemic involvement, especially of the cardiopulmonary system, should also be evaluated, since such complications can affect the risk of exertion and the ability to exercise.[24,34] Generally, exercise should be aimed at maximizing flexibility, strength, and cardiorespiratory endurance. The Steinbrocker functional class differences may be of use for exercise prescription. Patients in functional class I should be able to perform almost any activity except those associated with high impact to diseased joints, such as intense running and racquet and contact sports.[24] Patients in class II should be able to perform bicycling, walking and, if involvement of weightbearing joints is minimal, slow jogging. Proper footwear is especially important for patients with RA.[38]

Class III patients often are at greater risk of systemic involvement and must be more closely monitored. Exercising in water and bicycling have been shown to be safe and effective activity modes for this group.[24,26,33] Class IV patients require assistance, and exercise in the water is probably preferred. Activities performed in the water have the advantages of warmth and buoyancy.[5] Thus, movement may be made with little stress, and certain muscle groups may be exercised in a manner not possible without such support.[35] Even severely debilitated patients can perform 5 minutes of water therapy exercise consisting of active ROM exercises, and this time can be slowly increased as improvement occurs.[5] Exercise should be done at the time of day the patient feels the best.[2,36]

CASE: M.T., a 32-year-old woman, was initially examined 3 years ago with a complaint of pain and stiffness in her hands for 8 months. The pain and stiffness was preceded by fatigue, which interfered with her ability to accomplish daily activities. Her stiffness was predominant in the morning, lasting up to 4 hours. She had synovitis of her wrists and second and third metacarpal joints bilaterally. M.T. met the diagnostic criteria for RA and was treated with a nonsteroidal anti-inflammatory drug. Six months later, morning stiffness was still lasting 1½ hours each morning; she had pain and swelling in her knees and continued to feel fatigued. Radiographs revealed bony decalcification and early erosions of the right wrist. M.T. was then started on a second-line agent. Two years after initiating that treatment, her morning stiffness lasts only 15 minutes. Fatigue continues to be a major problem.

Prior to onset of symptoms, she jogged 3 to 4 miles two to three times each week. Although M.T. was participating in therapy consisting of ROM exercises and joint protection activities, she did no endurance exercise. Before a conditioning program was suggested, evaluation by a 6-minute walk test found her to have very poor aerobic capacity.

Because of her deconditioned state and knee involvement, it was decided that low-impact activities would be most appropriate. M.T. chose walking. Initially the program consisted of walking half a mile in 15 minutes four times a week. This prescription reflected a very low intensity and duration, a level she was confident that she would be able to accomplish. A plan for inclement weather was to walk in the local shopping mall for 15 minutes without stopping. After 2 to 3 weeks of getting accustomed to regular walking, she was prescribed the program found in Table 4–4.

This program was provided to her as a guide. Should she experience a symptom flare in her lower extremities, she was told to stop the walking and perform daily isometric exercises to minimize muscle atrophy. She could ride a stationary cycle without resistance when the acute phase

Table 4−4 **A WALK PROGRAM FOR PERSONS WHO ARE DECONDITIONED**

Week	Pace (mph)	Distance (in miles)	Time (min:sec)
1,2	3.0	1.5	30:00
3,4	3.5	1.5	25:42
5,6	3.5	2.0	34:16
6,7	3.5	2.5	42:50
8,9	3.75	2.5	40:00
10−12	3.75	2.75	44:00
12+	4.0	3.0	45:00

Adapted from Pollock, Wilmore, Fox: *Exercise in Health and Disease*. Philadelphia: WB Saunders, 1984. p. 264, with permission.

had passed. She also was instructed to continue the ROM exercises that she had been doing, even after adding the endurance component to her exercise therapy.

Overall, pain must be respected, but patients need to be aware that few people ever exercise without a mild degree of transient discomfort. Initially, exercise performed by deconditioned patients (particularly if begun at a level of intensity that exceeds 50% of their maximum heart rate) causes discomfort in about 85% of patients with RA. Three fourths of these patients relate that the discomfort lasts up to 24 hours. However, this experience of discomfort lessens as training continues.[31]

During times of greater inflammatory activity, local rest of the involved joints is recommended. However, since patients tend to avoid exercise during times of high disease activity, some loss of function is likely to occur. With inactivity, muscle strength decreases by 1.5% to 5% per day.[36] Isometric exercise, during which the muscle is contracted but the joint does not move, may be preferred during acute joint-disease activity. The isometric contraction should be maximal and held for 5 to 6 seconds.[2] Stationary cycling without resistance may also be recommended as long as no acute process is occurring at the hip or knee joints.[5,25,26,33] However, resistive strength training during high disease activity is not recommended.[2,24,26]

Ankylosing Spondylitis

Ankylosing spondylitis is an inflammatory disease distinguished by stiffening of the spine, with the characteristic lesion occurring in the sacroilium.[7] Ankylosing spondylitis may be primary if associated with no other rheumatic disorder, or secondary if sacroiliitis occurs in association with psoriatic arthritis, Reiter's syndrome, or inflammatory bowel disease. It may involve the peripheral joints as well.

Current evidence[37] suggests that ankylosing spondylitis is far more common than previously thought, and frequently exists in a subclinical form. The reported prevalence is from 0.2% to 2% of the white U.S. population, with a mean age at onset of 20 years.[7,38,39,40] It was once thought to be almost exclusively a male disorder, but the current estimate of the male-to-female ratio is 3:1. Women are less likely to have progressive spinal disease but are more likely to have peripheral joint manifestations. Because of this atypical presentation, ankylosing spondylitis is occasionally misdiagnosed as seronegative RA in female patients.[7,41]

DIAGNOSTIC CRITERIA

A diagnosis of ankylosing spondylitis is suggested by a history of insidious onset of low-back discomfort persisting longer than 3 months and worsened by rest but relieved by exercise, in a patient younger than age 40.[7,40] The history should include pain, morning stiffness, and functional disability. Diagnosis depends on an adequate history and examination, which should include an assessment of spinal mobility, muscle spasm, loss of lumbar lordosis, and reduced chest expansion.[42] The most useful single measure of spinal mobility is the Schober test (Figure 4–1).

The primary pathologic site for ankylosing spondylitis is the enthesis (site of insertion of ligaments and capsules into bone). Enthesopathic changes explain findings of syndesmophyte formation, squaring of vertebral bodies, Achilles tendinitis, plantar fasciitis, and heel spurs.[43,44]

The symptoms eventually progress to constant pain and early-morning awakening due to discomfort and stiffness in the back. The symptom that best differentiates anklyosing spondylitis from noninflammatory back pain is nocturnal pain and stiffness that paradoxically forces the patient out of bed. The vertebral spine may be severely involved and, when ankylosed, is vulnerable to injury from even trivial trauma. The most common site of fracture is the

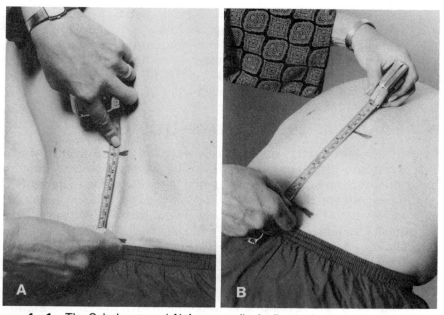

Figure 4–1   The Schober test. (*A*) A perpendicular line is drawn midpoint between the posterior iliac spines; another line is drawn 10 cm above the first line. (*B*) With the patient in anterior flexion, the distance between these two lines is measured. Normally, the distance should increase from 10 cm to 16.22 cm.

lower cervical spine, and the most common mechanism of fracture is hyperextension.[45,46]

Fatigue, weight loss, low-grade fever, hypochromic anemia, and an elevated erythrocyte sedimentation rate (ESR) are common systemic manifestations and findings. In the later stages of severe involvement, aortic regurgitation, spinal cord compression, and upper lobe pulmonary fibrosis may occur. Alves and associates[47] suggest that cardiovascular changes are more common than usually acknowledged, reporting that among 40 patients with a mean duration of disease of 11 years, 22.5% had significant changes in conduction resulting in sinus bradycardia, while 20% had systemic hypertension. However, Calin[40] states that 3.5% of patients with a 15-year duration of disease, and 10% with a 30-year history, will have cardiovascular involvement. Aortic incompetence, cardiomegaly, and conduction defects are the most common cardiovascular findings.

There are no pathognomonic tests for ankylosing spondylitis, but it is strongly associated with HLA-B27 in more than 95% of cases. However, HLA-B27 should not be used for diagnosis, which depends on clinical and radiologic evidence of the disease. Ankylosing spondylitis should not be diagnosed without radiographic evidence of sacroiliitis, although this finding may be subtle.[7,40,48]

COURSE OF DISEASE

The likelihood that ankylosing spondylitis is the underlying cause of back pain, and the course of the disease for any one patient, are difficult to predict. Sixty-six patients presenting with low back pain lasting more than 3 months, who also had at least one of peripheral arthritis, heel pain, anterior uveitis, or an elevated ESR, were evaluated 5 years later. Sacroiliitis was initially equivocal. After 5 years, ankylosing spondylitis was diagnosed in 24 patients; after 10 years an additional 8 patients were found to have the disease. Thus, approximately 50% of those with a diagnosis suspicious for ankylosing spondylitis went on to develop definite disease.[41] However, the natural history of disease for any individual remains undefined.[7,49]

EXERCISE AND ANKYLOSING SPONDYLITIS

Despite the therapeutic use of exercise, the number of studies evaluating the fitness of patients with ankylosing spondylitis or documenting training's benefits is small. A few investigators have attempted to quantify fitness among these patients. Hopkins and coworkers[50] evaluated 20 patients with ankylosing spondylitis as defined by the New York criteria.[42] All had back involvement, and 13 had disease of either the hip or knee. Muscle biopsy of the quadriceps femoris revealed nonspecific atrophic changes commonly found with disuse; 10 of the 20 had reduced quadriceps muscle strength.[50] In another study,[51] no differences in grip force or shoulder flexion strength were found between AS patients and normal controls, although patients with ankylosing spondylitis were found to develop fatigue more rapidly in the descending part of the trapezius muscle. No studies have evaluated the aerobic capacity of patients with ankylosing spondylitis.

Improving or preventing the loss of flexibility is of great importance to these patients. Bulstrode and colleagues[52] assessed the effects of daily passive stretching of the hip joints to determine if increased ROM could be achieved. Of 39 patients admitted to a 15-day physiotherapy course, 12 were assigned to a usual care control group and 27 to a passive-stretching group. Initially, the two groups had comparable ROM. At the conclusion of the study, the stretching group had a significantly greater increase in flexion and abduction. The authors concluded that passive stretching of the hip flexors may prevent contractures and thereby prevent deformities.

TREATMENT

The goals of therapy are to relieve pain, maintain flexibility, and prevent deformity.[37] Medications for pain relief and reduction of inflammation are indicated, but salicylates are not effective.[38,53,54] Phenylbutazone is generally considered to be most effective, but concerns over its potential bone marrow toxicity have made indomethacin the preferred medication.[37,40,55]

Exercise traditionally has been upheld as the cornerstone of treatment for ankylosing spondylitis, based on empirical evidence, despite lack of a strong research base demonstrating efficacy. Because patients attempt to ease back pain by adopting a flexed position, exercise regimens often are designed to counteract the excessive pull of the abdominal flexor muscles. Back extension exercises of 10 to 20 repetitions each session, with two to four sessions per day, are suggested.[56] Also, three to five repetitions of ROM exercises of all involved areas, including stretching of the hamstring muscles, are encouraged on a daily basis[55] (Figure 4–2). Lying facedown with the feet extended over the edge of

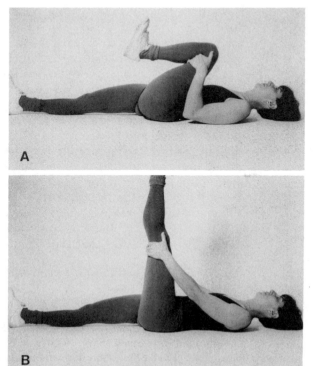

Figure 4–2 Hamstring stretch. The patient should lie on the floor or bed with knees bent, or with the legs straight for greater stretch. (*A*) One leg is brought up toward the chest and the patient grasps the back of the thigh. (*B*) The leg is straightened at the knee as much as possible. The patient then slowly pulls the thigh toward the chest, keeping the knee as straight as possible, and holds the position for 5 seconds. The patient then relaxes to the starting position and repeats with the opposite leg, for a total of five times with each leg.

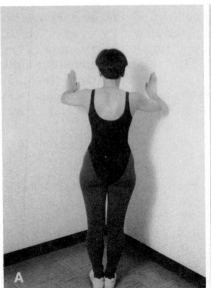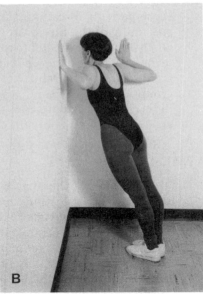

Figure 4–3 Pectoral stretch. (*A*) The patient should stand facing a corner with his or her feet in a position of comfort, and places the hands on opposite walls. (*B*) The patient slowly leans forward, keeping the body straight and breathing in, and holds the position for 5 seconds before returning to the starting position. This can be repeated, initially five to ten times, then up to 20 times, three times each day. Adapted from Swezey.[57]

the bed for 15 minutes daily is advised as one of the best ways to keep hip joints stretched.[56] An exercise to stretch the upper chest and shoulder muscles, such as the pectoral stretch (Figure 4–3), is also recommended, and may help to retard the reduced chest expansion seen in ankylosing spondylitis.

Since ankylosing spondylitis exists in many forms, from very mild sacro-iliitis to severe multiorgan disease, therapeutic exercise must be tailored to each patient, considering the degree of spine and peripheral joint involvement and the presence of systemic effects. Swimming is suggested as the most appropriate endurance exercise mode.[37,40,55] However, breathing technique may be difficult during swimming for persons with decreased neck range of motion unless assistive devices are used; for example, 11 of 12 patients enrolled in a swimming program were able to use a mask and snorkel for freestyle swimming.[58] Jogging usually is not endorsed due to the impact load on the lower spine and peripheral joints. Also, bicycling in a flexed (trunk flexion) position is discouraged.[40,55,57] Patients are encouraged to exercise daily, to walk erect, and to avoid activities that require forward flexion.

CASE: T.R., a 49-year-old man, was diagnosed as having ankylosing spondylitis at the age of 18. T.R. is married with two children, works in a canning factory doing clerical work, and spends most of the day sitting at a desk. He has never been an active person, even though exercise has seemed to benefit his back pain and stiffness. T.R. is a 20-pack-year smoker and has a family history of coronary artery disease. Over the past 5 weeks, he has been concerned about a mild chest pain that occurs when he walks uphill on his way home from work. He assumes this is another manifestation of his ankylosing spondylitis, but his wife made an appointment with his physician for him against his wishes. His physician observes normal findings on cardiovascular examination, but notes a reduced lumbar flexion (with Schober's test going from 10 to 11.5 cm), a severely restricted rotation of the cervical spine, a chest expansion of 2 cm, and a moderately stooped posture due to a thoracic kyphosis. His chest x-ray, electrocardiogram (ECG), and complete blood count (CBC) were normal, but a Westergren ESR was elevated at 35 mm/h and his total cholesterol level was 289 mg/dL.

The exercise ECG revealed a 1-mm depression of the ST segments in the anterolateral leads. His measured Vo_{2max} was only 19 mL/kg/min, and he achieved 75% of his maximum heart rate. A subsequent thallium stress test showed a small area of reduced myocardial perfusion; a coronary angiogram did not reveal any significant lesions, and no further investigations were thought to be indicated. This incident served to underline T.R.'s vulnerability to ischemic heart disease and helped him to focus on improving his general health.

After he quit smoking, T.R. gained 8 pounds. He was advised to swim, but was unable to do so due to his restricted neck movement; jogging was no better, as it exacerbated his back pain. He was instructed in the use of snorkel and mask; after 3 weeks he was able to swim a quarter of a mile twice a week, attaining a pulse rate of about 70% maximum. As he could not always make it for lap swims at his local pool, he purchased a stationary cycle and began 25 minutes of cycling at 75% of his maximum heart rate 2 to 3 times a week, and swimming up to half a mile once a week. He was instructed in cycling without assuming a flexed position. After 1 year of this regimen he was 11 pounds lighter, felt more energetic, and had been free of chest pain for the past 4 months. Furthermore he noted an increased suppleness in his back and a slight increase in the mobility of his neck.

COMMENT: This program was designed to meet the specific needs of T.R., based on the limited range of motion of his neck and back. He found that a stationary cycle that allowed him to sit behind the cycle and pedal reduced his tendency to flexion while cycling.

Fibromyalgia

Fibromyalgia is a common disorder characterized by diffuse, generalized aching and fatigue. The term "fibrositis," originally coined in 1904 by Sir William Gowers, is a misnomer, since no evidence of inflammation is found.[59] Many now prefer the term "fibromyalgia syndrome" (FMS). FMS also has been called fibromyositis, muscular rheumatism, myofascial pain syndrome, and many other names.[60,61]

Fibromyalgia syndrome is the second most common rheumatic condition seen by rheumatologists.[60] It is estimated to affect 5% of the general medical population and 10% to 20% of the patients seen in a rheumatology practice.[62] The typical patient is a woman who had the onset of symptoms between ages 25 and 55,[61-64] with a duration of symptoms at time of diagnosis of at least 5 years.[65-67]

DIAGNOSTIC CRITERIA

Diagnostic criteria have emphasized chronic, diffuse aches and pains, disturbed sleep, morning fatigue and stiffness, and the characteristic tender points.[61,62,62a,64] In 1979 Smythe[65] proposed the presence of a specified number of tender points in order to make the diagnosis of FMS. Wolfe and colleagues[62a] found that the number of tender points better differentiated patients with FMS from those with other rheumatic disorders than did any historical data. This recent multicenter study[62a] has developed simple and effective criteria for diagnosis of FMS: a history of whole body pain (in all four quadrants) of greater than 3 months' duration and unexplained by another diagnosis, plus 9 or more of a possible 18 tender points. These criteria were found to be 88% sensitive and 81% specific when tested against a control group of patients with other painful conditions. Since the diagnosis of FMS cannot be made without the presence of these tender points, clinicians should include this evaluation as a routine part of the physical examination.[68] Campbell and associates[67] found that patients with FMS differed from normal subjects on all the tender points but did not differ on the "control points" (see Figure 4-4). By including the control points in the examination, a clinician can differentiate a true FMS patient from one who has a psychogenic or pain-modulation disorder.[61]

Since laboratory and radiographic investigations reveal no abnormalities, many physicians have doubted the existence of FMS. Earlier investigators were inclined to believe that FMS was a pain-modulation syndrome or a form of psychogenic rheumatism. Other investigations have disputed this notion, and several studies demonstrate that no distinctive psychopathology is associated with FMS, and it should not be considered a primary psychiatric condition.[67,69,70,71] Although other considerations such as hypothyroidism or polymyalgia rheumatica must be ruled out, FMS is not merely a diagnosis of exclusion and should be diagnosed based on its own characteristics.[61,62,72,73]

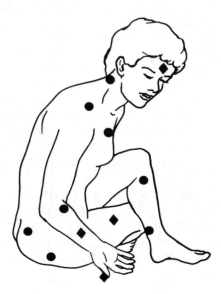

Figure 4-4 Tender and control points in FMS. (♦ Control; • FMS tender points.)

COURSE OF DISEASE

Fibromyalgia is not a deforming disease,[59] but patients may consider the pain of FMS to be disabling.[72,74] Symptoms tend to be unrelenting, with most patients reporting little change in a 3-year follow-up study.[75] Remissions are rare and, if they occur, are transitory. The natural course of FMS appears to lead to functional disability and chronic disease.[76,77]

EXERCISE CAPACITY OF FMS PATIENTS

Objective data can assess the work capacity of patients with FMS.[77] Exercise capacity is related to functional disability, psychologic status, and pain. Upper-body exercise capacity, as measured by five standardized work tasks, has been shown to be 58.6% of that performed by normal controls.

The fatigue from which FMS patients suffer led early investigators to explore a loss of sleep as a potential explanation. A loss of non-REM (specifically, delta [slow-wave]) sleep was found among those with FMS.[78] Normal subjects deprived of only delta sleep developed a typical fibrositis syndrome,[79] but three physically fit subjects, when deprived of delta sleep, did not develop this syndrome, providing a clue to a potential relationship between fitness and FMS.

Patients with FMS have been shown to have decreased muscle strength. In one study,[80] 15 patients and controls matched for age, sex, height, and weight used an isokinetic dynamometer. The fibrositis group's performance was one third of the control values. Whether this was due to muscle pathology is unknown. Muscle biopsies have shown swollen mitochondria, "moth-eaten" myofilaments, endothelial swelling, and dissolution of contractile elements in type I and type II fibers.[81-85] However, these findings are nonspecific and are also found with disuse.[86]

Bengtsson and colleagues[83] found decreased levels of high-energy phosphates while evaluating specific tender points, although results of ischemic forearm tests were without abnormality. Lower phosphate concentrations, however, may be found in tissues with inadequate oxygen supply to meet metabolic demands. Other researchers[87] reported that the oxygen tension in the trapezius muscle of FMS patients was lower than that of normal controls, indicating a maldistribution of capillary blood flow. Supporting this concept, muscle blood flow was found by ^{133}Xe clearance to be lower in FMS patients than in controls matched by age, sex, and maximal oxygen consumption.[88] When performing a symptom-limited exercise test, 80% of fibromyalgia patients were aerobically unfit when compared to published normal values of predicted maximal oxygen consumption.[89]

These studies demonstrating exacerbation of pain by strenuous exertion provide further evidence that skeletal muscle may be the end organ responsible for FMS symptoms.[61] Similar findings have been reported following unaccustomed exercise that causes delayed-onset muscle soreness. This muscle soreness is characterized by aching and is associated with abnormal muscle ultrastructure; changes include myofibril disorganization, sarcolemmal disruption, and Z-line smearing. The severity of these problems appears related to the intensity of the exercise and to the proportion of eccentric contractions. The best preventive treatment for delayed-onset muscle soreness is activity, especially exercise that results in noneccentric training and stretching of the involved muscle groups.[90]

TRAINING STUDIES

Two studies[91,92] have examined the effect of a training program for patients with fibromyalgia. Although methods differed, both used a randomized, controlled design to compare patient groups involved in endurance exercise with non–endurance-trained control groups. Both independently found that patients with FMS have low levels of aerobic fitness when compared to normal individuals, but that the level of fitness can be improved with a cycle ergometer endurance training program. Readings using a dolorimeter (a spring-loaded gauge) over the tender points improved in both experimental groups, while no improvements were found in the control groups. No adverse effects due to the exercise occurred. Thus endurance exercise appears to play a therapeutic role in decreasing pain and improving overall feelings of well-being in FMS patients.

TREATMENT

The goals of treatment in FMS are to relieve pain and to retain or regain normal function.[92] A tool for measuring functional ability is shown in Table 4–5.

Table 4–5 **FIBROMYALGIA IMPACT QUESTIONNAIRE**

Name _____

Date _____

Directions: For questions 1 through 10, please circle the number that best describes how you did **overall** for the **past week**. If you don't normally do something that is asked, cross the question out.

	Always	Most times	Occasionally	Never
Were you able to:				
1. Do shopping?	0	1	2	3
2. Do laundry with a washer and dryer?	0	1	2	3
3. Prepare meals?	0	1	2	3
4. Wash dishes and cooking utensils by hand?	0	1	2	3
5. Vacuum a rug?	0	1	2	3
6. Make beds?	0	1	2	3
7. Walk several blocks?	0	1	2	3
8. Visit friends or relatives?	0	1	2	3
9. Do yard work?	0	1	2	3
10. Drive a car?	0	1	2	3

11. Of the 7 days in the past week, how many days did you feel good?

    0 1 2 3 4 5 6 7

12. How many days last week did you miss work because of your fibromyalgia? If you don't have a job outside the home, leave this item blank.

    0 1 2 3 4 5

Table 4–5   FIBROMYALGIA IMPACT QUESTIONNAIRE—Continued

Directions: For the remaining items, place a mark like this (|) at the point on the line that best indicates how you felt **overall** for the past week.

13. When you did work, how much did pain or other symptoms of your fibromyalgia interfered with your ability to do your job?

•· ·•

No problem   Great difficulty
with work   with work

14. How bad has your pain been?

•· ·•

No   Very severe
pain   pain

15. How tired have you been?

•· ·•

No   Very
tiredness   tired

16. How have you felt when you got up in the morning?

•· ·•

Awoke   Awoke
well rested   very tired

17. How bad has your stiffness been?

•· ·•

No   Very
stiffness   stiff

18. How nervous or anxious have you felt?

•· ·•

Not   Very
anxious   anxious

19. How depressed or blue have you felt?

•· ·•

Not   Very
depressed   depressed

Adapted from Burckhardt et al.,[95] with permission.

With the exception of low-dose tricyclic antidepressants for sleep restoration (amitriptyline hydrochloride 10 mg h.s.), medications have little role in the treatment of FMS. However, exercise programs increase physical fitness and may alleviate symptoms.[91,92] Patients with FMS do not typically complain of pain during the exercise bout, but rather complain of delayed-onset muscle soreness, usually 12 to 48 hours after the training period. Beginning an exercise program at a low intensity level will help to alleviate this soreness, as will stretching following exercise (Figure 4–5).

There is no known contraindication to any endurance activities, but clinical experience has shown that walking, bicycling, low-intensity jogging, and swimming with a paddleboard (to eliminate the upper-body requirements) are best tolerated.[72,76,91,94] An interesting clinical observation is that patients do not tolerate low-impact aerobic classes that rely on upper-body muscle contractions to keep the heart rate within a target range, nor do they tolerate the eccentric contractions required in weight training. The emphasis for FMS patients should be on prolonging the duration of an exercise bout rather than increasing intensity.

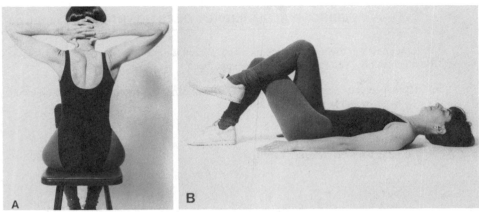

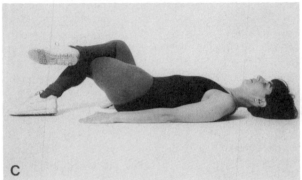

Figure 4–5 (*A*) Upper back stretch. While seated or lying on the floor, the hands are placed behind the head. The shoulder blades are pulled towards each other and elbows extended to the side. The patient holds the position for 10 seconds, repeating three to five times. (*B, C*) Secretary stretch. Lying on the floor, the patient brings the knees together with the soles of the feet on the floor, then lifts the right leg over the left leg. The right leg is used to pull the left leg towards the floor until a stretch is felt, and the position is held for 30 seconds. The stretch should be repeated three to four times on each side.

CASE: G.W. is a 55-year-old sedentary women who makes the following complaint: "I wake up in the morning feeling as tired as when I go to bed, I can barely get things done and I ache all over." These symptoms have been present for 9 years, and she has been evaluated by four physicians, including a psychiatrist, in an attempt to obtain relief. Treatment has included a variety of pain medications, tranquilizers, and even prednisone, with little to no relief. An exercise history is elicited. G.W. has not performed any exercise on a regular basis for the past 5 years due to the generalized pain. Also, she feels very tired after exercising. She is uncertain whether she can do any exercise. On examination she has 14 tender points but no tender control points. Findings for other components of the examination, with the exception of Heberden's nodes (indicating primary osteoarthritis of the hands), are normal. Results of laboratory studies, including thyroid function tests and ESR, are normal.

G.W. is diagnosed with FMS and started on a low-dose tricyclic antidepressant (amitriptyline 10 mg h.s.). An exercise program is considered. She is evaluated with maximal cycle ergometry with expired gas analysis. Her maximal oxygen uptake is 17 mL/kg/minute (70% of the expected value). She achieves 90% of predicted maximum heart rate, has no ECG changes, and stops the test due to leg pain and fatigue. Her back and hamstring flexibility is 11⅛ inches, and she is only able to lift 7.5 pounds above her head. Each of these values place G.W. in a category of poor fitness.

She believes that she can ride a stationary cycle for a few minutes each day. Because of upper back pain, stretching this area is an additional exercise. She cycled for 5 minutes twice a day, followed by the stretching program after each exercise bout.

After 3 weeks, G.W. complains that a headache develops following exercise. She has had no other adverse experience. Examination reveals a "trigger point" that reproduced the headache, and when injected, relief is obtained. This finding is common, and the "trigger point" must be differentiated from the generalized tender points of FMS.

G.W. gradually increases her exercise duration until she is training for 30 minutes, three times per week. She follows each session by stretching. Initially she is resistant to "working harder," and the goal is to have her exercise regularly. When she has achieved a duration of 30 minutes and is able to express that she is "feeling improved," her training is evaluated. During exercise the intensity was 40% of maximal. Since she does not believe that she has the ability to increase intensity or duration, she adds another exercise session each week.

COMMENT: Starting at a low intensity is important for patients with FMS, who may be easily dissuaded from complying with an exercise program. Deconditioned individuals may improve exercise capacity with minimal training and increase confidence in their ability to exercise. As conditioning occurs, further improvements will require greater duration, intensity, or frequency. Negotiating training goals and the exercise prescription should be based on what the individual believes he or she can achieve.

Summary

Recent findings support exercise as a therapeutic modality in the management of rheumatic conditions. Lack of endurance exercise is now proposed to be one of the factors in the deterioration of health status frequently seen early in rheumatic disorders. Contrary to earlier fears, exercise has not resulted in worsening of symptoms, nor in a more rapid progression of joint destruction.

It is important that systemic involvement be evaluated prior to starting any exercise program; although exercise is not ruled out as treatment, it may require modifications. Rheumatoid arthritis and ankylosing spondylitis both have an increased incidence of cardiac involvement, which may alter the intensity at which the patient may exercise. Fibromyalgia has no known underlying systemic disorder. Since muscle pain may increase following eccentric work, however, exercise should be prescribed so that eccentric work is minimized.

The state of disease activity is particularly important in rheumatic conditions, since they are prone to a pattern of remission and exacerbation. Even during a flare of the disease, light exercise should still be performed. The buoyancy factor makes water exercise particularly appealing for rheumatic patients during these times. Intermittent exercise and rest (3 minutes exercise followed by 3 minutes rest and then repeated) has been shown to cause no worsening of symptoms during a flare of rheumatoid arthritis. Patients need to be encouraged to accept that exercise is as important as other forms of therapy for the long-term management of their condition.

REFERENCES

1. *Acute Conditions: Incidence and Associated Disability, U.S 1974-1975.* Vital and Health Statistics Series 10, Number 114, 1977. Washington, D.C.: U.S. Dept. of Health, Education, and Welfare publication (HRA) 77-1541.
2. Banwell BF: Exercise and mobility in arthritis. *Nurs Clin North Am* 1984; 19:605-616.
3. Lightfoot RW Jr: Treatment of rheumatoid arthritis. In McCarty DJ, ed: *Arthritis and Allied Conditions A Textbook of Rheumatology*, ed 11. Lea & Febiger: Philadelphia, 1989.
4. Smith RD, Polley HF: Rest therapy for rheumatoid arthritis. *Mayo Clin Proc* 1978; 53:141-145.
5. Bardwick PA, Swezey RL: Physical therapies in arthritis; Which to choose, when to use, how not to abuse. *Postgrad Med* 1982; 72:223-234.
6. Kottke TE, Caspersen CJ, Hill CS: Exercise in the management and rehabilitation of selected chronic diseases. *Prev Med* 1984; 13:47-65.
7. Schumacher HR Jr, ed: *Primer on the Rheumatic Diseases*, ed 9. Arthritis Foundation: Atlanta, 1988.
8. Sharp JT, et al.: Methods of scoring the progression of radiologic changes in rheumatoid arthritis: Correlation of radiologic, clinical and laboratory abnormalities. *Arthritis Rheum* 1971; 14:706-720.
9. McKenna F: Clinical and laboratory assessment of outcome in rheumatoid arthritis. *Brit J Rheumatol* 1988; 27(suppl 1):12-20.
10. Steinbrocker O, Traeger CH, Batterman RC: Therapeutic criteria in rheumatoid arthritis. *JAMA* 1949; 140:659-662.
11. Meenan RF, Gertman PM, Mason JH: Measuring health status in arthritis: The arthritis impact measurement scales. *Arthritis Rheum* 1980; 23:146-152.
12. Wolfe F: Arthritis and musculoskeletal pain. *Nurs Clin North Am* 1984; 19: 565-574.
13. Kaarela K, Lehtinen K, Luukkainen R: Work capacity of patients with inflammatory joint diseases. *Scand J Rheum* 1987; 16:403-406.
14. Kramer JS, Yelin EH, Epstein WV: Social and economic impacts of four musculoskeletal conditions: A study using national community-based data. *Arthritis Rheum* 1983; 26:901-907.
15. Pincus T, et al.: Severe functional declines, work disability, and increased mortality in seventy-five rheumatoid arthritis patients studied over nine years. *Arthritis Rheum* 1984; 27:864-872.
16. McFarlane AC, Brooks PM: Determinants of disability in rheumatoid arthritis. *Br J Rheumatol* 1988; 27:7-14.
17. Sherrer YS, et al.: The development of disability in rheumatoid arthritis. *Arthritis Rheum* 1986; 29:494-500.
18. Halla JT, et al.: Rheumatoid mystosis: Clinical and histologic features and possible pathogenesis. *Arthritis Rheum* 1984; 27:737-743.
19. Herbison GJ, Ditunno JF, Jaweed M: Muscle atrophy in rheumatoid arthritis. *J Rheumatol* 1987; 14:78-81.
20. Ekblom B, et al.: Physical performance in patients with rheumatoid arthritis. *Scand J Rheumatol* 1974; 3:121-125.
21. Burckhardt CB, Clark SR, Nelson DL: Assessing physical fitness of women with rheumatic disease. *Arthritis Care Res* 1988; 1:38-44.
22. Price LG, et al.: Five-minute walking test of aerobic fitness for people with arthritis. *Arthritis Care Res* 1988; 1:33-37.
23. Minor MA, et al.: Exercise tolerance and disease-related measures in patients with rheumatoid arthritis and osteoarthritis. *J Rheumatol* 1988; 15:905-911.
24. Lyngberg K, Danneskiold-Samsoe B, Halskov O: The effect of physical training on patients with rheumatoid arthritis: Changes in disease activity, muscle strength and aerobic capacity. A clinically controlled minimized cross-over study. *Clin Exper Rheumatol* 1988; 6:253-260.
25. Hsieh LF, et al.: Isokinetic and isometric testing of knee musculature in patients with rheumatoid arthritis with mild knee involvement. *Arch Phys Med Rehabil* 1987; 68:294-297.
26. Beals CA, et al.: Measurement of exercise tolerance in patients with rheumatoid arthritis and osteoarthritis. *J Rheumatol* 1985; 12:458-461.
27. Ekblom B, Nordemar R: Rheumatoid arthritis. In Skinner JS (ed). *Exercise Testing and Exercise Prescription For Special Cases*. Lea & Febiger: Philadelphia, 1987.
27a. Nordemar R: Physical training in rheumatoid arthritis: A controlled long-term study. *Scand J Rheumatol* 1981; 10:25-30.
28. Lightfoot RW Jr: Treatment of rheumatoid arthritis. In McCarty DJ, ed: *Arthritis and Allied Conditions: A Textbook of Rheumatology*, ed 9. Lea & Febiger: Philadelphia, 1979.
29. Ekblom B, et al.: Effect of short-term physical training on patients with rheumatoid arthritis. I. *Scand J Rheumatol* 1975; 4: 80-86.
30. Ekblom B, et al.: Effect of short-term physical training on patients with rheumatoid arthritis. II. *Scand J Rheumatol* 1975; 4: 87-91.
31. Nordemar R, et al.: Physical training in rheumatoid arthritis: A controlled long-term study. *Scand J Rheumatol* 1981; 10:17-23.
32. Nordemar R, Edstrom L, Ekblom B: Changes in muscle fiber size and physical performance in patients with rheumatoid arthritis after short-term physical training. *Scand J Rheumatol* 1976; 5:70-76.

33. Harkcom TM, et al.: Therapeutic value of graded aerobic exercise training in rheumatoid arthritis. *Arthritis Rheum* 1985; 28:32–39.
34. American College of Sports Medicine: *Resource Manual for Guidelines for Exercise Testing and Prescription.* Lea & Febiger: Philadelphia, 1988.
35. Basmajian JV: Therapeutic exercise in the management of rheumatic diseases. *J Rheumatol* 1987; 14:22–25.
36. Swezey RL: Rehabilitation Medicine and Arthritis. In McCarty DJ, ed: *Arthritis and Allied Conditions: A Textbook of Rheumatology*, ed 11. Lea & Febiger: Philadelphia, 1989.
37. Ball GV: Ankylosing spondylitis. In McCarty DJ, ed: *Arthritis and Allied Conditions: A Textbook of Rheumatology.* ed 11. Lea & Febiger: Philadelphia, 1989.
38. Shah BC, Khan MA: Review of ankylosing spondylitis. *Compr Ther* 1987; 13: 52–59.
39. Moller P: Seronegative arthritis: Etiology and diagnosis. *Scand J Rheumatol* 1987; 66:119–127.
40. Calin A: Ankylosing spondylitis. In Kelley WN, et al., eds: *Textbook of Rheumatology,* ed 3. WB Saunders: Philadelphia, 1989.
41. Mau W, et al.: Clinical features and prognosis of patients with possible ankylosing spondylitis: Results of a 10-year follow-up. *J Rheumatol* 1988; 15:1109–1114.
42. Goie The HS, et al.: Evaluation of diagnostic criteria for ankylosing spondylitis: A comparison of the Rome, New York and modified New York criteria in patients with a positive clinical history screening test for ankylosing spondylitis. *Br J Rheumatol* 1985; 24:242–249.
43. Revell PA, Mayston V: Histopathology of the synovial membrane of peripheral joints in ankylosing spondylitis. *J Rheumatol* 1982; 2:296.
44. Dougados M, et al.: Evaluation of a functional index and an articular index in ankylosing spondylitis. *J Rheumatol* 1988; 15:302–307.
45. Fast A, Parikh S, Marin EL: Spine fractures in ankylosing spondylitis. *Arch Phys Med Rehabil* 1986; 67:595–597.
46. Hunter T, Dubo HI: Spinal fractures complicating ankylosing spondylitis: a long-term followup study. *Arthritis Rheum* 1983; 26:751–759.
47. Alves MG, et al.: Cardiac alterations in ankylosing spondylitis. *Angiology— The Journal of Vascular Diseases* 1988; 567–571.
48. van der Linden S, Valkenburg HA, Cats A: Evaluation of diagnostic criteria for ankylosing spondylitis: A proposal for modification of the New York criteria. *Arthritis Rheum* 1984; 27:361–368.
49. Wordsworth BP, Mowat AG: A review of 100 patients with ankylosing spondylitis with particular reference to socio-economic effects. *Br J Rheumatol* 1986; 25: 175–180.
50. Hopkins GO, et al.: Muscle changes in ankylosing spondylitis. *Br J Rheumatol* 1983; 22:151–157.
51. Hagberg M, Hagner IM, Bjelle A: Shoulder muscle strength, endurance and electromyographic fatigue in ankylosing spondylitis. *Scand J Rheumatol* 1987; 16:161–165.
52. Bulstrode SJ, et al.: The role of passive stretching in the treatment of ankylosing spondylitis. *Br J Rheumatol* 1987; 26: 40–42.
53. Kelsey J, Pastides H, Bisbee G: *Musculoskeletal Disorders: Their Frequency of Occurrence and Their Impact on the Population of the United States.* Prodist: New York, 1978.
54. Calabro JJ: The seronegative and spondyloarthropathies: A graduated approach to management. *Postgrad Med* 1986; 80: 173–188.
55. Calabro JJ, Eyvazzadeh C, Weber CA: Contemporary management of ankylosing spondylitis. *Compr Ther* 1986; 12: 11–18.
56. Yunus MB: Current therapeutic practices in spondyloarthropathies. *Compr Ther* 1988b; 14:54–64.
57. Swezey RL, ed: *Straight Talk on Ankylosing Spondylitis,* ed 2. Ankylosing Spondylitis Assoc: Sherman Oaks, CA, 1988.
58. Aponte J: A swimming program for patients with ankylosing spondylitis (abstract). *Scientific Abstracts American Rheumatism Association* 1987; s205.
59. Bennett RM: Fibrositis: Misnomer for a common rheumatic disorder. *West J Med* 1981; 134:405–413.
60. Hench PK, Mitler MM: Fibromyalgia: Review of a common rheumatologic syndrome. *Postgrad Med* 1986; 80:47–56.
61. Bennett RM, Goldenberg DL: The fibromyalgia syndrome. *Rheum Dis Clin North Am* 1989; 15:1–191.
62. Wolfe F: Fibromyalgia: The clinical syndrome. *Rheum Dis Clin North Am* 1989; 15:1–18.
62a. Wolfe F, et al.: The American College of Rheumatology 1990 Criteria for the Classification of Fibromyalgia: Report of the Multicenter Criteria Committee. *Arthritis Rheum* 1990; 33:160–172.
63. Bennett RM: Current issues concerning management of the fibrositis/fibromyalgia syndrome. *Am J Med* 1986; 81:15–18.
64. Yunus MB, et al.: Primary fibromyalgia (fibrositis): Clinical study of 50 patients with matched normal controls. *Semin Arthritis Rheum* 1981; 11:151–171.
65. Smythe HA: Non-articular rheumatism and psychogenic musculoskeletal syndromes. In McCarty DJ, ed: *Arthritis and Allied Conditions: A Textbook of Rheumatology,* ed 9. Lea & Febiger: Philadelphia, 1979.
66. Dinerman H, Goldenberg DL, Felson DT: A

prospective evaluation of 118 patients with the fibromyalgia syndrome: Prevalence of Raynaud's phenomenon, sicca symptoms, ANA, low complement, and Ig deposition at the dermal-epidermal junction. *J Rheumatol* 1986; 13:368–373.

67. Campbell SM, et al.: Clinical characteristics of fibrositis: A 'blinded,' controlled study of symptoms and tender points. *Arthritis Rheum* 1983; 26:817–824.

68. Goldenberg DL: Research in fibromyalgia: Past, present and future. *J Rheumatol* 1988; 15:992–996.

69. Payne TC, et al.: Fibrositis and psychologic disturbance. *Arthritis Rheum* 1982; 25: 213–217.

70. Ahles TA, Yanus MB, Masi AT: Is chronic pain a variant of depressive diseases? The case of primary fibromyalgia syndrome. *Pain* 1987; 29:105–111.

71. Clark S, et al.: Clinical characteristics of fibrositis, II: A "blinded," controlled study using standard psychological tests. *Arthritis Rheum* 1985; 28:132–137.

72. Yunus MB: Diagnosis, etiology and management of fibromyalgia syndrome: An update. *Compr Ther* 1988; 14:8–20.

73. Campbell SM, and Bennett RM: Fibrositis. *Dis Mon* 1986; 32:653–722.

74. Cathey MA, et al.: Socioeconomic impact of fibrositis: A study of 81 patients with primary fibrositis. *Am J Med* 1986; 81: 78–84.

75. Felson DT, Goldenberg DL: The natural history of fibromyalgia. *Arthritis Rheum* 1986; 92:1522–1526.

76. Hench PK, Mitler MM: Fibromyalgia: Management guidelines and research findings. *Postgrad Med* 1986; 80:57–69.

77. Cathey MA, Wolfe F, Kleinheksel SM: Functional ability and work status in patients with fibromyalgia. *Arthritis Care Res* 1988; 1:85–98.

78. Moldofsky H, et al.: Musculoskeletal symptoms and non-REM sleep disturbance in patients with "fibrositis syndrome" and healthy subjects. *Psychosom Med* 1975; 37:341–351.

79. Moldofsky H, Scarisbrick P: Induction of neurasthenic musculoskeletal pain syndrome by selective sleep stage deprivation. *Psychosom Med* 1976; 38:35–44.

80. Jacobsen S, Danneskiold-Samsoe B: Isometric and isokinetic muscle strength in patients with fibrositis syndrome. *Scand J Rheumatol* 1987; 16:61–65.

81. Kaylan-Raman UP, et al.: Muscle pathology in primary fibromyalgia syndrome: A light microscopic, histochemical and ultra- structural study. *J Rheumatol* 1984; 11: 808.

82. Henriksson KG: Muscle pain in neuromuscular disorders and primary fibromyalgia. *Eur J Appl Physiol Occup Physiol* 1988; 57:348–352.

83. Bengtsson A, Henriksson KG, Larsson J: Reduced high-energy phosphate levels in the painful muscles of patients with primary fibromyalgia. *Arthritis Rheum* 1986; 29:817–821.

84. Bengtsson A, et al.: Primary fibromyalgia: A clinical and laboratory study of 55 patients. *Scand J Rheumatol* 1986; 15: 340–347.

85. Bengtsson A, Henriksson KG, Larsson J: Muscle biopsy in primary fibromyalgia: Light-microscopical and histochemical findings. *Scand J Rheumatol* 1986; 15:1–6.

86. Bortz WM: Disuse and aging. *JAMA* 1982; 248:1203–1208.

87. Lund N, Bengtsson A, Thorborg P: Muscle tissue oxygen pressure in primary fibromyalgia. *Scand J Rheumatol* 1986; 15: 165–173.

88. Bennett RM, et al.: Aerobic fitness in patients with fibrositis: A controlled study of respiratory gas exchange and ^{133}xenon clearance from exercising muscle. *Arthritis Rheum* 1989; 32:454–460.

89. Klug G, McAuley E, Clark S: Factors influencing the development and maintenance of aerobic fitness: Lessons applicable to the fibrositis syndrome. *J Rheumatol* 1989; 19(Suppl 16):30–39.

90. Armstrong RB: Mechanisms of exercise-induced delayed onset muscular soreness: A brief review. *Med Sci Sports Exerc* 1984; 16:529–538.

91. McCain GA, et al.: A controlled study of the effects of a supervised cardiovascular fitness training program on the manifestations of primary fibromyalgia. *Arthritis Rheum* 1988; 31:1135–1141.

92. Clark SR, Burckhardt C, Nelson D: Prospective evaluation of the effect of physical conditioning on fibrositis patient outcomes (abstract). *Scientific Abstracts American Rheumatism Association* 1987; s207.

93. Burckhardt CB, et al.: Assessment of dysfunction in the fibrositis syndrome. *Arthritis Rheum* 1988; 31(suppl 14):s100.

94. Sheon RP: Regional myofascial pain and the fibrositis syndrome (fibromyalgia). *Compr Ther* 1986; 12:42–52.

95. Burckhardt CS, Clark SR, Bennett RM: The fibromyalgia impact questionnaire: Development and validation. *J Rheumatol* 1991; 18:728–733.

CHAPTER 5

EXERCISE AND NEUROMUSCULAR DISEASE

DIANE L. ELLIOT, MD, and LINN GOLDBERG, MD

Neuromuscular disorders are a heterogeneous group of problems. Their pathophysiology can relate to neurologic illnesses, alterations in energy production, and loss of muscle mass due to inflammation or metabolic abnormalities. The direct relationship between the muscular system and exercise suggests that physical training might have a beneficial role in treating neuromuscular disease. Although exercise, in the context of physical therapy, is an important component of rehabilitation programs for many conditions,[1-4] concern about overuse injuries and variability in the progression of many neuromuscular diseases has limited assessment of the therapeutic potential of conditioning.

In this chapter, we review an approach to assessing individuals with muscular complaints and outline the available tests of muscle function. These tests can define abilities, index disease progression, and evaluate therapy. In addition, we discuss exercise training as management for neuromuscular disease, and present recommendations based on these findings.

Evaluation of Individuals with Muscular Complaints

GENERAL DIAGNOSTIC APPROACH

Fatigue, weakness, inability to exercise, and muscle pain are common complaints. Each are nonspecific and can be due to a variety of problems, including functional disorders, metabolic abnormalities, muscular dystrophies, degenerative neuromuscular disorders, and inflammatory myopathies. For some patients, the history and physical examination can suggest a disorder and lead the evaluation toward a diagnosis that does not directly involve the neuromuscular system. Laboratory evaluation is used to exclude endocrine disorders and electrolyte abnormalities. Additional laboratory assessment often involves a complete blood count, erythrocyte sedimentation rate (ESR), and serum creatine kinase (CK) level.

Among patients with muscular complaints referred to a clinic for muscle disorders, the ESR and CK level have been reported to have relatively high specificity (90% and 80%, respectively) in indicating muscle disease; that is, an elevated value often is predictive of muscle disease. However, the sensitivity of these tests were found to be low (30% and 60%, respectively).[5] Thus, although an abnormal value indicates the need for further testing, a normal test does not exclude a myopathy, and additional evaluation may be indicated.

Muscle biopsy for histology and in vitro testing often is considered the gold standard for assessing muscle disorders.[6-9] However, not all processes are distributed uniformly throughout muscle. Based on results of multiple forms of testing, the sensitivity of biopsy is estimated at only 80%.[10] In addition, definitive diagnosis of metabolic abnormalities may require an open biopsy for in vitro testing of fresh tissue or a highly specialized histologic assessment.

Because their results can guide subsequent open muscle biopsy,[11] exercise testing and needle biopsy have been advocated as appropriate initial diagnostic steps. Needle biopsy techniques, using a Bergstrom needle and local anesthesia,[6,9] can allow diagnosis without the need for open muscle biopsy.[8,12] Even in referral centers, with access to extensive diagnostic evaluation, a significant percentage of patients with muscular complaints will have no abnormality diagnosed.[5,11]

Our approach to patients with potential muscular disorders is to perform a history, physical examination, and selected laboratory studies. The subsequent test sequence is a graded exercise test using expired gas analysis, followed by a needle muscle biopsy. Additional studies are guided by results of that evaluation. Features of disorders that can present as muscular weakness are discussed in the following section.

DISORDERS RESULTING IN MUSCULAR COMPLAINTS

Metabolic Myopathies

The term metabolic myopathy includes many disorders. Some are characterized by localization of the biochemical defect (e.g., glycogenolytic defect myopathies),[13] localization of pathophysiology to a specific organelle (mitochondrial myopathies),[14] or histologic appearance (lipid myopathy, nemaline myopathy, multicore disease).[15,16] In certain patients with metabolic myopathies, findings during exercise testing indicate the underlying disorder. Table 5–1 presents results of testing in patients with various muscular disorders.

Mitochrondrial Myopathies

The final reactions of oxidative metabolism occur along the mitochondrial inner membrane. Defects in several components of the respiratory chain have been identified.[17,18] The term *mitochondrial encephalomyopathy* has been used to describe the conditions characterized by abnormal mitochondrial respiration in both muscle and the central nervous system (CNS). These disorders can present at any time, from the neonatal period to adulthood, with varying clinical manifestations.[17,19,20] Interest in mitochondrial disorders is increasing as their unique genetics are becoming better understood.[14,21] At present, it is not clear how the biochemical and genetic abnormalities relate to the spectrum of abnormalities.[14,20]

Affected individuals often present with symptoms of muscular fatigue. Although some patients with mitochrondrial abnormalities have CNS dysfunction or progressive ophthalmoplegias, results of the clinical examination also can be normal, without abnormalities in muscular strength or muscle enzyme levels. If the individual is severely affected, the resting serum lactate level may be elevated. Staining of muscle biopsy reveals ragged red fibers that contain peripheral aggregates of abnormal mitochondria.[22] Moderate-to-severe reductions in maximal oxygen uptake have been reported in these disorders,[11,23] and in one kindred, reduced oxygen consumption correlated with clinical and biochemical abnormalities.[24]

CASE: C.S. a 17-year-old girl with a mitochrondrial myopathy, was referred for evaluation. She had been well until age 9, when decreased exercise tolerance was noted. At age 10, muscle cramps and vomiting occurred after limited exertion, and ventricular ectopy also was observed. Results of a cardiac examination and echocardiography were normal. By age 15, her symptoms had progressed, and she was dyspneic after slowly walking less than 100 yards.

At the time of exercise testing, she was a small, slender girl (height, 157 cm [5'3"]; weight, 50 kg); results of physical examination were normal except for skeletal muscle weakness, which was graded 4+ in proximal muscle groups. Her resting serum lactate level was elevated at 3.4 mEq/L.

Results of the exercise test are shown in Figure 5–1. The patient was only able to exercise for 4 minutes at the lowest work load on the cycle ergometer (approximately 3 watts). Beta blocker therapy probably contributed to the low maximal heart rate. The patient's maximum oxygen uptake was 450 ml/min, with a predicted normal level of 2,300 mL/min. At maximal exercise, she was exhausted, and her respiratory exchange ratio (R) value was 2.39.

Muscle biopsy obtained at that time demonstrated a ragged-red-fiber myopathy, and electron microscopy revealed abnormal mitochondria with crystalline inclusions. Biochemical analysis indicated deficits in multiple components of complex III of the respiratory chain, with succinate : cytochrome c reductase activity being less than 5% of normal. Treatment included sodium bicarbonate (300 mEq/d), vitamin C, and menadione 40 mg/d. Propranolol hydrochloride was prescribed for the ventricular arrhythmia. Response to therapy was documented by clinical improvement and by ^{31}P nuclear magnetic resonance (NMR) spectroscopy (see page 119).[25]

Table 5−1 DIAGNOSTIC FEATURES OF MYOPATHIES

	Creatine Kinase	Maximum Oxygen Uptake	RER at End Exercise	EMG	Biopsy	Other
Metabolic Myopathies						
Mitochondrial myopathy	Normal	Greatly reduced	Normal to increased	Normal or nonspecific	"Ragged red" fibers	± elevated resting serum lactate
McArdle's disease	Normal to increased	~70% predicted	<1.0	Normal or nonspecific	Histochemical absence enzyme	Abnormal ischemic forearm test
Inflammatory Myopathies						
Polymyositis	Increased in 70%–75%	NK	NK	90% abnormal with myopathic pattern	Necrosis fibers, inflammatory infiltrate	
Inclusion body myositis	Usually normal	NK	NK	Both myopathic and neuropathic components	Necrosis and inflammation with eosinophilic inclusions	
Muscular Dystrophies						
Duchenne's	Increased	Reduction reflects atrophy	Normal	~85% abnormal	Fibrosis, necrosis, basophilic fibers	XR inheritance
Facioscapulohumeral	Usually increased	Reduction reflects atrophy	Normal	~85% abnormal	Abnormal	AD inheritance
Limb-girdle	Normal	Reduction reflects atrophy	Normal	~85% abnormal	Abnormal	AR inheritance; sporadic

Key: RER = respiratory exchange ratio, EMG = electromyography, NK = not known, XR = X-linked recessive, AD = autosomal dominant, AR = autosomal recessive.

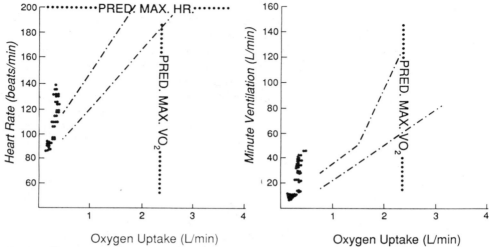

Figure 5–1 The response to exercise testing of the patient with a mitochondrial myopathy. The dashed lines are the predicted normal range, and the dots are the patient's data.

COMMENT: Mitochondrial myopathies are treated by minimizing energy demands, including avoidance of temperature elevation and drugs that inhibit the respiratory system (barbiturates, phenytoin) or mitochondrial protein metabolism (tetracycline).[20,26] Among certain patients, mitochondrial defects have responded to treatment with vitamins. Riboflavin, a precursor of flavin mononucleotide and flavin-adenine dinucleotide (part of complexes I and II), has been effective for patients with complex-I defects.[27] Additional management attempted for individuals with complex-I disorders includes carnitine, thiamine, and vitamin K_3 (menadione). Disorders of complex III may be bypassed by vitamin C and menadione, due to their ability to bridge deficits in electron transport.[28] Management of complex II or IV disorders is unclear, and use of similar supplements has been attempted. For this patient, management was followed and benefits documented by NMR measurements, although her oxygen consumption remained depressed.

Glycogenolytic Defect Myopathies

A second group of metabolic disorders are the glycogenolytic defects. These are characterized by a moderate reduction in total oxygen consumption and failure of the respiratory exchange ratio to increase to greater than 1.0.[11,23,28,29] Because of the inability to break down glycogen or glucose to produce pyruvate, the normal increase in lactate level is not seen on ischemic forearm testing.[30] Individuals with these disorders develop muscle pain with exertion, sometimes associated with rhabdomyolysis and myoglobinuria.[31] Although progressive proximal weakness can be seen as the individual ages, muscle strength and bulk usually are normal.

Lipid Myopathies

Lipid myopathies are a group of disorders in which lipid accumulates within muscle fibers.[32,33] Examples include carnitine palmitoyl transferase

(CPT) deficiency, systemic or muscle carnitine deficiency, and other lipid-storage myopathies.[34] An early ventilatory threshold, consistent with limitations in fat metabolism and early reliance on carbohydrates, has been noted in an individual with CPT deficiency.[11] A twofold increase in oxygen consumption was observed in an individual with a lipid myopathy who favorably responded to riboflavin treatment.[35] In addition, patients have been reported who responded clinically to supplemental SC/L-carnitine. Peak oxygen uptake can markedly increase coincident with the clinical improvement,[36] but more data are required before recommending exercise testing to diagnose and follow patients with this group of disorders.

Muscular Dystrophies

Unlike the metabolic myopathies, muscular dystrophies (e.g., facioscapulohumeral, Duchenne's, limb-girdle) result in muscle fiber loss. Oxygen consumption is decreased in patients with these disorders. This reduction reflects loss of muscle tissue, rather than the alteration in muscular metabolism seen with mitochondrial myopathies.[23,37-39]

Inflammatory Myopathies

The inflammatory myopathies[40-44] include polymyositis or dermatomyositis and inclusion-body myositis. Inflammatory myopathies vary in their clinical manifestations; a common finding is the inflammatory lesions seen on muscle biopsy. The utility of exercise testing in diagnosing these disorders has not been determined.

Muscular Fatigue and the Chronic Fatigue Syndrome

Fatigue is a common complaint in ambulatory care.[45,46] The physiologic basis of muscle fatigue is a complex combination of peripheral and central factors.[47-49] In general, fatigue that occurs both at rest and during exertion is not typical of muscular disorders.[50]

A small subset of fatigued patients meet the explicit diagnostic criteria proposed for chronic fatigue syndrome (CFS).[51] Most who complain of fatigue do not meet these criteria,[52] but instead have symptoms due to psychiatric diagnoses (depression, anxiety, and somatization).[53] Patients who have CFS must have fatigue for at least 6 months, with no other diagnoses to explain the problem. In addition, they must have 8 of the 11 symptoms or 6 symptoms and 2 of the 3 physical findings listed in Table 5-2.

CASE: M.P., a 47-year-old woman, was referred for evaluation of a year of fatigue. The symptoms were gradual in onset, and unassociated with any viral illness, toxic exposures, or change in medication. She worked as a clerk in a department store, and she had to shorten her shifts because of progressive fatigue such that she would go directly to bed after coming home. She also noticed trouble concentrating and reported palpitations, wherein her heart would beat rapidly but regularly following minimal exertion.

She denied weight loss or other specific complaints. Her family history was negative for neuromuscular disease. Prior to development of these symptoms, her health was reported as "good." Many physicians had been consulted in her attempt to find successful therapy.

Table 5–2 **SYMPTOMS AND SIGNS OF THE CHRONIC FATIGUE SYNDROME**

Symptoms*
Headache
Myalgia
Mild fever
Sore throat
Painful cervical or axillary lymphadenopathy
Arthralgias
Muscle weakness
Postexertional generalized fatigue
Neuropsychiatric complaints
Sleep disturbances
Rapid onset of fatigue
Signs†
Low-grade fever
Nonexudative pharyngitis
Cervical or axillary adenopathy

*To qualify as a symptom, the complaint must have begun at or after the onset of fatigue and persisted for at least 6 months.
†Signs must be documented on at least two occasions, at least a month apart.

Results of her general physical examination (including evaluation for trigger-point tenderness), neurologic assessment, and mental status evaluation were normal. Results of a number of tests were normal, including muscle enzyme levels, ESR, thyroid function test, computed tomography (CT) scan of the head, ambulatory Holter monitoring, and exercise thallium scintigraphy.

During exercise testing with expired gas analysis, her blood pressure increased appropriately, and a maximum heart rate of 170 bpm was achieved. Maximal oxygen consumption was depressed, reaching a value of only 14 ml/kg (normal for a 47-year-old woman, 24 to 30 ml/kg). This result was not a reflection of poor effort, because her heart rate reached near the predicted maximum and her respiratory exchange ratio was 1.5 at the end of the exercise test.

Because of the low oxygen consumption, a muscle biopsy was performed. Fiber size and grouping were normal, and no muscle fiber necrosis, inflammation, or increased lipid concentrations were found. Likewise, no ragged red fibers were seen on the trichrome preparation. Adenylate deaminase was present, and a Congo red stain for amyloid was negative. Because of the normal findings on biopsy, management was directed toward anxiety, depression, and somatization disorder.

COMMENT: Expected normal values for oxygen consumption have been reported for adults and children.[54–57] As illustrated by this patient, although a reduced oxygen uptake suggests a metabolic myopathy, it also may be "normal" and reflect a deconditioned state.

Fatigue has been difficult to analyze by traditional muscle testing. Postexertional fatigue and an exacerbation of myalgias are criteria for the diagnosis of CFS, and these complaints have suggested a muscle metabolic disorder among CFS patients. Interest in the association of a biochemical abnormality with CFS was heightened by a report of excessive intracellular acidosis discovered by NMR testing in a single patient with post-varicella fatigue.[58] In addition, analysis of biopsy specimens demonstrated enterovirus-specific RNA in approximately 25% of patients with chronic post-viral fatigue syndrome.[59]

Some degree of cardiac limitation may contribute to CFS, as reduced maximal heart rates have been noted among patients with CFS.[60] However, oxygen uptake, minute ventilation, respiratory exchange ratio, and lactate levels were not measured in that study to document maximal effort.

Volition also may be a factor limiting exertion among those with CFS, as was suggested in a study by Stokes and colleagues.[61] These investigations evaluated chronically fatigued patients' muscular function with both involuntary strength tests (electrical stimulation) and maximal voluntary isometric contraction. Fatigued subjects' results were lower than controls only during voluntary exercise, which suggested that the contractile properties of the muscle were normal. However, these findings did not exclude a peripheral etiology for fatigue nor do they justify an unsympathetic approach to patients' symptoms.

Other investigations have found normal results on muscle testing among fatigued individuals. Byrne and Trounce[62] evaluated 11 patients with chronic fatigue and myalgia that were exacerbated by exercise. Results of ischemic forearm testing were normal in each subject tested, as was muscle biopsy histology. Special staining for glycogenolytic and mitochondrial muscle myopathies were negative, as were levels of muscle carnitine.

No consistent histologic or metabolic abnormality has been associated with CFS. A role for exercise in management of these patients also has not been established. Anecdotal reports suggest improvement among patients who began a gradual program of aerobic conditioning, while others do not find exercise therapy useful.[63] Psychological benefits and an increased sense of well-being can occur with training (Chapter 16), and a therapeutic trial may be indicated in selected individuals. Finally, the findings in CFS and fibromyalgia can overlap[64] and, as discussed in chapter 4, exercise can benefit the latter patient group. Assessing for trigger-point tenderness should be a component of examination of the fatigued individual, and gradual, low-impact aerobic conditioning is appropriate for those whose illness has features of fibromyalgia.

EXERCISE TESTING OF PATIENTS WITH NEUROMUSCULAR COMPLAINTS

The term *exercise test* usually refers to an incremental treadmill test. This type of progressive exertion is enhanced by assessment of expired oxygen and carbon dioxide concentrations, and ventilatory volumes. However, several other types of exercise tests are available. Knowing about available tests will enhance the clinician's use of the tests and interpretation of them when evaluating patients with neuromuscular complaints.

Strength Assessment

Several methods are available to measure muscle strength.[65] The selection of the most appropriate test is made depending on the disease, its distribution, and the extent of disability. During the clinical examination, strength often is determined by the 0- to 5-point Kendall system, with grade 5 = active resistance, 3 = full range of motion against gravity only, and 0 = no contraction.[66] Grade 4 can be subdivided as 4−, 4, and 4+, to indicate motion against slight, moderate, and strong resistance, respectively.[67] Defining a patient's ability to perform certain common activities also can add to strength assessment (Table 5–3).[68] Measuring joint range of motion is a further method to longitudinally follow muscular strength, as reduction (contractures) can occur with decreasing function.[65]

To quantitate strength more reliably, investigators have used functional tests, wherein the patient performs a task repeatedly over a certain time. Examples include timed tests of carrying a given weight for a specified distance, climbing a specific number of stairs, or repeatedly standing from a sitting position.[69] Although these tests are landmarks of severity, the end points are

Table 5–3 STRENGTH ASSESSMENT USING FUNCTIONAL ABILITIES

Arms and shoulders
1. Starting with arms at the sides, patient can abduct the arms in a full circle until they touch above the head.
2. Can raise arms above head only by flexing the elbow (i.e., shortening the circumference of the movement) or by using accessory muscles.
3. Cannot raise hands above head but can raise an 8-ounce glass of water to mouth (using both hands if necessary).
4. Can raise hands to mouth but cannot raise an 8-ounce glass of water to mouth.
5. Cannot raise hand to mouth but can use hands to hold pen or pick up pennies from table.
6. Cannot raise hands to mouth and has no useful function of hands.

Hips and legs
1. Walks and climbs stairs without assistance.
2. Walks and climbs four standard stairs with aid of railing (< 12 seconds).
3. Climbs four standard stairs slowly (> 12 seconds).
4. Walks unassisted and rises from chair but cannot climb stairs.
5. Walks unassisted but cannot rise from chair or climb stairs.
6. Walks only with assistance or walks independently with long-leg braces.
7. Walks in long-leg braces but requires assistance for balance.
8. Stands in long-leg braces but is unable to walk even with assistance.
9. Is in wheelchair.
10. Is confined to bed.

From Brooke et al.,[68] p 476, with permission.

subjective,[70] interrater reliability is limited,[71] and findings are not precise measurements of muscle function.[72,73]

Muscular strength can be more accurately assessed by determining contractile force. Isometric force is quantified by maximum voluntary contraction (MVC). A simple method of isometric testing is handgrip strength with a dynamometer.[74] An apparatus can be used to measure MVC in other muscle groups.[70,74] When evaluated over time, this technique can provide reliable testing for normal individuals. However, the test's reliability is reduced twofold to threefold in those with neuromuscular dysfunction, with a coefficient of variation of up to 27%.[74,75] In addition to voluntary contraction, direct electrical stimulation of muscle can measure contractile force and allows isolation of particular muscles, eliminating effects of patient effort.[75,76]

The force a muscle develops is dependent on joint angle. Thus, for accuracy, strength must be measured over a range of motion. Because tension is inversely proportional to movement velocity, that variable must be held constant. Isokinetic dynamometry holds velocity constant, measuring force through a joint's motion at a constant speed of movement. The prototype device is the Cybex II, although other systems are available (Figure 5–2). These systems are used extensively in rehabilitation of musculoskeletal injuries. Isokinetic devices use an electromagnetic or hydraulic apparatus to maintain a constant movement speed. Although many technical issues affect interpretation of results,[77] normal values are available for both adults and children.[78-81] However, isokinetic testing has only fair reliability, which is further reduced among patients with neuromuscular disease.[65]

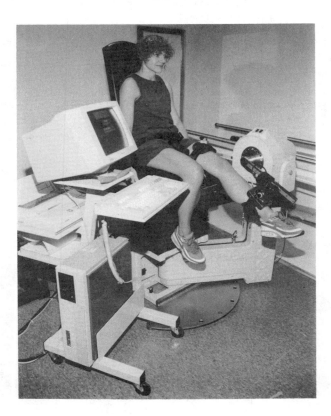

Figure 5–2 Measuring quadriceps strength with an isokinetic dynamometer.

Ischemic Forearm Testing

In 1951 McArdle[82] first used the ischemic forearm test to evaluate a patient who developed exertional muscle cramps. During this testing, forearm ischemia is induced by applying an upper-arm sphygmomanometer cuff and inflating it above systolic pressure. While blood flow and oxygen delivery are prevented, the subject squeezes a handgrip dynamometer every 2 seconds for 2 minutes. The cuff is then deflated, and a blood sample is obtained from the antecubital vein immediately and at 1, 3, 5, and 7 minutes (in addition to a baseline sample before testing). Failure to produce lactate indicates a glycogenolytic defect.[83]

Measuring serum ammonia from the same specimens allows assessment for myoadenylate deaminase deficiency. This metabolic block prevents generation of adenosine triphosphate through the purine nucleotide cycle during anaerobic metabolism. Patients with myoadenylate deaminase deficiency do not develop the normal increase in serum ammonia after ischemic forearm testing.[84] Myoadenylate deaminase deficiency was discovered when muscle biopsies were examined for this enzyme's activity.[85] The clinical significance of the biochemical abnormality is not clear. Although some affected individuals have myalgias, exertional fatigue, or both,[86] others are asymptomatic.

Electromyography

The electromyogram (EMG) can help differentiate weakness caused by primary muscle disease, neuromuscular junction abnormalities, and lower motor neuron dysfunction.[10,87–89] When used to evaluate patients with symptoms of weakness or muscle pain, EMG findings can indicate both the presence of an abnormality and its location.

Decreased firing of muscle cells (decreased motor unit action potentials and submaximal interference pattern) and signs of reinnervation (polyphasic giant waves of long duration) indicate a peripheral neuropathy. Results from patients with a myopathy reflect smaller or fewer muscle cells (small or short-duration action potentials or polyphasic action potentials) and increased nerve stimulation with a low work load (full interference pattern at 30% maximal force). Both denervation and a primary myopathy can show insertion irritability, positive sharp waves, and fibrillation potentials at rest. Although EMG results may indicate a myopathy, findings are rarely diagnostic of a specific disorder, and additional testing often is required to establish a diagnosis.

Graded Exercise Testing with Expired Gas Analysis

When exertion is not limited by cardiopulmonary dysfunction, measuring oxygen uptake during progressive exercise can evaluate muscular metabolism.[90] The specific response pattern of minute ventilation, oxygen consumption, and CO_2 production can indicate abnormalities in aerobic and anaerobic metabolism and assist in the evaluation of muscular weakness and fatigue.[11]

Energy sources of the muscle vary as exercise intensity increases. The ventilatory response reflects both changes in these substrates and the amount of aerobic and anaerobic metabolism. During low-intensity activity, free fatty acids are oxidized aerobically as the primary fuel source, resulting in a respiratory exchange ratio (CO_2 produced divided by O_2 consumed) that is relatively low at approximately 0.7. As exertion increases, more carbohydrates also are metabolized. When exercising at the ventilatory or anaerobic threshold, the muscle cell is utilizing approximately equal proportions of free fatty acids and carbohydrates (muscle glycogen and blood glucose). During high-intensity exercise, carbohydrates also are metabolized anaerobically, resulting in lactate production. Initially, lactate is cleared from the blood and does not accumulate, but levels increase with additional production.

There is a linear relationship between increased minute ventilation and oxygen consumption below the ventilatory threshold (Figure 5–3). The line's slope changes as a greater amount of ventilation occurs for increases in oxygen uptake. The inflection point is termed the ventilatory threshold. Beyond this threshold, it is theorized that additional ventilation is required to compensate for excess CO_2 produced by bicarbonate buffering of accumulating lactic acid.

$$\text{lactate (H}^+\text{)} + HCO_3 \longrightarrow H_2CO_3 \rightarrow H_2O + CO_2$$

Thus, this point coincides with accumulation of lactate from anaerobic metabolism. Prior to the ventilatory threshold, minute ventilation relates to blowing off CO_2 produced from aerobic metabolism. Beyond the ventilatory threshold, additional ventilation is needed to respond to the CO_2 resulting from buffering of lactic acid. Working above this threshold will lead to progressive acidemia and the need to stop exercise. Accordingly, the optimal aerobic training point is at the ventilatory threshold, which is the highest intensity achieved before lactate begins to accumulate.

The respiratory exchange ratio is an additional index of lactate accumulation. During progressive aerobic exertion, increasing reliance on glucose as a fuel causes the ratio to approach 1.0. As lactate begins to increase, this ratio becomes greater than 1.0 (from CO_2 produced from buffering lactic acid), usually reaching 1.2 to 1.4 at maximal exertion.[91]

Disorders of muscle metabolism affect normal values at maximal exertion and the response pattern (see Table 5–1). For example, during maximal exercise, those with glycogenolytic defects (glycogen storage diseases) will not

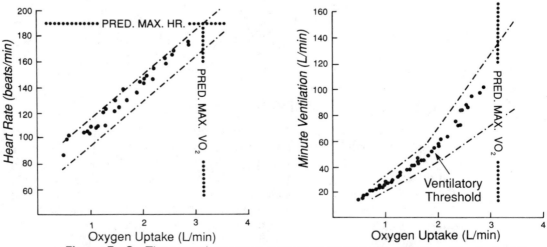

Figure 5–3 The normal response pattern to progressive exertion. The dashed lines are the predicted normal response range. From Elliot et al,[11] p. 165, with permission.

achieve a respiratory exchange ratio greater than 1.0, as glycogen cannot be used as a fuel substrate and lactate is not produced. Alternatively, those with mitochondrial defects have reduced aerobic metabolism and oxygen consumption, while they produce high respiratory exchange ratios, even at very low exercise work loads.

Nuclear Magnetic Resonance

NMR spectroscopy can be used to evaluate muscle energy metabolism.[92,93] Abnormal findings have been reported in myopathies,[92] and the testing has been used to detect disordered carbohydrate[92,94] and mitochondrial[95] function, as well as overuse muscle injury.[5,96] However, the technique is not widely available and presently has greatest utility as a research tool.

Exercise as Management for Neuromuscular Disease

Physical therapy is a component of rehabilitation both following nervous system injury and in cases of primary neuromuscular disease. Several texts[2,3] are available that present comprehensive rehabilitation guidelines. However, only limited information is available concerning therapeutic exercise training for patients with neuromuscular disease. Investigations were hampered by concern that overuse would lead to deterioration in muscle function. In 1915, Lovett[97] reported that exercise following poliomyelitis caused a decrement of muscle strength. In the late 1950s, a similar phenomenon was described, noting that patients with post-poliomyelitis weakness could permanently lose strength with physical exertion.[98] In addition to these detrimental effects among individuals with denervation weakness, adverse consequences from exercise were thought to occur in patients with muscular dystrophies. In 1971, Johnson and Braddom[99] reported on members of a family with facioscapulohumeral muscular dystrophy. All individuals demonstrated asymmetric weakness, with the weaker side being the most-often-used arm. Thus, overuse was felt to have accelerated the dystrophic degeneration.

Although these reports raised concern about exercise training and overwork, the potential benefits of improved strength, aerobic capacity, and cardiovascular performance led to several carefully supervised small studies to determine the efficacy of physical conditioning. However, their conclusions are limited because the number of investigations with any disorder is small, and findings are difficult to interpret due to variability in the disorders' natural history.

Muscular Dystrophy

Muscular dystrophies vary in their distribution and progression.[100] Duchenne's dystrophy, an X-linked recessive disorder, is rapidly progressive, with individuals usually wheelchair-bound by age 12. New understanding of its genetics and biochemical abnormality has clarified its inheritance and clinical variability.[101] A second group of dystrophies (limb-girdle and facioscapulohumeral muscular dystrophy) are later in onset and more slowly progressive.

Cardiomyopathy can occur with certain muscular dystrophies,[102] but usually is seen late in the disease and does not compromise the ability to exercise when training is applicable.

As shown in Table 5–4, six studies have evaluated exercise training among individuals with muscular dystrophy. In an early study, Hoberman[103] strength-trained hospitalized boys with Duchenne's dystrophy for 4 months. Although strength initially increased, as the disease progressed over 9 months, an overall decrement in strength occurred. In the mid-1960s, Vignos and Watkins[104] assessed 24 individuals with various dystrophies (14 with Duchenne's, 6 limb-girdle, and 4 facioscapulohumeral), who followed a 1-year home resistance program of strength training. Strength (by manual muscle tests) improved over the first 4 months and then plateaued. The greatest benefit occurred in those with slowly progressive forms of dystrophy. De Lateur and Giaconi[105] trained one leg of four ambulatory boys with Duchenne's dystrophy, using submaximal exercise on an isokinetic dynamometer for 4 or 5 days per week for 6 months. No evidence of overwork weakness was observed. Although no increase in strength was seen during training, the exercised leg was stronger than the control limb 3 months later.

Individuals with more slowly progressive muscular dystrophies were strength-trained with a regimen of resistance exercises.[106] Training progressed over a 9-week period to four sets of 10 repetitions at 50% to 70% of maximum. Gains in strength were demonstrated, and results suggested that neuromuscular adaptation, rather than hypertrophy of existing muscle, accounted for the increased strength. That is, the force generated by a muscle depends on both the number and size of muscle fibers and on synchronization of motor units.[107] It appears that the latter adaptation occurs in patients with muscular dystrophies.[106] Milner-Brown and coworkers[108] also strength-trained patients with slowly progressive dystrophies. Strength increased in selected muscle groups after training, and the absolute gain was related to initial strength. No improvement was observed in severely weakened muscles.

In addition to weakness due to muscle loss, individuals with dystrophies also have reduced aerobic capacity.[23,37–39] Florence and Hagberg[109] trained patients with slowly progressive dystrophies using cycle exercise. Exercise occurred 3 days per week and consisted of six 5-minute exercise periods (at 70% maximum heart rate), separated by 2-minute rests. Following 3 months of conditioning, maximal oxygen consumption was increased 25%.

Maintaining function is an important objective for individuals with muscular dystrophies. Several reviews have outlined the comprehensive care of individuals with muscular dystrophies.[110–113] Although the absence of controls and the variability of the disease process limit evaluation of exercise rehabilitation, it appears that training has a limited role in Duchenne's dystrophy. Physical conditioning's greatest effects have been demonstrated in slowly progressive dystrophies, especially when it is implemented before marked decrements in strength have occurred.

POST-POLIOMYELITIS SYNDROME

Acute poliomyelitis now is rare in the United States. However, approximately 400,000 adults have had childhood poliomyelitis and are at risk for post-poliomyelitis sequelae. Post-poliomyelitis syndrome is a poorly under-

Table 5–4 **EXERCISE TRAINING AND MUSCULAR DYSTROPHY**

Author	Number of Subjects	Age Range (yr)	Diagnosis	Training	Controls	Outcome
Hoberman 1955[103]	10	9–13	D	Strength training for 4 months	No	Initial improvement, but overall decrement over 9 months
Vignos and Watkins 1966[104]	14 6 4	5–10 8–39 22–44	D LG FSH	Home strength training for 1 year	Yes No No	Improved; greatest benefit with stronger muscles and slowly progressive disease
Florence and Hagberg 1984[109]	6	20–46	Nonprogressive or slowly progressive MD	Aerobic training 3X/wk for 12 weeks	Yes	25% increase in maximum oxygen uptake
de Lateur and Giaconi 1979[105]	4	4–11	D	Strength training 4–5X/wk for 6 months	Contralateral side	No adverse effect; on average, isokinetic strength greater in exercised leg
McCartney et al. 1988[106]	5	20–62	4 FSH, 1 B	Strength training 3X/wk for 9 weeks	Contralateral side	Improved strength
Milner-Brown and Miller 1988[108]	8	20–53	6 FSH, 1 B, 1 myotonic	Strength training 4X/wk for 4 to 24 months	No	Improvement averaged 80% of baseline; improvement when initial strength >10% normal

Key: D = Duchenne's dystrophy, LG = limb-girdle muscular dystrophy, FSH = facioscapulohumeral muscular dystrophy, MD = muscular dystrophy, B = Becker type muscular dystrophy.

stood disorder characterized by fatigue, decreased endurance, joint and muscle pain, respiratory difficulties, limb discoloration, and progressive weakness.[114] Its pathogenesis is unclear. Reinnervation may result in anterior horn cells[115] or neuromuscular junctions that are unable to meet metabolic demands,[116] resulting in premature degeneration. Although exercise in the initial weeks to months following poliomyelitis was reported to exacerbate weakness,[97,98] training of patients 1 to 49 years after their illness indicates that strength increases are possible.[117,118]

Aerobic conditioning has been attempted among individuals with post-poliomyelitis syndrome. In a controlled study,[119] 16 subjects were trained three times a week for 6 weeks. Heart rate was used to guide training intensity, and initial bouts of exertion were as brief as a few minutes. During the first month of exercise, duration was slowly increased to 20 minutes. This gradual increase in exercise time allowed individuals to attain a more traditional training schedule. The exercised group experienced no adverse consequences and significantly increased their maximum oxygen consumption. However, further study will be needed to assess the long-term impact of training on the manifestations and progression of this disorder.

> **CASE:** E.G., a 44-year-old woman, sought medical help to improve her physical condition and lose weight. Past history was significant for childhood poliomyelitis with residual weakness in her left leg, requiring a short-leg brace. In addition, she had a 5-year history of hypertension, which was controlled with a diuretic. Other than hypertension, she had no risk factors for atherosclerosis.
>
> Her physical examination revealed height of 165 cm (5'6"), weight 83 kg (162 pounds) (32% body fat), blood pressure 112/80 mm Hg, and heart rate of 76. The cardiovascular examination was normal, and neurologic findings included atrophy, weakness, and hyporeflexia of the muscles of her left lower leg.
>
> The patient began a program of bicycling three times a week for 15 minutes at a heart rate of 100 bpm. Training duration increased by 5 minutes per week. When she was able to bicycle for 30 minutes, her intensity was gradually increased to achieve a heart rate of 130 bpm. She tolerated the program well. Over the next 4 months, with exercise and mild caloric restriction, she was able to lose 5.4 kg (12 pounds) of body fat.
>
> **COMMENT:** Training modes should be individualized for patients with neuromuscular limitation. Because of concerns about exacerbating the underlying process, the initially prescribed programs are of low intensity and short duration, with gradual increases in training parameters. Individuals are instructed to assess their abilities and to reduce training if persistent muscular symptoms are present at the time of the next scheduled exercise bout.

AMYOTROPHIC LATERAL SCLEROSIS

Amyotrophic lateral sclerosis (ALS) is due to degeneration of both the upper and lower motor neurons. Lower motor neuron loss results in flaccid weakness and atrophy; spasticity predominates with upper motor neuron loss. Exercise has been advocated as a component of the comprehensive therapy of individuals with ALS.[120]

Early in the course of the illness, low-intensity aerobic exercise of unaffected muscles may assist maintenance of joint mobility. In an uncontrolled case study,[120] aerobic training increased oxygen consumption, and results suggested that individuals with upper motor neuron involvement may benefit more than those with combined upper and lower motor neuron dysfunction. Spasticity in ALS, as with other disorders, may be reduced through muscle stretching and exercise.[121,122]

As function becomes limited, several brief exercise periods each day are preferred, rather than usual aerobic conditioning, to maintain function-limiting fatigue.[120] When patients become wheelchair-dependent, breathing exercises and range-of-motion exercises can be continued.[123]

MULTIPLE SCLEROSIS

Fatigue is a common complaint among patients with multiple sclerosis (MS). Reduced exercise efficiency and low fitness levels may contribute to the fatigue and exertional dyspnea observed among patients with MS.[124] These individuals may be prone to deconditioning, as exercise often exacerbates their fatigue. Survey data[125] indicated that vigorous physical activity worsened symptoms in approximately 80% of individuals, although 15% noted that moderate exercise reduced their fatigue. Thus, for selected individuals, exercise may lessen fatigue and may be incorporated into management of MS. Because an increase in body temperature can exacerbate MS symptoms, however, aquatic exercise in cool water (24–27.5°C) may be a preferred training method.[126] Patients with MS can increase strength with aquatic exercise. Gehlsen and colleagues[127] evaluated 20 MS patients following 20 weeks of aquatic exercise and demonstrated an increase in isokinetic strength and the ability to maintain peak torque.

Summary

Muscular complaints include pain, weakness, and limited endurance. History, physical examination (including muscle bulk, strength, and sensory evaluation) and initial laboratory testing (electrolyte levels, thyroid function test, complete blood count, ESR, and CK level) can suggest a diagnosis, such as a peripheral neuropathy, metabolic disorder, or inflammatory myopathy. Some patients will have trigger-point tenderness and meet criteria for fibromyalgia (see Chapter 4). However, these parameters all can be normal among individuals with an underlying metabolic myopathy. Further diagnostic information can be obtained by graded exercise testing with expired gas analysis and needle muscle biopsy. These results can guide subsequent evaluation and provide information for prescribing physical conditioning programs. Strength testing has limited utility in diagnosis but can be useful in following disease progression. Ischemic forearm testing can characterize certain metabolic myopathies.

Physical conditioning (both strength training and aerobic conditioning) has received limited study in individuals with neuromuscular disease. Data suggest that slowly progressive regular exercise has benefits, especially when begun early in the disease process. Because of the potential for symptom exacerbation, close follow-up and enlistment of a physical therapist, or a supervised rehabilitation program, is useful when exercise is prescribed for patients with neuromuscular disease.

REFERENCES

1. Reding MJ, McDowell F: Stroke rehabilitation. *Neurol Clin* 1987; 5:601–630.
2. DeLisa JA: *Rehabilitation Medicine: Principles and Practice.* JB Lippincott: Philadelphia, 1988.
3. Goodgold J: *Rehabilitation Medicine.* Mosby Year-Book: St Louis, 1988.
4. Pollack SF, et al.: Aerobic training effects of electrically induced lower extremity exercises in spinal cord injured people. *Arch Phys Med Rehabil* 1989; 70:214–219.
5. Mills KR, Edwards RH: Investigative strategies for muscle pain. *J Neurol Sci* 1983; 58:73–78.
6. Edwards R, Young A, Wiles M: Needle biopsy of skeletal muscle in the diagnosis of myopathy and the clinical study of muscle function and repair. *N Engl J Med* 1980; 302:261–269.
7. Banker BQ, Engel AG: Basic reaction of muscle, In Engel AG, Banker BQ, eds: *Myology.* McGraw-Hill Book Co: New York, 1986, pp 865–907.
8. Engle WK: The essentiality of histo and cytochemical studies of skeletal muscle in the investigation of neuromuscular disease. *Neurol* 1962; 12:778–793.
9. Heckmatt JZ, et al.: Diagnostic needle muscle biopsy: A practical and reliable alternative to open biopsy. *Arch Dis Child* 1984; 59:528–532.
10. Buchthal F, Kamieniecka Z: The diagnostic yield of quantified electromyography and quantified muscle biopsy in neuromuscular disorders. *Muscle Nerve* 1982; 5:265–280.
11. Elliot DL, et al.: Metabolic myopathies: Evaluation by graded exercise testing. *Medicine* (Baltimore) 1989; 68:163–172.
12. Mastaglia FL, Walton J: *Skeletal Muscle Pathology.* Churchill Livingstone: London, 1982.
13. Servidei S, DiMauro S: Disorders of glycogen metabolism of muscle. *Neurol Clin* 1989; 7:159–178.
14. Zeviani M, et al.: Mitochondrial diseases. *Neurol Clin* 1989; 7:123–156.
15. Bodensteiner J: Congenital myopathies. *Neurol Clin* 1988; 6:499–518.
16. Verity MA: Infantile Pompe's disease, lipid storage, and partial carnitine deficiency. *Muscle Nerve* 1991; 14:435–440.
17. DiMauro S, et al.: Mitochondrial myopathies. *Ann Neurol* 1985; 17:521–538.
18. DiMauro S, et al.: Mitochondrial myopathies. *J Inher Metab Dis* 1987; 10(suppl 1):113–128.
19. Sengers RC, Stadhouders AM, Trijbels JM: Mitochrondrial myopathies: Clinical, morphological and biochemical aspects. *Eur J Pediatr* 1984; 141:192–207.
20. Peterson PL, Martens ME, Lee CP: Mitochondrial encephalomyopathies. *Neurol Clin* 1988; 6:529–544.
21. Moraes CT, et al.: Mitochondrial DNA deletions in progressive external ophthalmoplegia and Kearns-Sayre syndrome. *N Engl J Med* 1989; 320:1293–1299.
22. Olson W, et al.: Oculocraniosomatic neuromuscular disease with "ragged-red" fibers. *Arch Neurol* 1972; 26:193–211.
23. Carroll JE, et al.: Bicycle ergometry and gas exchange measurements in neuromuscular diseases. *Arch Neurol* 1979; 36:457–461.
24. Wallace DC, et al.: Familial mitochondrial encephalomyopathy (MERRF): Genetic, pathophysiological, and biochemical characterization of a mitochondrial DNA disease. *Cell* 1988; 55:601–610.
25. Eleff S, et al.: ^{31}P NMR study of improvement in oxidative phosphorylation of vitamins K_3 and C in a patient with a defect in electron transport at complex III in skeletal muscle. *Proc Natl Acad Sci* 1984; 81:3529–3533.
26. Przyrembel H: Therapy of mitochondrial disorders. *J Inher Metab Dis* 1987; 10(suppl 1):129–146.
27. Arts WF, et al.: NADH-CoQ reductase deficient myopathy: Successful treatment with riboflavin. *Lancet* 1983; 2:581–582.
28. Haller RG, et al.: Hyperkinetic circulation during exercise in neuromuscular disease. *Neurology* 1983; 33:1283–1287.
29. Hagberg JM, et al.: Exercise hyperventilation in patients with McArdle's disease. *J Appl Physiol* 1982; 52:991–994.
30. McArdle B: Myopathy due to a defect in muscle glycogen breakdown. *Clin Sci* 1951; 10:13–33.
31. Layzer RB, Lewis SF: Clinical disorders of muscle energy metabolism. *Med Sci Sports Exerc* 1984; 16:451–455.
32. DiMauro S, Trevison C, Hays A: Disorders of lipid metabolism in muscles. *Muscle Nerve* 1980; 3:369–388.
33. Carroll JE: Myopathies caused by disorders of lipid metabolism. *Neurol Clin* 1988; 6:563–574.
34. DiLiberti JH, Weleber RG, Budden S: Ruavalcaba-Myhre-Smith syndrome: A case with probable autosomal-dominant inheritance and additional manifestations. *Am J Med Genet* 1983; 15:491–495.
35. Carroll JE, et al.: Riboflavin-responsive lipid myopathy and carnitine deficiency. *Neurology* 1981; 31:1557–1559.
36. Elliot DL, et al.: Carnitine responsive lipid myopathy: Report of a family. *Med Sci Sports Exerc* 1992; 24:S56.
37. Sockolov R, et al.: Exercise performance in 6-to-11-year-old boys with Duchenne muscular dystrophy. *Arch Phys Med Rehabil* 1977; 58:195–201.
38. Haller RG, et al.; Hyperkinetic circulation during exercise in neuromuscular disease. *Neurology* 1983; 33:1283–1287.
39. Haller RG, Lewis SF: Pathophysiology of exercise performance in muscle disease. *Med Sci Sports Exerc* 1984; 16:456–459.
40. Banker BQ, Engel AG: The polymyositis

and dermatomyositis syndromes. In Engel AG, Banker BQ, eds: *Myology*. McGraw-Hill: New York, 1986, pp 1385–1421.

41. Mikol J: Inclusion body myositis. In Engel AG, Banker BQ, eds: *Myology*. McGraw-Hill: New York, 1986, pp 1423–1437.

42. Bohan A, Peter JB: Polymyositis and dermatomyositis. *N Engl J Med* 1975; 292:344–347, 403–407.

43. Plotz PH, et al.: Current concepts in the idiopathic inflammatory myopathies: Polymyositis, dermatomyositis, and related disorders. *Ann Intern Med* 1989; 111:143–157.

44. Dalakas MC: Polymyositis, dermatomyositis and inclusion-body myositis. *N Engl J Med* 1991; 325:1487–1498.

45. Kroenke K, et al.: Chronic fatigue in primary care: Prevalence, patient characteristics, and outcome. *JAMA* 1988; 260:929–934.

46. Buchwald D, Sullivan JL, Komaroff AL: Frequency of 'chronic active Epstein-Barr virus infection' in a general medical practice. *JAMA* 1987; 257:2303–2307.

47. Human muscle fatigue: Physiological mechanisms. *CIBA Foundation Symposium* 1981; 82:1–314.

48. Gibson H, Edwards RHT: Muscular exercise and fatigue. *Sports Med* 1985; 2:120–132.

49. Maclaren DP, et al.: A review of metabolic and physiological factors in fatigue. *Exerc Sport Sci Rev* 1989; 7:1–66.

50. Milner-Brown HS, Mellintrium M, Miller RG: Quantifying human muscle strength, endurance and fatigue. *Arch Phys Med Rehabil* 1986; 67:530–535.

51. Holmes GP, et al.: Chronic fatigue syndrome: A working case definition. *Ann Intern Med* 1988; 108:387–389.

52. Manu P, Lane TJ, Matthews DA: The frequency of the chronic fatigue syndrome in patients with symptoms of persistent fatigue. *Ann Intern Med* 1988; 109:554–556.

53. Mann P, Matthews DA, Lane TJ: The mental health of patients with a chief complaint of chronic fatigue: A prospective evaluation and follow-up. *Arch Intern Med* 1988; 148:2213–2217.

54. Sue DY, Hanson JE: Normal values in adults during exercise testing. *Clin Chest Med* 1984; 5:89–98.

55. Jones NL, Campbell EJM, eds: *Clinical Exercise Testing*. WB Saunders: Philadelphia, 1982, p 249.

56. Cooper DM, et al.: Aerobic parameters of exercise as a function of body size during growth in children. *J Appl Physiol* 1984; 56:628–634.

57. Bar-Or O: *Pediatric Sports Medicine for the Practitioner*. Springer-Verlag: New York, 1983, pp 303–304.

58. Arnold DL, et al.: Excessive intracellular acidosis of skeletal muscle on exercise in a patient with a post-viral exhaustion/fatigue syndrome: A 31P nuclear magnetic resonance study. *Lancet* 1984; 1:1367–1369.

59. Archard LC, et al.: Postviral fatigue syndrome: Persistence of enterovirus RNA in muscle and elevated creatine kinase. *J Roy Soc Med* 1988; 81:326–329.

60. Montague TJ, et al.: Cardiac function at rest and with exercise in the chronic fatigue syndrome. *Chest* 1989; 95:779–784.

61. Stokes MJ, Cooper RG, Edwards RH: Normal muscle strength and fatigability in patients with effort syndromes. *BMJ* 1988; 297:1014–1017.

62. Byrne E, Trounce I: Chronic fatigue and myalgia syndrome: Mitochondrial and glycolytic studies in skeletal muscle. *J Neurol Neurosurg Psychiat* 1987; 50:743–746.

63. Eichner ER: Chronic fatigue syndrome: Searching for the cause and treatment. *Phys Sportsmed* 1989; 17:142–152.

64. Goldenberg DL: Fibromyalgia and other chronic fatigue syndromes: Is there evidence for chronic viral disease? *Semin Arthritis Rheum* 1988; 18:111–120.

65. Cook JD, Glass DS: Strength evaluation in neuromuscular disease. *Neurol Clin* 1987; 5:101–123.

66. Kendall HO, Kendall FP: Care during recovery period in paralytic poliomyelitis. *US Public Health Bull* 1938; 242:1–92.

67. *Aids to the Examination of the Peripheral Nervous System*. Oxford: Bailliere Tindall, 1986.

68. Brooke MH, et al.: Duchenne muscular dystrophy: Patterns of clinical progression and effects of supportive therapy. *Neurology* 1989; 39:475–481.

69. Csuka M, McCarty DJ: Simple method for measurement of lower extremity muscle strength. *Am J Med* 1985; 78:77–81.

70. Hosking GP, et al.: Tests of skeletal muscle function in children. *Arch Dis Child* 1978; 53:224–229.

71. Brooke MH, et al.: Clinical trial in Duchenne dystrophy, I: The design of the protocol. *Muscle Nerve* 1981; 4:186–197.

72. Vignos PJ Jr, Archibald KC: Maintenance of ambulation in childhood muscular dystrophy. *J Clinic Dis* 1960; 12:173–190.

73. Resnick JS, et al.: Muscular strength as an index of response to therapy in childhood dermatomyositis. *Arch Phys Med Rehabil* 1981; 62:12–19.

74. Wiles CM, Karni Y: The measurement of muscle strength in patients with peripheral neuromuscular disorders. *J Neurol Neurosurg Psych* 1983; 46:1006–1013.

75. Edwards RG, Wiles GM, Mills KR: Quantitation of muscle contraction and strength. In Dyck P, Thomas P, et al., (eds): *Neuropathy*. WB Saunders: Philadelphia, 1984, pp 1093–1101.

76. Edwards RHT, et al.: Human skeletal muscle function: Description of tests and normal values. *Clin Sci Molecular Med* 1977; 52:283–290.

77. Rothstein JM, Lamb RL, Mayhew TP: Clinical uses of isokinetic measurements: Critical issues. *Phys Ther* 1987; 67:1840–1844.
78. Molnar GE, Alexander J: Development of quantitative standards for muscle strength in children. *Arch Phys Med Rehabil* 1974; 55:490–493.
79. Molnar GE, Alexander J, Gutfeld N: Reliability of quantitative strength measurements in children. *Arch Phys Med Rehabil* 1979; 60:218–221.
80. Tabin GC, Gregg JR, Bonci T: Predictive leg strength values in immediately prepubescent and postpubescent athletes. *Am J Sports Med* 1985; 13:387–389.
81. Nicholas JJ, et al.: Isokinetic testing in young nonathletic able-bodied subjects. *Arch Phys Med Rehabil* 1989; 70:210–213.
82. McArdle B: Myopathy due to a defect in muscle glycogen breakdown. *Clin Sci* 1951; 10:13–35.
83. Munsat TL: A standardized forearm ischemic exercise test. *Neurology* 1970; 20:1171–1178.
84. Fishbein WN, Abmbrustmacher VW, Griffin JL: Myoadenylate deaminase deficiency: A new disease in muscle. *Science* 1978; 200:545–548.
85. Keleman J, et al.: Familial myoadenylate deaminase deficiency and exertional myalgia. *Neurology* 1982; 32:857–863.
86. Coleman RA, et al.: The ischemic exercise test in normal adults and in patients with weakness and cramps. *Muscle Nerve* 1986; 9:216–221.
87. Warmolts JR: Electrodiagnosis in neuromuscular disorders. *Ann Intern Med* 1981; 95:599–608.
88. Daube JE: Electrodiagnosis of muscle disorders. In Engel AG, Banker BQ, eds: *Myology*. McGraw-Hill: New York, 1986, pp 1081–1121.
89. Buchthal F: Electromyography in the evaluation of muscle disease. *Neurol Clin* 1985; 3:573–598.
90. Neuberg GW, et al.: Cardiopulmonary exercise testing: The clinical value of gas exchange data. *Arch Intern Med* 1988; 148:2221–2226.
91. Hansen JE, Sue DY, Wasserman K: Predicted values for clinical exercise testing. *Am Rev Respir Dis* 1984; 129(Suppl):49–55.
92. Chance B, et al.: Magnetic resonance spectroscopy of normal and diseased muscles. *Am J Med Genet* 1986; 25:659–679.
93. Sapega AA, et al.: Phosphorus nuclear magnetic resonance: A non-invasive technique for the study of muscle bioenergetics during exercise. *Med Sci Sports Exerc* 1987;19:410–420.
94. Ross BD, et al.: Examination of a case of suspected McArdle's syndrome by ^{31}P nuclear magnetic resonance. *N Engl J Med* 1981; 304:1338–1342.
95. Argov Z, et al.: Bioenergetic heterogeneity of human mitochondrial myopathies: Phosphorus magnetic resonance spectroscopy study. *Neurology* 1987; 37:257–262.
96. McCully KK, et al.: Detection of muscle injury in humans with ^{31}P magnetic resonance spectroscopy. *Muscle Nerve* 1988; 11:212–216.
97. Lovett RW: The treatment of infantile paralysis. *JAMA* 1915; 64:2118.
98. Bennett RL, Knowlton GC: Overwork weakness in partially denervated skeletal muscle. *Clin Orthop* 1958; 12:22–29.
99. Johnson EW, Braddom R: Over-work weakness in facioscapulohumeral muscular dystrophy. *Arch Phys Med Rehabil* 1971; 52:333–336.
100. Furnkawa T, Peter JB: The muscular dystrophies and related disorders. *JAMA* 1978; 239:1537–1542, 1654–1659.
101. Worton RG, Thompson MW: Genetics of Duchenne muscular dystrophy. *Ann Rev Genet* 1988; 22:601–629.
102. Perloff JK: Cardiomyopathy associated with heredofamilial neuromyopathic disease. *Mod Concepts Cardiovas Dis* 1971; 40:23–26.
103. Hoberman M: Physical medicine and rehabilitation: Its value and limitations in progressive muscular dystrophy. *Am J Phys Med* 1955; 34:109–115.
104. Vignos PJ, Watkins MP: The effect of exercise in muscular dystrophy. *JAMA* 1966; 197:843–848.
105. de Lateur BJ, Giaconi RM: Effect on maximal strength of submaximal exercise in Duchenne muscular dystrophy. *Am J Phys Med* 1979; 58:26–36.
106. McCartney N, et al.: The effects of strength training in patients with selected neuromuscular disorders. *Med Sci Sports Exerc* 1988; 20:362–368.
107. Milner-Brown HS, Stein RB, Lee RG: Synchronization of human motor units: Possible roles of exercise and supraspinal reflexes. *Electroenchephalog Clin Neurophysiol* 1975; 38:245–254.
108. Milner-Brown HS, Miller RG: Muscle strengthening through high-resistance weight training in patients with neuromuscular disorders. *Arch Phys Med Rehabil* 1988; 69:14–19.
109. Florence JM, Hagberg JM: Effect of training on the exercise responses of neuromuscular disease patients. *Med Sci Sports Exerc* 1984; 16:460–465.
110. Fowler WM Jr, Gardner GW: Quantitative strength measurements in muscular dystrophy. *Arch Phys Med Rehabil* 1967; 48:629–644.
111. Siegel IM: The management of muscular dystrophy: A clinical review. *Muscle Nerve* 1978; 1:453–460.
112. Fowler WM Jr: Rehabilitation management of muscular dystrophy and related disorders, II: Comprehensive care. *Arch Phys Med Rehabil* 1982; 63:322–328.
113. Vignos PJ Jr: Physical models of rehabilita-

tion in neuromuscular disease. *Muscle Nerve* 1983; 6:323–328.

114. Jubelt B, Cashman NR: Neurological manifestations of the post-polio syndrome. *Crit Rev Neurobiol* 1987; 3:199–220.

115. Feldman RM: The use of EMG in the differential diagnosis of muscle weakness in post-polio syndrome. *Electromyog Clin Neurophysiol* 1988; 28:269–272.

116. Wiechers DO, Hubbell SL: Late changes in the motor unit after acute poliomyelitis. *Muscle Nerve* 1981; 4:524–528.

117. Delorme TL, Schwab RS, Watkins AL: The response of the quadriceps femoris to progressive-resistance exercises in poliomyelitic patients. *J Bone Joint Surg* 1948; 30A:834–847.

118. Muller EA: Influence of training and of inactivity on muscle strength. *Arch Phys Med Rehabil* 1970; 51:449–462.

119. Jones DR, et al.: Cardiorespiratory responses to aerobic training by patients with postpoliomyelitis sequelae. *JAMA* 1989; 261:3255–3258.

120. Sanjak M, Reddan W, Brooks BR: Role of muscular exercise in amyotrophic lateral sclerosis. *Neurol Clin* 1987; 5:251–268.

121. Davis R: Spasticity following spinal cord injury. *Clin Orthop* 1975; 112:66–75.

122. deVries HA, et al.: Fusimotor system involvement in the tranquilizer effect of exercise. *Am J Phys Med* 1982; 61:111–122.

123. Janiszewski DW, Caroscio JT, Wisham LH: Amyotrophic lateral sclerosis: A comprehensive rehabilitation approach. *Arch Phys Med Rehabil* 1983; 64:304–307.

124. Olgiati R, Jacquet J, De Prampero PE: Energy cost of walking and exertional dyspnea in multiple sclerosis. *Am Rev Respir Dis* 1986; 134:1005–1010.

125. Freal JE, Kraft GH, Coryell KL: Symptomatic fatigue in multiple sclerosis. *Arch Phys Med Rehabil* 1984; 65:135–138.

126. Wainapel SF: Rehabilitation of the patient with multiple sclerosis: In Goodgold J, (ed): *Rehabilitation Medicine.* Mosby Yearbook: St. Louis, 1988, pp 343–362.

127. Gehlsen GM, Grigsby SA, Winant DM: Effects of an aquatic fitness program on the muscular strength and endurance of patients with multiple sclerosis. *Phys Ther* 1984; 64:653–657.

CHAPTER 6

REHABILITATION OF ORTHOPEDIC INJURIES

MARK R. COLVILLE, MD

Problems related to the musculoskeletal system comprise over 20% of office visits to primary care physicians.[1] Because individuals of all ages are becoming more physically active, overuse injuries are seen with increasing frequency.[2] This chapter's purpose is to identify common overuse injuries and outline methods for management of these injuries. Therapeutic exercise for the rehabilitation of selected acute orthopedic injuries is also presented.

Management Principles for Overuse Injuries

Two management principles apply to all overuse injuries: (1) activity modification to allow healing, and (2) therapeutic exercise to help the patient return to his or her preinjury level of performance.[3]

Overuse injuries commonly are caused by an exercise regimen or activity pattern that traumatizes soft tissue or bone at a rate greater than the body is able to repair or recover. The most common overuse injury is inflammation of a musculotendinous unit, that is, tendinitis. When muscle contraction causes shortening of the musculotendinous unit, it is called a *concentric contraction*. An *eccentric contraction* occurs when this unit actively contracts against a lengthening force. For example, when an athlete lands after jumping, the quadriceps muscles contract. The muscle is loaded eccentrically, as it opposes the flexion force of impact and prevents the knee from buckling. Because greater force is applied during eccentric contractions, injuries more commonly result from repetitive eccentric overloading. Examples include patellar tendinitis due to jumping and posterior rotator cuff tendinitis due to throwing.

The first principle of rehabilitation requires resting the injured musculotendinous unit. Elimination of eccentric loading and the repetitive stresses that led to the injury will allow the reparative process to begin. Although complete rest is tolerable for some, many individuals will want an alternative training program to maintain fitness while exercising the injured body part in a different, less traumatic manner. As the principle of cross-training becomes more widely accepted by recreational athletes, a decrease in the injury rate should result, as well as an increase in the effectiveness of postinjury rehabilitation.[2] Specific therapeutic exercises are discussed in the following sections, which are arranged anatomically.

Neck and Cervical Spine Injuries

Cervical pain may be associated with acute injury or exacerbation of a chronic process. Overuse injuries of the neck and cervical spine are rare. When athletes older than age 50 experience neck pain during exercise, it often is secondary to degenerative changes in the cervical spine. Symptoms frequently are characterized by pain located to one side of the spine, without definite point tenderness. The ipsilateral paraspinal muscles are usually in spasm, and neck motion away from the involved side is painful and restricted. Although pain can radiate to the top of the ipsilateral shoulder, it should not extend to the arm, forearm, or hand. Radiographs may show degenerative changes with osteophyte formation in the cervical spine, with narrowing of disk spaces, commonly at the C5-6 space. Oblique views may show osteophytic encroachment of the cervical nerve root foramina.

Rest, heat, and gentle stretching that does not cause pain accelerate recovery. A soft cervical collar may facilitate relief during periods of severe pain. Physical therapy with home cervical traction, with instruction and supervision by a physical therapist, can be effective in relieving muscle spasm and reducing pain. Since the pain is secondary to degenerative cervical spine changes, however, a more vigorous exercise program is contraindicated.

Pain or weakness that extends into the upper extremity may indicate nerve root compression. This often is due to either osteophyte encroachment on neural foramina or acute cervical disk herniation. Patients with signs of peripheral nerve involvement should be urgently referred to a neurologist, orthopedist, or neurosurgeon.

Individuals without osteoarthritis may sustain acute neck strains and sprains secondary to trauma.[4,5] Significant osteoligamentous injury must be excluded prior to initiating a rehabilitation program. Significant cervical spine injury is suggested by persistent midline neck pain, with associated neck weakness and loss of motion. In these cases, conventional cervical spine radiographs are indicated, with a lateral film visualizing the C7-T1 junction. Also, flexion–extension lateral radiographs are needed to evaluate for ligamentous injury. Patients with clinical or radiographic evidence of bone or ligament injury should be urgently referred to either an orthopedic surgeon or neurosurgeon for further diagnostic evaluation and treatment.

When the acute pain from cervical sprain subsides, flexibility can be regained with the aid of gentle passive stretching, heat, and massage. Significant residual weakness secondary to pain may persist even after motion is regained. Individuals involved in contact sports must not participate in those sports until pain is eliminated and normal neck strength, as determined by manual muscle testing, returns. Manual muscle testing is performed by having the patient push his or her head against resistance offered by the examiner's hand in flexion, extension, and lateral bending. Equal strength, without pain, should be present in all directions.[3,5,6]

Shoulder Injuries

Table 6–1 illustrates the differential diagnosis and treatment of various shoulder disorders.

Table 6–1 **DIAGNOSIS AND TREATMENT OF SHOULDER PAIN**

Diagnosis	Symptoms and Signs	Treatment
Rotator cuff tendinitis	Pain with foward elevation; positive impingement test	Cessation of repetitive forward elevation; rotator cuff strengthening and stretching program; NSAIDs and corticosteroid injection.
Rotator cuff tear	Night pain; weakness in forward elevation and external rotation	Surgical repair of rotator cuff or symptomatic management, including NSAIDs, corticosteroid injection, and activity modification
Adhesive capsulitis	Gradual loss of motion following period of pain; motion restricted in all planes	Gradual passive and active stretching program; surgical manipulation in some patients
Calcific tendinitis	Acute onset of severe shoulder pain, point tenderness, painful motion; calcium deposits on radiographs	Rest, NSAIDs, and corticosteroid injections
Recurrent subluxations	Sudden pain or "dead arm" with throwing or other specific movements; no pain between episodes	Rotator cuff strengthening exercises; surgical stabilization in patients who remain symptomatic after exercise program

Key: NSAIDs = nonsteroidal anti-inflammatory drugs.

ROTATOR CUFF DISEASE

The rotator cuff is particularly susceptible to both athletic and occupational overuse injuries, which can be due to repetitive forward elevation above shoulder level, causing wear and tear of the supraspinatus tendon as it passes underneath the bony acromion. In those younger than age 40, the supraspinatus tendon can become inflamed and edematous. The edema increases the impingement, creating a cycle of trauma, edema, impingement, and further trauma.[7,8,9] In athletic overuse injuries, specific training regimens may be altered to avoid such weight training exercises as the military press, upright flyes, and inclined bench press.[10] Fortunately, these injuries rarely progress to rotator cuff tears in younger patients.[7] For occupational injuries, an important rehabilitation step is to modify the patient's work situation to stop the offending repetitive motion.

In individuals older than 40, chronic attritional changes of the rotator cuff can occur. In addition, increased bony impingement of the overlying acromion can result from osteophyte formation. These circumstances can cause progression to rotator cuff tear.[9,11]

In the early stages of rotator cuff tendinitis (prior to signs of a tear), a therapeutic exercise program is helpful. Pendulum movements should be initiated (Figure 6–1). These exercises provide gentle mobilization of the rotator cuff without impingement, trauma, or excessive tendon strain. When instructing an individual, it is important to explain that this exercise is relatively

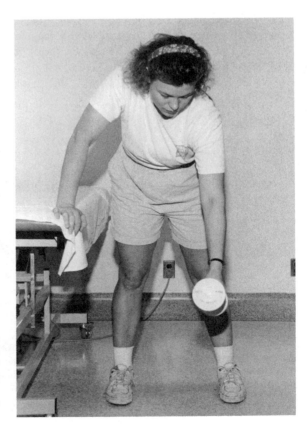

Figure 6–1 Pendulum exercises: passive gentle circular motion is emphasized, with the body supported parallel to the floor and the arm in a dependent position. Weights may or may not be used.

passive and is assisted by gravity. The patient bends over at the waist, so that the treated arm is perpendicular to the floor. The patient then traces gentle circular arcs, both clockwise and counterclockwise, with the arms in the palm-up and palm-down positions. Positioning is important, because if the patient does not bend over far enough, the motion becomes active forward elevation, which could aggravate the tendinitis. Pendulum movements are performed for 10 minutes, three times a day.[3]

Once the initial pain has decreased, gentle internal and external rotation is begun, while the patient stands with the extremity at the side (Figures 6–2 and 6–3). These exercises can be performed with lightweight elastic bands (Theraband) to gradually strengthen the subscapular, infraspinous, and teres minor muscles. With external rotation, the supraspinous muscle is exercised to a lesser extent, but the impingement position is avoided. This rehabilitation program should be performed daily, with light resistance (2 to 5 lbs). Progressive resistive exercises in forward elevation above shoulder level are harmful and should be avoided.

Many young patients with rotator cuff tendinitis have mild degrees of shoulder instability. This instability leads to a secondary impingement as the shoulder subluxates superiorly and anteriorly against the undersurface of the acromion. In these individuals, a controlled rotator cuff exercise program to aid dynamic stability can be beneficial. Once the patient is pain-free, he or she can begin progressive resistive exercises, emphasizing internal and especially external rotation strength in the shoulder.[12]

During the course of rehabilitation, nonsteroidal anti-inflammatory drugs (NSAIDs) can be used. Subacromial injection of a long-acting corticosteroid can reduce inflammation in the rotator cuff and therefore decrease impingement. However, repetitive subacromial corticosteroid injections are contraindicated.

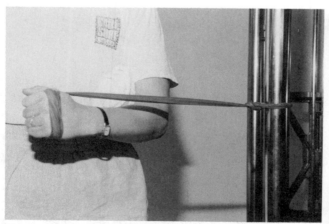
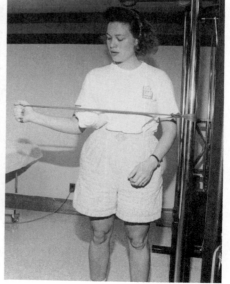

Figures 6–2 and 6–3 Internal and external rotation exercises may be performed while standing using elastic bands, or while lying on one's side using light free weights. Three sets of 20 repetitions generally are performed for each muscle group.

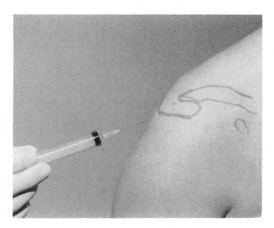

Figure 6-4 Access to the subacromial space is easy at the posterolateral border of the acromion. Starting 1 cm below the acromion, the needle is angled upward parallel to the under surface of the acromion and into the subacromial space.

This injection most easily is performed with a posterolateral approach, with the patient in a sitting position (Figure 6-4).

Also, those with rotator cuff tendinitis frequently complain of pain along the superior medial border of the scapula, radiating to the occiput on the involved side. This pain usually is increased by the end of the day or after vigorous activities and may be associated with severe headaches. The medial scapular and trapezial pain results from overuse of the muscles that rotate and elevate the scapula. This overuse compensates for reduced glenohumeral motion caused by the rotator cuff tendinitis. As the primary injury is treated, these secondary problems usually resolve. Occasionally, an individual will benefit from a stretching and strengthening program for the periscapular musculature, under the supervision of a physical therapist.

> **CASE:** W.S., a 35-year-old man, presented with a 4-week history of increasing pain in the right shoulder. He noticed that the pain developed approximately 1 week after he was transferred to a new position on the assembly line. His new work involved removing a 1-pound object from an overhead bin every 45 seconds. He described the pain as a dull ache on the lateral aspect of the right shoulder, extending down to the deltoid insertion and anteriorly near the coracoid process. The pain did not radiate into the forearm or hand, and he did not complain of neck pain. He had no previous shoulder difficulties.
>
> Examination of the neck revealed full range of motion without pain. Results of neurovascular examination of both upper extremities were normal. Inspection of the shoulders revealed no atrophy or asymmetry. Palpation revealed tenderness over the anterior acromion and over the coracoacromial ligament. Shoulder range of motion was relatively unrestricted: external rotation with the arms at the side to 70° bilaterally; internal rotation to the T-10 spinous process on the right versus T-7 on the left. Forced forward elevation of the right arm, causing impingement of the greater tuberosity under the acromion, was painful (positive impingement test). No increased laxity was detected to anterior, inferior, and posterior stress testing. Radiographs were normal, with no evidence of calcific deposit or osteophyte formation above the shoulder joint.
>
> A diagnosis of supraspinatus tendinitis secondary to repetitive overuse was made. The patient temporarily was transferred to another job, which involved minimal use of the right upper extremity. He was

instructed to do pendulum exercises, and a 2-week course of NSAIDs was prescribed. Three weeks later, his symptoms and signs were greatly diminished. He continued with his exercise program, and after discussion with the patient's employer, arrangements were made to lower the overhead parts bin to waist level. Within 6 weeks after initial presentation, W.S. was back on the job at the modified work station without symptoms.

FROZEN SHOULDER (ADHESIVE CAPSULITIS)

Adhesive capsulitis can be triggered by a variety of causes. Immobilization after injury, a lengthy hospitalization with ventilator assistance, irritation due to increased activity, or prolonged abnormal shoulder position, such as during a surgical procedure, all can lead to the condition. In many instances, there is no known antecedent event. The patient initially complains of shoulder pain, which is diffuse and increases with motion (i.e., forward elevation, abduction, and internal and external rotation). Over the ensuing weeks, glenohumeral motion is lost due to gradual obliteration of the redundant inferior joint capsule. An arthrogram may show a dramatic loss in joint capsular volume. Although pain generally decreases within a few weeks, loss of motion remains, and mobility may take up to 2 years to return. Despite improvement, most patients experience some residual motion loss.[9,13]

A majority of patients will respond to a gradual stretching and exercise program. Because resolution of symptoms is prolonged, the physical therapist should be cautioned against unnecessary vigor during stretching. Too aggressive stretching can result in pain and further loss of motion. Stretching is easier and safer when the patient is supine. Forward elevation and external rotation are aided by gravity (Figures 6–5 and 6–6). The shoulder is stretched gradually into forward elevation, as well as external and internal rotation. Also, pendulum exercises are initiated. Both the pendulum and stretching exercises should be performed several times a day for short periods (10 to 15 minutes). However, abduction of the shoulder initially is not emphasized, because of pain.

A weight training or resistive exercise program is inappropriate for these individuals. Corticosteroid injections generally are not helpful, although trig-

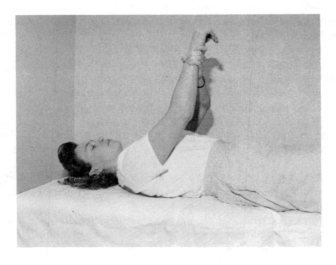

Figure 6–5 Gravity is used to assist the patient in gaining forward elevation when passive assistive exercises are performed in the supine position.

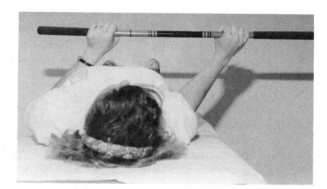

Figure 6–6 The patient uses a cane to assist in gaining external rotation. The elbow is kept at the side to ensure that humeral rotation is achieved.

ger-point injection with a local anesthetic may allow greater progress during rehabilitation exercises. Manipulation of the frozen shoulder while the patient is under anesthesia has been advocated by some authors,[13,14] but these patients are generally younger or are those who fail to improve after several weeks of a controlled exercise program.

BICEPS TENDINITIS

Inflammation of the long head of the biceps tendon as it passes through the bicipital groove commonly is associated with rotator cuff disease and early degenerative changes in the shoulder joint. A rehabilitation program similar to that outlined for rotator cuff tendinitis may be helpful in decreasing symptoms and allowing healing. Since significant rotator cuff disease can co-exist, a rotator cuff tear should be ruled out in those with persistent symptoms.

CALCIFIC TENDINITIS

Calcific tendinitis is characterized by pain associated with amorphous calcium deposits in the rotator cuff tendons, especially the supraspinatus tendon. The pain is due to an acute inflammatory reaction. Avoidance of overhead motion, along with use of pendulum exercises and NSAIDs (usually indomethacin) can control symptoms during the first 2 to 4 days. Occasionally subacromial injection of corticosteroid with a local anesthetic may be required to control severe discomfort. The majority of individuals with an acute flare of calcific tendinitis will have their pain resolve within a few weeks, and surgical excision of the calcium deposits is rarely required.[9]

INSTABILITY

The shoulder has the greatest range of motion of all human joints and also is the least stable. Recurrent dislocation or subluxation may be classified as traumatic or atraumatic, voluntary or involuntary, and unidirectional or multidirectional. Approximately 80% of patients younger than age 20 who sustain traumatic dislocation experience subsequent recurrent dislocation.[9] Surgery often is needed for traumatic unidirectional recurrent dislocation; multidirectional, atraumatic, and voluntary dislocations usually are treated with activity modification and a therapeutic exercise program. These exercises, aimed at controlling shoulder instability, are designed to strengthen the rotator cuff and scapular rotational muscles while avoiding positions of instability. In general, external rotation and internal rotation exercises with the arm at the side are instituted. These activities are progressive, with use of increased weights as strength is gained.[3]

Depending on the direction of instability, certain movements and positions should be avoided. Patients with anterior shoulder instability should avoid abducted, externally rotated arm positions, whereas those with posterior shoulder instability should eliminate horizontally adducted positions with forward arm elevation. The majority of those with multidirectional and posterior shoulder instability can be managed successfully with patient education, activity modification, and specific exercises. If a patient's symptoms do not improve after 6 to 9 months in a carefully outlined exercise program, referral to an orthopedic surgeon is appropriate.

Elbow Injuries

LATERAL EPICONDYLITIS (TENNIS ELBOW)

Overuse of the wrist extensor muscles may lead to tendinitis at the lateral epicondyle of the humerus, with symptoms of pain directly over, or just distal to, the lateral epicondyle. Pain is increased with resisted wrist dorsiflexion or forearm supination and occasionally with finger extension. Those at risk for this condition include tennis players, carpenters (from using a hammer), weight lifters with a power grip and wrist extension, and those who carry heavy suitcases or similar loads. Histologic examination has shown degenerative changes in the musculotendinous origin at the lateral epicondyle.

After initial symptoms subside, use of a tennis elbow strap decreases stress on the extensor origin. A night volar wrist splint that holds the wrist in moderate extension also can be helpful if the patient is prone to sleeping with the wrist in forced volar flexion. NSAIDs and corticosteroid injections can decrease symptoms. Care must be used to place any corticosteroid injection beneath the fascia. Skin and subcutaneous tissue are thin in this area, and extravasation of drug may result in atrophy, thinning of the skin, and worse pain than the original problem.

A progressive resistive exercise program for wrist extensions and supinations is undertaken only after the patient is pain-free. Low-resistance exercises are initiated, and weights are increased gradually over time. Ice after exercise is indicated.[6,15,16]

MEDIAL EPICONDYLITIS

Overuse of the wrist and finger flexion muscles may result in tendinitis at the medial epicondyle of the elbow. Symptoms and signs are similar to those for lateral epicondylitis, but occur on the medial side. Medial epicondylitis is seen in throwing athletes and tennis players who use backhand topspin techniques. Treatment is similar to that for lateral epicondylitis, but the object is to decrease concentric and eccentric loading of the forearm flexor–pronator muscle group.

Table 6–2 **DIAGNOSIS AND TREATMENT OF HIP PAIN**

Diagnosis	Symptoms and Signs	Treatment
Degenerative joint disease	Groin pain; loss of hip extension and internal rotation	NSAIDs; cane in opposite hand; consultation for hip arthroplasty
Greater trochanteric bursitis	Lateral hip pain over greater trochanter	NSAIDs; stretching exercises; occasional steroid injection
Adductor strain	Pain with hip abduction; tenderness over inferior pubic ramus anteriorly	Rest, NSAIDs; avoidance of strenuous activity until fully reversed
Hamstring strain	Pain along course of hamstring, most commonly at ischial origin	Rest, ice, NSAIDs; avoidance of overstretching; after full ROM achieved, begin stretching program
Piriformis syndrome	Buttock pain during or after running, with occasional radiation down back of thigh; tenderness over sciatic notch	Rest, NSAIDs, internal rotational stretching; correction of any mechanical problems causing excessive hip rotation

Key: NSAIDs = nonsteroidal anti-inflammatory drugs, ROM = range of motion.

Hip and Pelvis Injuries

Table 6–2 illustrates the differential diagnosis and treatment of common hip disorders.

POSTOPERATIVE MANAGEMENT OF HIP FRACTURES

Hip fracture among the elderly is associated with a 50% death rate the first year after injury. Immobility and deconditioning contribute to the high morbidity after hip fracture, and mobilization to maintain both strength and endurance is an important aspect of care. Today most orthopedic internal fixation devices allow early weightbearing. Individuals can be sitting the day following surgery, and ambulation begun with appropriate assistive devices, such as a walker.

Since profound hip abductor weakness is present, a program emphasizing hip abduction strength is initiated as soon as pain permits. Hip motion is rarely a problem following hip fracture surgery, and range of motion (ROM) exercises should be undertaken, preferably two to three times daily in short, 10- to 15-minute sessions. In conjunction with strengthening the affected lower extremity, an upper-body exercise program should be instituted to maintain muscle strength.

ARTHRITIS VERSUS TROCHANTERIC BURSITIS

Pain attributed to the hip can be a manifestation of several problems. Pain due to the hip joint itself is most commonly referred to the groin. If its cause is arthritis, internal rotation and hip extension is lost as the disease progresses. Most younger patients who complain of hip pain localize their discomfort over

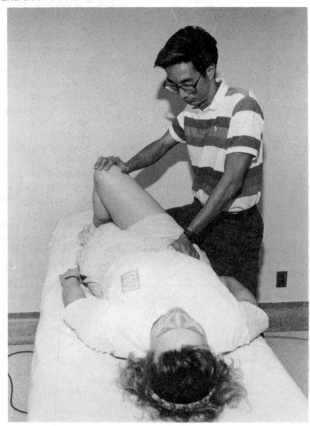

Figure 6–7 Iliotibial band stretching may be performed with assistance, as demonstrated, or may be performed alone in the sitting position with the patient pulling the knee across the midline in a similar fashion.

the lateral hip, in the area of the greater trochanter. This pain usually is due to inflammation of the greater trochanteric bursa, not the hip joint itself. Trochanteric bursitis is a frequent overuse injury in runners and walkers. Relief is achieved through an initial period of rest, followed by an iliotibial band stretching program (Figure 6–7). Hip abductor strengthening exercises can reduce recurrence of symptoms. Ice following exercise is prescribed, and occasionally corticosteroid injection in the greater trochanteric bursa is needed to relieve inflammation and pain.

Trochanteric bursitis and iliotibial band tendinitis can be aggravated by excessive or abnormal rotational movements of the femur and tibia while walking or running. These movements may be due to structural problems (internally rotated femur, externally rotated tibia, flat hyperpronated feet) that can be improved by an orthotic device. Therefore, those who fail to improve after a trial of exercise modification, stretching, and anti-inflammatory agents should be referred to a sports physician familiar with gait analysis and orthotic prescription[2,14,17]

ADDUCTOR AND HAMSTRING STRAINS

Adductor strain (groin pull) to the origin of the adductor longus tendon in the inferior pubic ramus is commonly seen in skaters and skiers, and after acute abduction injury. It is characterized by pain directly over the origin of the adductor muscle at the pelvis. Stress fractures of the inferior pubic ramus are not uncommon and should be ruled out before making this diagnosis.

Hamstring strains commonly occur after a sudden sprint by a deconditioned athlete, such as a weekend softball player running to first base. They are characterized by severe pain in the posterior thigh, usually either in the muscle or at the ischial origin of the hamstring. Occasionally, a palpable defect will be appreciated. Severe ecchymoses in the thigh, descending down into the calf, are not unusual.

Both adductor and hamstring strains are prone to reinjury if initial treatment is not appropriate. Rest and avoidance of stretching after initial injury are essential to prevent further bleeding and muscle tearing. Once this pain has subsided, gentle motion is undertaken. Passive stretching should not cause pain. When full painless hip and knee range of motion are achieved, high-speed progressive resistive exercises, such as isokinetic training, can be initiated. The athlete should not return to competition until full motion and strength, without pain, have returned and the individual is able to run at full speed without difficulty.[4,6,18,19] Warm-up and stretching reduce the incidence of hamstring and adductor muscle injuries.[20] Static stretching for 10 to 15 minutes prior to exercise will increase the elasticity of the musculotendinous unit (Figure 6–8).

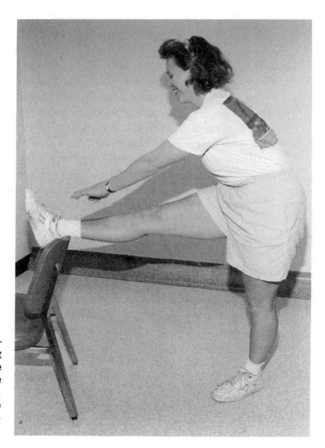

Figure 6–8 While stretching the hamstrings, a straight back is maintained. Raising the height of the heel will increase the stretch on the hamstrings. These exercises may also be performed in the sitting position.

PIRIFORMIS SYNDROME

Piriformis syndrome is tendinitis of the short hip external rotators occasionally observed in patients with excessive hip rotation while running. Symptoms are characterized by buttock pain and palpable tenderness approximately halfway between the ischium and the greater trochanter. Alteration of running gait and an exercise program to strengthen the external rotators can improve symptoms. A stretching program to increase internal rotation also is advocated. Rarely, sciatic nerve irritation in the area of the piriform muscle is secondary to swelling and fibrosis of the muscle. This may be characterized by radiating pain similar to, although not specific for, a particular nerve root.[21]

SACROILIAC PAIN

Sacroiliac joint pain may be seen in runners with significant leg length discrepancy (greater than 1/2"). Correction of leg length inequality, using a heel lift, can improve symptoms. Low-back exercises, with a flexibility program for hamstrings and calf muscles, also can decrease sacroiliac joint symptoms (see also Chapters 4 and 7).

Knee Injuries

PATELLOFEMORAL PAIN SYNDROME

Chronic anterior knee pain is the single most common overuse symptom related to this joint. Patients with patellofemoral difficulties note pain with prolonged bent knee position, such as sitting in a theater (positive theater sign). Pain and grinding will accompany ascending and especially descending stairs, and a feeling of catching and giving way can be a prominent complaint. The pain is poorly localized and somewhat diffuse at the anterior of the knee. There are several possible causes of patellofemoral pain. Even in a normal patellofemoral joint, high compressive forces are present during impact activities. For instance, up to 10 times the body weight is transmitted across the joint when jumping, and a fourfold increase is transmitted when climbing stairs. Conditions that can lead to chondromalacia patellae also may cause patellofemoral pain without articular cartilage damage.

CHONDROMALACIA PATELLAE

Impact sports, such as running and jumping, can cause a stress reaction in the patellar subchondral bone, leading to pain and softening of the articular cartilage (chondromalacia). Chondromalacia describes an anatomic finding and should not be used as a wastebasket diagnosis for patients with patellofemoral pain.

Lateral subluxation of the patella or lateral malposition is a common cause of patellofemoral pain and is more commonly seen in patients with a small, high-riding patella. A low patella also is characterized by abnormal joint forces, with increased patellofemoral contact pressures. Another condition, lateral patellar facet syndrome, occurs when the lateral fascia of the patellofemoral joint is excessively tight, resulting in increased contact pressures on the lateral aspect of the patellofemoral joint (Table 6-3).

Table 6–3 **DIAGNOSIS AND TREATMENT OF CHONDROMALACIA PATELLAE**

Cause	Symptoms and Signs	Treatment
Lateral subluxation	History of "giving way"; positive apprehension test	Quadriceps strengthening program, patella brace; can require surgery
Lateral facet syndrome	History of anterolateral pain with repetitive sports; evidence of lateral tilt on tangential radiographs	Quadriceps strengthening, hamstring stretching; correction of lower-extremity alignment problems such as hyperpronation; can require surgical release
Trauma	History of direct injury; pain and grinding following injury	Avoidance of stairs; knee brace, NSAIDs
Repetitive overuse	History of running or jumping, gradual-onset anterior knee pain, occasional chronic knee effusion	Change in exercise routine to decrease patellofemoral impact; hamstring stretching, ice, NSAIDs

Key: NSAIDs = nonsteroidal anti-inflammatory drugs.

To assess patellar position and tracking, the clinician observes the standing patient, noting whether the patella points medially, indicating excessive internal femoral rotation. Then, while the patient performs a deep knee bend, the patella is palpated, feeling for any crepitus. When the patient is seated, patellar tracking should be observed during knee extension. The patella can subluxate laterally at 20° to 30° during active extension.

While the patient is supine, gentle attempts to laterally subluxate the patella will result in apprehension and pain. Attempts to subluxate the patella medially indicate the degree of lateral extensor fascia tightness. Hamstring tightness commonly accompanies patellofemoral disease. With the hip flexed to 90°, note the amount of knee extension possible (Figure 6–9).

Treatment of patellofemoral conditions that can lead to chondromalacia is aimed at correcting the underlying problem. In the case of lateral subluxation or maltracking, a program to strengthen the vastus medialis muscle and correct tracking is initiated. Exercises are performed that avoid excessive patellofemoral excursion, commonly including straight-leg raises and short arch quadriceps exercises. Daily straight-leg raises are performed with ankle weights. Enough weight is prescribed so that the patient can perform three sets of 20 repetitions on each leg (Figure 6–10).[17,22,23] Ice cubes in a plastic bag are applied directly to the skin for up to 20 minutes following exercise. This decreases inflammation and swelling while providing pain relief. A hamstring, calf, and low-back stretching program is instituted to decrease quadriceps antagonist forces about the knee joint. A neoprene brace with a lateral patellar buttress occasionally is worn to aid in restoration of normal patellofemoral tracking. Failure to improve over the course of 6 to 8 months may necessitate surgical release of the lateral extensor retinaculum to correct tracking and abnormal patellofemoral contact pressures.

Chondromalacia can result from several other mechanisms. Direct trauma is a common initiator, and pain can persist for over a year. Post-traumatic chondromalacia is treated by decreasing load across the patellofemoral joint, that is, by avoiding stair climbing, running, and jumping. Cycling may be used

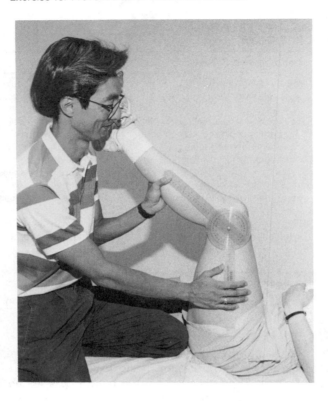

Figure 6–9 Hamstring tightness is frequently related to patellofemoral disorders and should be assessed during the knee examination.

with caution, provided resistance is low and seat position is arranged so that the arc of motion does not pass through the painful arc of the knee joint.

Overuse patellofemoral syndromes require activity modification to decrease repetitive impact and eccentric loading, with alternative cross-training activities such as swimming, low-intensity cycling, and isometric weight lifting programs. Corticosteroid injection of the knee joint is not helpful, nor is it indicated. Although NSAIDs are helpful, patellofemoral injuries frequently are chronic, and judicious use of these agents is advised.

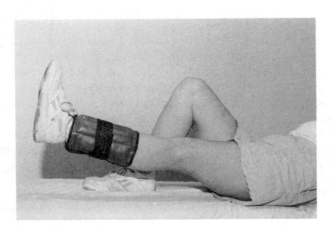

Figure 6–10 Straight leg raises employ isometric muscle contraction to strengthen the quadriceps muscles while minimizing patellofemoral trauma. Three sets of 20 repetitions can be used. As strength is increased, ankle weights are added.

CASE: J.B., a 36-year-old accountant who runs 50 miles a week, presented with knee pain. He had been increasing his jogging mileage over the past month in anticipation of an upcoming half-marathon. He felt pain in the anterolateral aspect of the knee, which began approximately 2 miles into his run. On arising in the morning, he experienced sharp anterior knee pain, especially when descending stairs.

On examination, the patient walked with a normal gait. Study of his lower-extremity alignment revealed mildly hyperpronated feet and external tibial torsion. The lateral extensor retinaculum was tight, and patellofemoral crepitus was noted bilaterally. With the hip flexed to 90°, the knee could be extended only to 45° (indicating significant hamstring tightness). Inspection of his running shoes revealed a worn shoe with minimal hindfoot and antipronation control. Because no history of trauma was reported, x-rays were deferred. The patient was felt to have lateral patellar facet syndrome.

He was advised to decrease his mileage until he was pain-free. He cross-trained by running 4 days a week and bicycling 2 days a week, with 1 day of rest. He was instructed in static hamstring, calf, and low-back stretching exercises. He was started on a 2-week course of NSAIDs and iced his affected knee after exercise. He was instructed to purchase new shoes with a firm heel counter and adequate medial arch to resist hyperpronation.

PATELLAR TENDINITIS

Patellar tendinitis is a breakdown of tendon fibers at the distal patella, where tensile stress is maximal. This syndrome is commonly seen in jumping athletes, hence the name jumper's knee. On physical examination, the inferior pole of the patella is exquisitely tender. Although patellar tendinitis rarely progresses to tendon rupture, it can be disabling. Reduction of eccentric loading and impact activities is required. A patellar tendon strap may decrease eccentric stress and can be helpful. In addition, nonimpact progressive resistive quadriceps exercises, to strengthen the quadriceps mechanism, can be effective. Ice is helpful after exercise, but corticosteroid injections are contraindicated and may lead to patellar tendon rupture.[22]

POPLITEUS TENDINITIS, ANSERINE BURSITIS

Popliteus tendinitis and anserine bursitis also are common overuse injuries resulting in knee pain.[14] The popliteus tendon may be palpated posterolaterally in the lateral knee joint line. External rotation of the tibia can be painful due to stretching of the popliteus tendon. The anserine bursa is located on the medial aspect of the knee, approximately three fingerbreadths below the medial joint line. The bursa underlies the pes anserinus (the sartorius, gracilis, and semitendinosus tendons). Although external tibial rotation may aggravate the pain, there is no joint-line tenderness or locking, which would indicate medial meniscal injury.

Excessive downhill running can cause injury to the popliteus tendon, because it is overused while stabilizing the tibia against excessive posterolateral rotation. Anserine bursitis can be caused by excessive external rotation of the tibia during running. Both conditions are treated by cessation of the offending activities, followed by hamstring strengthening. Leg or hamstring curls are performed daily with enough weight so that three sets of 20 repetitions can be performed with each leg.

LIGAMENT INJURY

Early mobilization after knee ligament injuries is becoming standard treatment. After acute knee sprains, a careful knee examination must be done to exclude tears of the major ligaments.[24] Patients with joint effusion following trauma have a high likelihood of meniscus or cruciate ligament injury and should be referred to an orthopedist. Ligament injuries are graded according to their severity. Grade I represents minor trauma to the ligament with no fiber disruption or increased laxity during stress testing. Grade II sprains represent a partial disruption of the ligament. Laxity is increased, but stress testing reveals a solid end point; that is, part of the ligament remains intact and is noted with anterior and posterior manipulation of the joint. In grade III sprains, the ligament is completely disrupted, and no end point is appreciated during stress testing.

The site and severity of injury will define the need for referral and prescription for rehabilitation. The anterior cruciate ligament is assessed by attempting to subluxate the tibia anteriorly relative to the femur. This test is performed with the knee flexed 20°, where the anterior cruciate ligament is the primary restraint to anterior tibial subluxation. The posterior cruciate ligament is assessed by attempting to subluxate the tibia posteriorly while the knee is flexed 70° to 90°. The medial and lateral collateral ligaments are assessed by exerting a valgus or varus stress, respectively, with the knee at 30° flexion.

All patients with suspected tears of the cruciate ligaments should be referred to an orthopedic surgeon, because they usually require surgical treatment. If the cruciate ligaments are intact and there is no meniscal injury, medial and lateral collateral ligament injuries may be treated with early joint mobilization and progressive resistive exercises.[25]

Careful early protected motion is permitted after isolated collateral ligament injury. In grade I and II collateral ligament injuries, immobilization is not necessary and early active motion is emphasized until full movement without pain is achieved. After approximately 3 to 4 weeks, full motion is usually regained. The emphasis then turns to progressive resistive exercises for the quadriceps and hamstring muscle groups.[3,6] Full return to sport after grade I and II injuries is allowed in 4 to 6 weeks, provided a brace is worn to prevent excessive varus and valgus stresses. If no brace is prescribed or possible, then 8 weeks should be allowed for healing.

Grade III collateral ligament injuries require application of a cast brace or a removable brace that allows flexion and extension but prevents against excessive varus and valgus angulation. Hinges are initially set in the pain-free arc, which usually is approximately 30° to 90° of flexion. After 3 weeks, hinges are reset to allow motion from 0° to full flexion. The patient can begin to put weight on the affected leg as knee extension returns (approximately 3 weeks after injury). A brace to prevent reinjury during athletic activities should be worn for 6 months following a grade III collateral ligament injury. Prior to return to sport, isokinetic exercises are helpful to regain speed and strength; thus, referral to a facility with equipment to perform these exercises is helpful.

Full-speed running and agility drills are carried out prior to return to unrestricted activity.[3]

MENISCAL INJURY

Meniscal tears usually occur during flexion and rotation injuries to the knee. Patients with meniscal injuries will be tender to palpation in the joint line, and pain is elicited with knee hyperflexion and tibial rotation (the McMurray test).[26] Most acute meniscal injuries will not respond to nonoperative management. In many circumstances, however, surgical treatment of degenerative meniscal tears is not indicated. Among those not requiring surgery are elderly individuals and those undergoing nonimpact exercise programs such as bicycling or swimming. This type of activity will allow improvement of quadriceps and hamstring muscle strength without causing further trauma to the meniscus. Also, many patients with degenerative tears will see their symptoms subside over time without the need for surgical debridement. Continued avoidance of impact activities may be necessary to minimize recurrent episodes of pain and swelling. A double upright cartilage brace can provide functional improvement for a patient with a degenerative meniscal tear by decreasing knee motion and gently compressing soft tissues.

Leg Injuries

SHIN SPLINTS

Repetitive foot pronation during running can lead to traction (eccentric) injury to the tibial muscle along the posteromedial tibia. Runners with flat feet are particularly susceptible to developing shin splints, due to their hyperpronation.[14] This syndrome is characterized by tenderness to palpation along the posteromedial border of the tibia about two thirds of the way down the leg. The primary cause of shin splints is an alteration in training, most commonly an increase in mileage or a sudden change in running terrain.

If the problem occurs, runners with hyperpronated feet (flexible flat feet) should use a high-quality running shoe with a firm heel counter and arch support. Occasionally, when symptoms persist and the condition becomes chronic, a custom orthotic to prevent excessive pronation is indicated.[2,17,23] During recovery, mileage should be increased by no more than 10% per week. Approximately 3 months is required for complete rehabilitation.

EXERTIONAL COMPARTMENT SYNDROME

Chronic exertional compartment syndrome of the anterior tibial compartment is characterized by deep muscle pain lateral to the tibia after running. Unlike shin splints or sore muscles, pain subsides with the cessation of activities, and there usually is no residual soreness the following day. Occasionally pain will be accompanied by acute onset of foot-drop and numbness in the superficial and deep peroneal nerve distribution. Exertional compartment syndrome should be differentiated from overuse tendinitis of the anterior compartment muscles. Surgical decompression of the anterior tibial compartment often is required if the patient desires to continue the athletic activities that caused the injury.[27]

GASTROCNEMIUS STRAIN, ACHILLES TENDON RUPTURE

Acute strain of the medial or lateral head of the gastrocnemius muscle commonly is caused by sudden, explosive push-off movements, such as in tennis and baseball. Patients complain of pain with push-off and are unable to walk on their toes. Pain is localized to the origin of the medial or lateral head of the gastrocnemius muscle or the musculotendinous junction. A defect in the muscle belly rarely is palpable. Straightening the knee joint also may elicit pain because the gastrocnemius muscle crosses the knee joint and originates on the lateral and medial condyles of the femur. Ruptures of the Achilles tendon can be excluded by squeezing the calf while the patient is prone. If the Achilles tendon is intact, passive plantar flexion of the foot is noted (Figure 6–11).[26] It is necessary to remember that voluntary plantar flexion still is possible with Achilles tendon rupture, using the posterior tibial muscle, the long flexor muscle of the great toe, and the long flexor muscle of the toes. Suspected ruptures of the Achilles tendon should be referred to an orthopedic surgeon, because they can require surgical intervention.

Initial treatment for gastrocnemius strains consists of avoidance of placing weight on the affected limb, rest, ice, and occasionally a compressive dressing for comfort. After 24 to 48 hours, gentle active ankle motion is undertaken. Excessive stretching is avoided, to prevent further bleeding into the injured muscle. A heel lift is prescribed to prevent excessive dorsiflexion of the ankle and relieve strain on the musculotendinous unit. Early motion is prescribed, emphasizing that movement should not elicit pain. As pain subsides and motion increases, the patient progresses to a flat-soled shoe and begins gentle stretching (Figure 6–12). When full motion returns without pain, progressive resistive exercises for the calf muscles, such as toe raises, are undertaken.[3] Return to sport is preceded by a gradual running program, and the patient is allowed full activity when able to sprint at full speed without pain.

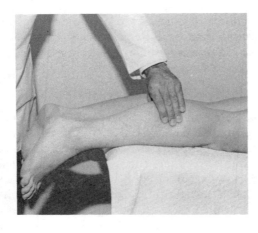

Figure 6–11 The Thompson test is used to detect rupture of the Achilles tendon. Lack of passive plantar flexion of the foot when the calf muscles are compressed is evidence of an Achilles tendon rupture.

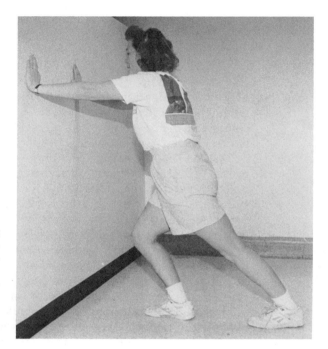

Figure 6–12 Calf stretches with the knee flexed will emphasize soleus muscle stretching. With the knee extended, both the soleus and the gastrocnemius muscles are stretched. After a warm-up, these exercises can continue for approximately 10 minutes.

ACHILLES TENDINITIS

Inflammation of the peritendineum, or peritendinous sheath, is the most frequent cause of Achilles tendinitis.[28] This injury usually is due to overuse. The patient is tender along the tendon, and the gastrocnemius–soleus complex is excessively tight. A heel lift and a stretching program are prescribed. Occasionally, excessive foot pronation will lead to Achilles tendinitis; in these cases, an orthotic device may be useful. Corticosteroid injection can lead to tendon rupture and is contraindicated. Achilles tendinitis rarely progresses to acute rupture. Rest and cross-training activities, which avoid eccentric loading of the Achilles tendon, are instituted. Ice massage after exercise and NSAIDs also are used to control the inflammatory response.

Foot and Ankle Injuries

ANKLE SPRAINS

Because ankle sprains are common, they are frequently overlooked as trivial injuries with little or no treatment or rehabilitation prescribed. However, up to 20% of patients sustaining a severe inversion sprain of the ankle complain of long-term residual dysfunction.[29] Therefore, careful evaluation and treatment are important to prevent recurrent injury and facilitate return of function.[30]

Inversion sprains are graded according to the degree of injury. A grade I sprain is a minor capsular sprain without ligament disruption. Grade II injuries imply partial tearing of the anterior talofibular ligament, and a grade III sprain is complete disruption of the anterior talofibular ligament, occasionally with associated disruption of the calcaneofibular ligament.

Initial treatment for grade I ankle sprains consists of ice, elevation, and a compressive wrap. After 48 hours, early joint motion is begun, and the patient may place weight on the foot as pain permits. Individuals return to athletics when they are able to run without pain. Taping or an ankle brace provides comfort in the first few weeks after injury, and most patients return to unlimited sport by 2 weeks.

Grade II ankle sprains should be immobilized in a position of eversion to prevent continued stretching of torn structures. A removable ankle support or brace facilitates rehabilitation. The brace is removed after initial swelling subsides (4 to 5 days), and exercises consisting of ankle dorsiflexion and plantar flexion while avoiding inversion and eversion of the ankle are initiated. Weight bearing is allowed as tolerated while in the brace.

Grade III ankle sprains require immobilization in dorsiflexion and eversion to ensure healing of the ligaments in their shortest position. However, because of the severity of the swelling, frequent changes of the cast or compressive dressing are required to provide continuous compressive support to the lateral ankle structures. Limited ankle dorsiflexion and plantar flexion, without inversion and eversion, are allowed as swelling permits. These exercises should not cause pain. For patients for whom it is not possible to reapply a compressive splint, a below-the-knee plaster cast with the foot in dorsiflexion and eversion is applied for 3 weeks. The patient is allowed to put weight on the foot in the cast as tolerated.

After cast removal, a vigorous rehabilitation program is initiated.[3] Generally, rehabilitation after ankle inversion sprains consists of active ROM exercises to regain ankle dorsiflexion and plantar flexion. Inversion and eversion exercises are started as pain and motion permits (Figure 6–13). Progressive resistive exercises to strengthen the peroneal muscles are the key to successful ankle rehabilitation. Isometric exercises are added to increase strength. There

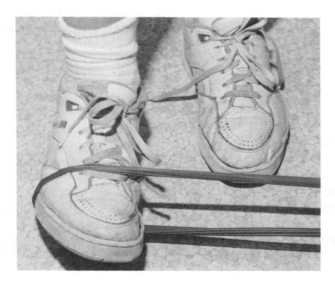

Figure 6–13 After inversion ankle sprains, the peroneal muscles are strengthened using both isometric and progressive resistive techniques, which can be performed daily. Three sets of 20 repetitions are attempted. Tension may be increased as rehabilitation progresses.

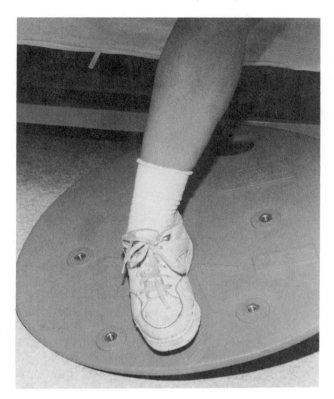

Figure 6–14 Ankle proprioceptive exercises have been shown to decrease the recurrence of inversion ankle sprains. Proprioceptive devices, such as the one shown, may be instituted under the direction of a physical therapist.

appears to be some loss of proprioception after severe ankle sprains, possibly due to damage of the stretch receptors in the anterolateral joint capsule.[29] As mobility is regained, proprioceptive exercises are used and have been shown to decrease recurrent injuries (Figure 6–14). Ice is used after exercise. For 6 months following a severe inversion sprain, a prophylactic ankle brace is worn during all cutting, pivoting, and jumping sports.[6,30]

External rotation, or eversion, ankle injuries are less common than inversion sprains. The deltoid ligament is injured, and with continued lateral rotation, disruption of the distal tibiofibular syndesmosis or fracture of the lateral malleolus is possible. Patients with flat feet are more prone to eversion or deltoid sprains, owing to the pronated and everted position of the weightbearing foot. On examination, pain and swelling are found over the anterior deltoid ligament.

Any patient with a suspected eversion and external rotation injury should be carefully examined for injury to the distal tibiofibular joint. Anteroposterior, lateral, and mortise radiographs should be taken in all ankle sprains to rule out fracture or distal tibiofibular joint disruption. If unexplained pain persists after normal recovery time (6 to 12 weeks), repeat radiographs should be taken to exclude an occult fracture. Magnetic resonance imagery is performed in patients with persistent pain and negative radiographs to assess occult articular cartilage or osteochondral injury.

Simple deltoid sprains usually heal uneventfully and do not require immobilization. Most patients recover and return to sport in 2 to 3 weeks. However, those with a distal tibiofibular syndesmosis injury can experience long-term pain and late degenerative changes due to diastasis of the ankle mortise. Patients with suspected distal tibiofibular syndesmosis sprains should not be allowed to put weight on the affected foot until the diagnosis is confirmed or ruled out, which can be accomplished in part by serial examinations during the first 2 weeks. Repeat radiographs and occasionally a bone scan may be required to diagnose injury to the distal tibiofibular ligaments.[31]

When the diagnosis of syndesmosis injury is made, the patient is kept off the affected foot for approximately 6 weeks, and this is followed by an aggressive rehabilitation program to emphasize inversion, eversion, dorsiflexion, and plantar flexion strength.

PLANTAR FASCIITIS

Heel pain is a common affliction of runners.[14] Symptomatic patients frequently will have a rather high-arched cavus foot. On examination, the hindfoot is inverted (varus) and rigid. The patient experiences tenderness over the plantar fascia medially, at its attachment to the calcaneus.[4,32] Toe walking increases the pain, owing to stretching of the plantar fascia. With the accompanying inflammation and edema, entrapment of the lateral plantar nerve may occur, causing symptoms of numbness in the lateral foot. Although heel pain is a predominant symptom, it is related to repetitive traction injury of the plantar fascia and is often not related to the heel itself.[32]

Effective treatment consists of arch support with a more rigid-soled shoe to decrease plantar fascia stretching. A slight heel lift also may decrease plantar fascial stretching, and a well-molded heel cup may provide relief by increasing the cushioning of the heel fat pad.[3,6]

Rehabilitation of plantar fasciitis consists of avoiding impact activities and stretching the plantar fascia. Occasionally, injection of corticosteroid deep into the fascia may relieve pain and swelling. However, caution is advised, as steroid extravasation into the subcutaneous fat pad over the heel may cause atrophy, with resultant functional disability.

STRESS FRACTURES

The most common lower-extremity stress fractures occur in the distal fibula and second metatarsal neck.[4] However, stress fractures are possible in all bones of the lower extremity and pelvis. Stress fractures are caused by repetitive loading of a bone unit at a rate greater than its ability to repair. Usually stress fractures occur 3 to 4 weeks following initiation of a new repetitive-loading activity, such as running or marching. Stress fractures are characterized by pain and swelling directly over the involved bone. Initial radiographs are frequently normal, but early detection of stress fractures is possible with the use of a technetium-99 bone scan.

Rehabilitation consists of elimination or reduction of the repetitive loading cycle, so that bone repair is possible. In lower-extremity injury, this unloading involves switching from higher-impact sports to bicycling or swimming. Occasionally, immobilization in a cast is required, and on rare occasions, it will be necessary to avoid placing any weight on the affected limb. Certain stress fractures are notorious for delayed healing and the need for protracted therapy or even surgical treatment. Other stress fractures, such as those to the fibula or second metatarsal neck, heal uneventfully within 6 to 8 weeks. Because of this variability, patients with stress fractures should be referred to an orthopedist. Following stress fracture healing, the patient's training activities are increased at a more gradual rate. Appropriate orthotics or shoes decrease the likelihood of future stress fracture in patients with a known anatomic abnormality.

Summary

Rehabilitation of the common orthopedic injuries seen in an outpatient setting has been described. Basically, their treatment involves rest to allow healing of the injured part followed by a controlled therapeutic exercise program. Cross-training will speed recovery and maintain the fitness of the injured patient.

REFERENCES

1. Kahl LE: Musculoskeletal problems in the family practice setting: Guidelines for curriculum design. *J Rheumatol* 1987; 14: 811–814.
2. Puffer JC, Zachazewski JE: Management of overuse injuries. *Am Fam Physician* 1988; 38:225–232.
3. Torg JS: *Rehabilitation of Athletic Injuries: An Atlas of Therapeutic Exercise.* Mosby Year-Book: St. Louis, MO, 1987.
4. Kulund DN: *The Injured Athlete,* ed 2: JB Lippincott: Philadelphia, 1988.
5. Torg JS, Wiesel SW, Rothman RH: Diagnosis and management of cervical spine injuries. In Torg JS, ed: *Athletic Injuries to the Head, Neck and Face.* Lea & Febiger: Philadelphia, 1982.
6. American Academy of Orthopedic Surgeons: *Athletic Training and Sports Medicine.* Chicago, 1984.
7. Hawkins RJ, Kennedy JC: Impingement syndrome in athletes. *Am J Sports Med* 1980; 8:151–158.
8. Matsen FA 3d, Kirby RM: Office evaluation and management of shoulder pain. *Orthop Clin North Am* 1982; 13:453–475.
9. Rowe CR, ed: *The Shoulder.* Churchill Livingstone: New York, 1988.
10. Zarins B, Andrews JR, Carson WG, eds: *Injuries to the Throwing Athlete.* WB Saunders: Philadelphia, 1985.
11. Post M, Silver R, Singh M: Rotator cuff tear: Diagnosis and treatment. *Clin Orthop* 1983; 173:78–91.
12. Jobe FW, Bradley JP: Rotator cuff injuries in baseball: Prevention and rehabilitation. *Sports Med* 1988; 6:378–387.
13. Crenshaw AH, ed: *Campbell's Operative Orthopaedics,* ed 7. Mosby Year-Book, St. Louis, 1987.
14. Lysholm J, Wiklander J: Injuries in runners. *Am J Sports Med* 1987; 15:168–171.
15. Kivi P: The etiology and conservative treatment of humeral epicondylitis. *Scand J Rehabil Med* 1983; 15:37–41.
16. Nirschl RP: Tennis elbow. *Orthop Clin North Am* 1973; 4:787–800.
17. Messier SP, Pittala KA: Etiologic factors associated with selected running injuries. *Med Sci Sports Exerc* 1988; 20:501–505.
18. O'Donoghue DH: *Treatment of Injuries to Athletes,* ed 4. WB Saunders: Philadelphia, 1984.
19. Cole WG, Gieck JH: An analysis of hamstring strain and their rehabilitation. *J Orthop Sports Phys Ther* 1987; 9:77–85.
20. Safran MR, et al.: The role of warmup in muscular injury prevention. *Am J Sports Med* 1988; 16:123–129.
21. Carer AT: Piriformis syndrome: A hidden cause of sciatic pain. *Athletic Training* 1988; 23:243–245.
22. Bourne MH, et al.: Anterior knee pain. *Mayo Clin Proc* 1988; 63:482–491.
23. Ireland ML: Patellofemoral disorders in runners and bicyclists. *Ann Sports Med* 1987; 3:77–84.
24. Zarins B, Adams M: Knee injuries in sports. *N Engl J Med* 1990; 318:950–960.
25. Indelicato PA: Non-operative treatment of complete tears of the medial collateral ligament of the knee. *J Bone Joint Surg [Am]* 1983; 65:323–329.
26. Hoppenfeld S: *Physical Examination of the Spine and Extremities.* Appleton & Lange: East Norwalk, CN, 1976.
27. Rorabeck CH, et al.: The role of tissue pressure measurement in diagnosing chronic anterior compartment syndrome. *Am J Sports Med* 1988; 16:143–146.
28. Leach RE, James S, Wasilewski S: Achilles tendinitis. *Am J Sports Med* 1981; 9:93–98.
29. Freeman MAR, Dean MRE, Hanhain IWF: The etiology and prevention of functional instability of the foot. *J Bone Joint Surg* 1985; 47B:678–685.

30. Jackson DW, Ashley RL, Powell JW: Ankle sprains in young athletes: Relation of severity and disability. *Clin Orthop* 1974; 101:201–215.

31. Marymont JV, Lynch MA, Henning CE: Acute ligamentous diastasis of the ankle without fracture: Evaluation by radionuclide imaging. *Am J Sports Med* 1986; 14:407–409.

32. Kosmahl EM, Kosmahl HE: Painful plantar heel, plantar fasciitis, and calcaneal spur: Etiology and treatment. *J Orthop Sports Phys Ther* 1987; 9:17–24.

CHAPTER 7

EXERCISE IN THE PREVENTION AND TREATMENT OF LOW BACK PAIN

RICHARD A. DEYO, MD, MPH

". . . many hospitals run a 'back class' at which spinal exercises are carried out under physiotherapists' supervision. Many hospitals order extension exercises only; others insist on flexion exercises; the chaos is complete."

—*James Cyriax, 1975*[1]

Low back pain is a pervasive problem, often estimated to afflict 60% to 80% of adults at some time in their lives.[2] Back problems are the second leading cause of all office visits to primary care physicians (internists and family physicians).[3] Back pain is the leading cause of work disability and results in

---

Supported in part by the Northwest HSR&D Field Program, Seattle VA Medical Center, and by Grant Number HS-06344 from the Agency for Health Care Policy and Research.

morbidity costs to industry (reduced productivity, absenteeism, and earnings losses) that exceed even those of ischemic heart disease.[4] Any successful intervention to prevent back pain or hasten recovery from it could have substantial economic and health impact.

Although back pain is a symptom caused by a wide variety of diseases,[5] the pathophysiology of pain is obscure in most patients.[6] Although pain can arise from many structures (e.g., ligaments, synovia, nerve roots, muscles, periostea), current diagnostic and imaging techniques rarely are successful in identifying a definite source. Fortunately, systemic diseases that cause back pain (e.g., neoplasm, infections, spondylitis) are rare and account for less than 2% of patients with back pain. Visceral causes of pain (e.g., aortic aneurysm, endometriosis, nephrolithiasis) also are relatively infrequent and that pain is not usually confused with mechanical pain. The majority of patients with back pain (probably 98%) have some form of mechanical pain, implying that there is no systemic disease or visceral etiology.[6] It is for this mechanical group that exercise may be an appropriate preventive or therapeutic intervention. The exercise recommendations discussed in this chapter are primarily intended for persons with uncomplicated mechanical pain, who have no neurologic deficits.

Mechanical pain syndromes are often subdivided according to the duration of pain into acute (0 to 6 weeks), subacute (6 weeks to 3 months), and chronic (over 3 months) types.[2] This distinction may have important therapeutic implications, assuming that systemic diseases and surgical problems (e.g., herniated disk with neurologic deficits) have been excluded. In particular, appropriate exercise recommendations may vary according to the duration of pain.

The recommendations for treatment of mechanical low back pain are currently undergoing important changes. These might be summarized as a shift from passive to active therapy.[7] The traditional view was that a patient with acute back pain required strict bed rest (for 1 to 2 weeks), subsequent activity limitations, and instructions to cut back or eliminate any activities that might cause discomfort. In contrast, the emerging view is that bed rest should be brief for most patients without neurologic deficits, that early return to activity is desirable,[8,9] and that increasing activity and exercise should be pursued even if they cause minor discomfort.[10]

The latter recommendation is supported by the work of Fordyce and colleagues,[10] who studied outpatients with acute back pain randomly assigned to one of two pain management methods. The first group was given pain-contingent instructions for medication and return to activity. The second group was given a fixed schedule for medication and activity, regardless of pain symptoms. The second group reported less pain behavior (symptoms and activity limitations) than the first. Similarly, two recent studies[8,9] from primary care practices have demonstrated no advantage of prolonged bed rest (4 to 7 days) over brief or no bed rest (0 to 2 days).

While there is a growing consensus in favor of increased activity and therapeutic exercise for persons with back pain, there is little consensus regarding the physiologic goals of exercise, the regimens to be employed, or their timing and duration. This confusion in turn reflects strong opinions and personalities in a field with a paucity of scientifically rigorous research. This chapter describes some of the competing regimens and rationales, and examines the best clinical evidence to date. It concludes with recommendations that cannot be strongly supported with evidence, but that appear reasonable given current knowledge.

Exercise Regimens, Rationales, and Physiologic Considerations

In general, exercise regimens have been designed to strengthen muscles (abdominal or paraspinal muscles), to stretch muscles and ligaments whose mobility may have been restricted by pain, or to improve overall aerobic fitness and endurance. An important theoretical concern for all regimens has been to avoid exacerbating back problems. It often has been assumed, for example, that exercise that increases pressure in the intervertebral disk may be counterproductive, since it could aggravate bulging or herniation of the nucleus pulposus. These concerns are discussed more fully below.

AEROBIC EXERCISE

Aerobic exercise often is prescribed to improve muscular endurance in patients with back pain. Persons who are not physically fit tend to fatigue rapidly when performing repetitive tasks and may therefore become more susceptible to back injury. While aerobic exercise is not primarily intended to increase strength, there is some cross-over effect, with strengthening of lower-extremity and abdominal muscles.[11]

Several secondary benefits also may accrue from aerobic exercise. First, as discussed in Chapter 10, exercise may help to reduce obesity, which is an independent risk factor for low back pain in general[12] and for disk herniation in particular.[13] Second, activities involving large muscle groups appear to increase plasma endorphins, the endogenous opiate-like substances that modulate pain perception.[14,15] However, intense or prolonged exercise may be needed to increase plasma endorphin levels,[16] and those levels may not reflect endorphin levels in the cerebrospinal fluid, which are probably more important with regard to pain reduction. Thus, this mechanism remains somewhat speculative. Third, aerobic exercise may have psychological effects that alter the perception of or response to pain. For example, as discussed in Chapter 16, exercise appears to reduce anxiety and depression,[17,18] which may prolong or amplify pain symptoms. A relaxation response follows aerobic exercise, with decreased peripheral muscle tension and electroencephalographic changes.[19] Cross-sectional data also suggest less subjective tension in more physically fit persons.[19,20] Thus, aerobic exercise may have a variety of benefits for the patient with low-back pain.

There is a theoretical concern that aerobic exercise should be chosen to avoid maneuvers that increase intradiskal pressure. On this basis, some authors caution against jogging or certain types of aerobic dance (which often requires torsion and forward flexion). Other experts argue that jogging is safe and causes no undue loading of the disk, an assertion with some physiologic support.[21,22] Furthermore, many back pain episodes may arise from lesions of the facet joints, muscles, or ligaments, in which case disk loading may be of minor importance.

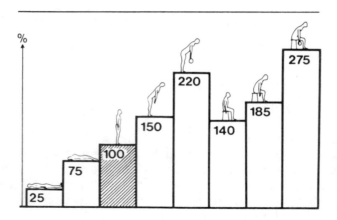

Figure 7–1 Relative pressure in the third lumbar disc, in various body positions. From Nachemson,[23] with permission.

Figure 7–1 shows intervertebral disk pressure measurements for several body positions. If we attribute some importance to these measurements, it is useful to note that disk pressure in the standing position is substantially less than in the sitting position.[23] Indeed, many patients are more comfortable standing than sitting, and resumption of sitting may be a clue that activity levels can be increased. An implication of this finding is that walking should be safer than sitting and can be prescribed even early in an acute episode of back pain. Swimming is a non-weightbearing activity that can also be prescribed with confidence.

STRETCHING EXERCISES

Several authors[24,25] have advocated stretching exercises with the rationale of improving spine mobility and limbering muscles and ligaments (in the spine and lower extremities) whose motion has been restricted in response to pain. Kraus[26,27] combined stretching exercises with relaxation exercises in a regimen that has been widely popularized by the Young Men's Christian Association (YMCA). Typical exercises from this regimen are illustrated in Figure 7–2.

FLEXION EXERCISES

Perhaps the most widely recognized exercises for back pain are the isometric flexion exercises. These were popularized by Williams[28] beginning in the 1930s. Examples of this regimen are illustrated in Figure 7–3.

The rationale for this regimen was fourfold: (1) to widen the intervertebral foramen and facet joints, reducing nerve root compression, (2) to stretch hip flexors and back extensors (thought often to be overdeveloped), (3) to strengthen the abdominal and gluteus muscles, and (4) to reduce posterior fixation of the lumbosacral junction. It was believed that abdominal muscle strengthening would create a muscular corset, reducing excessive loads on the lumbar disk. The original Williams flexion exercises have been modified and supplemented over the years, so that several variations are now common.

A theoretical concern again arises with this regimen in regard to elevations of intradiskal pressure. Direct measurements suggest that intradiskal pressure may be substantially elevated with certain flexion maneuvers,[23] as illustrated in Figure 7–4. This has led to the recommendation that isometric flexion exercises not be prescribed for patients with acute herniated disks.

EXTENSION EXERCISES

Extension principles have been most widely advocated by McKenzie.[29] McKenzie's teachings have gained popularity among physical therapists, many of whom now advocate this regimen as the primary treatment for low back pain. Again, the rationale for this program is multifaceted.

The McKenzie exercises (Figure 7–5) are intended to increase spinal mobility, to restore a normal lumbar lordosis, and to shift location of the gelatinous nucleus pulposus within the intervertebral disk. The assumption is that hyperextension produces compression of the posterior aspects of the disk, with a subsequent shift of nuclear material anteriorly, away from a bulging anulus.[30] This presumes not only that a shift of nuclear material occurs, but also that a

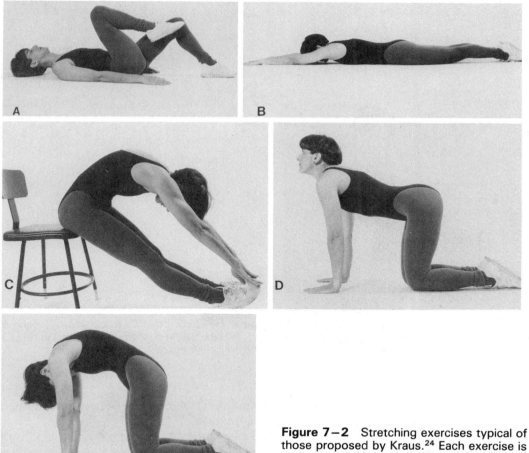

Figure 7–2 Stretching exercises typical of those proposed by Kraus.[24] Each exercise is performed two or three times, slowly. *(A)* Rotated leg stretch. *(B)* Prone stretch. *(C)* Hamstring stretch. *(D,E)* Cat back, at rest and flexed.

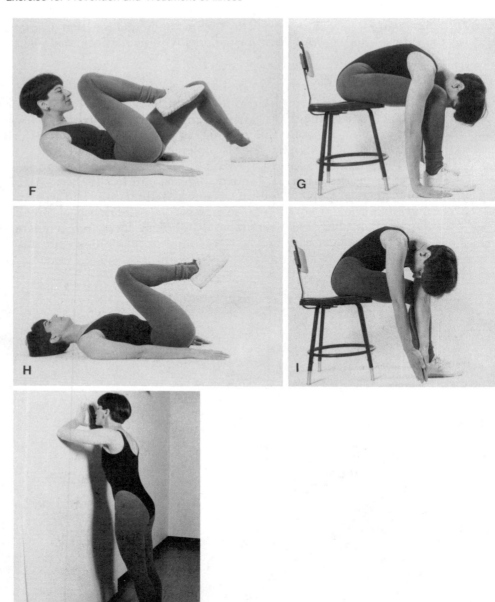

Figure 7−2, cont'd. *(F)* Knee kiss. *(G)* Bend sitting. *(H)* Double leg stretch. *(I)* Bend sitting rotation. *(J)* Heel cord stretch.

bulging disk is the cause of the pain and that reducing the bulge alleviates pain. The validity of these assumptions is unclear.

In some cases, spine extension can reduce or eliminate sciatic pain (in the leg), leaving only lumbar discomfort. This has been referred to as centralizing the pain, and suggests that extension exercises will be beneficial. If sciatica worsens with extension, the extension regimen would be contraindicated. In fact, the McKenzie program, although usually employing extension exercises, may also include flexion, lateral gliding, and rotation, depending on which direction centralizes and minimizes pain.[31] The exercise is passive and not intended for muscle strengthening.

Some investigators[30] have suggested that acute disk herniations may be successfully treated with extension exercises. Highlighting the controversy that exists over this (and most other) regimens, others[21] suggest that extension exercises are not indicated for acute disk herniations. Aside from the McKenzie program, other investigators have emphasized extension exercises for strengthening paraspinal and hip extensor muscles.

There is general agreement that extension forces the apophyseal (facet) joints into closer approximation and may be associated with some narrowing of the intervertebral foramen. Patients with spinal stenosis, lumbar scoliosis, and spondylolisthesis may have their pain aggravated by extension, and these conditions generally are contraindications to the extension regimen.

Clinical Trials of Exercise Regimens

Given the conflicting opinions about various regimens and the existence of a reasonable physiologic rationale for each opinion, it is essential to examine

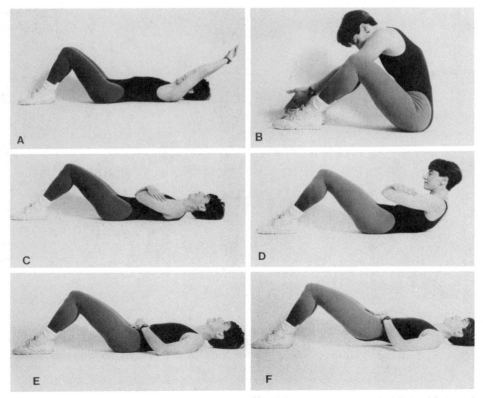

Figure 7–3 The Williams flexion exercises.[28] Williams recommended 5 to 40 repetitions of each exercise, depending on age, and one to three exercise sessions per day. *(A–D)* Starting and finishing positions of bent-leg situps, to be done either with the arms extended or folded across the chest. *(E,F)* Starting and finishing positions of hip raising.

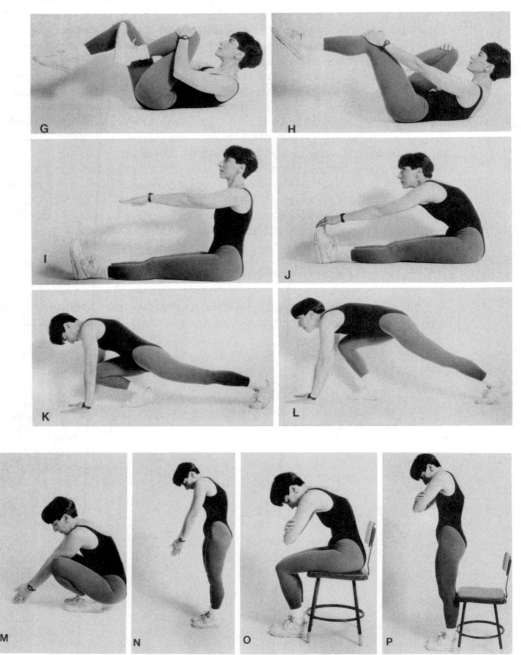

Figure 7–3, cont'd. (G,H) The trunk flexion positions, while alternately pulling the knees toward the chest. *(I,J)* From a position of sitting erect on the floor with the feet straight in front, reaching for the toes. *(K,L)* From the starting position shown, the hips are lifted, flexing the spine. *(M–P)* The upper back remains in forward flexion as the patient moves from crouching or sitting on a chair to standing.

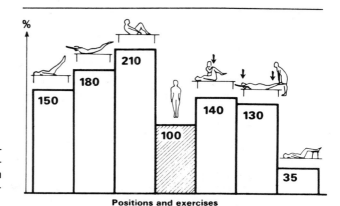

Figure 7–4 Relative intradiscal pressures during selected exercises. From Nachemson,[23] with permission.

clinical evidence for treatment efficacy. In doing so, we should acknowledge that clinician enthusiasm, encouragement, and placebo effects may all result in dramatic clinical improvements. Furthermore, the natural history of acute low back pain is to improve spontaneously in the majority of cases. At least two thirds of patients are substantially improved in 2 weeks,[32,33] and 75% to 90% are improved in 4 weeks.[33] To judge whether any treatment is better than placebo effect plus natural history, it is necessary to examine randomized, controlled trials.

Unfortunately, there are few controlled exercise trials for low back pain, and many published studies have substantial methodologic flaws that confuse their interpretation.[34] We have previously proposed a set of criteria by which to evaluate such trials, adapted from the suggestions of other methodologists.[35] We have evaluated most available randomized trials of exercise for back pain according to such criteria, and summarize their methodologic features in the following discussion.

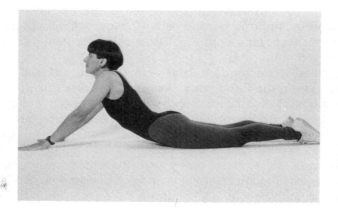

Figure 7–5 An example of an extension exercise similar to the McKenzie regimen. The program is highly individualized, depending on how the specific patient's pain responds to various exercises and positions. For this exercise, the arms are used to raise and lower the upper trunk, while the back and abdominal muscles are relaxed. The intent is to achieve passive, end-range, gravity-assisted lordosis.

AEROBIC EXERCISE

To date, no randomized trials of aerobic exercise for back pain have been reported. The growing enthusiasm for this regimen is largely based on the cohort studies of Cady and coworkers[36,37] among Los Angeles fire fighters. These studies addressed the efficacy of aerobic conditioning in the primary prevention of back pain or in prevention of recurrences of back pain. They reported fitness data for 1,652 fire fighters, based on cycle ergometry, isometric strength of selected muscle groups, and spine flexibility. After follow-up of uncertain duration, it was observed that in the one sixth who were most fit, only 0.8% suffered subsequent back injuries; in those of intermediate fitness, 3.2% had back injuries; and in the one sixth who were least fit, 7.1% had back injuries. Among a smaller group (of uncertain size) with previous back problems, no recurrences were observed among the most fit, while one third of the least fit had recurrences.

An ongoing trial of aerobic exercise in Sweden may provide support for this regimen as therapy for those with back pain. Although only preliminary results are available (in lay publications),[38] those results are promising. This study examined employees of a Volvo automotive assembly line who missed work because of back pain. Half received usual care and the other half were encouraged to promptly begin aerobic exercise, which could be walking, jogging, or swimming. Among the first 106 subjects enrolled, the active group returned to work an average of several weeks faster than the usual care group. After 2 years of follow-up, the usual care group missed an average of 20 weeks more from work than the active group.[38] Further details in a scientific report will be necessary to evaluate these findings critically.

STRETCHING EXERCISES

Again, few scientific reports of randomized trials have been reported for a regimen of stretching exercises. Some evidence for its value came from the 6-week YMCA program of group instruction. The regimen began with a sequence of relaxation exercises, followed by a program that was partly individualized, based on an initial series of strength and flexibility tests. Kraus and his colleagues[26,27] reported on pain ratings at the first and last session of the program for 11,809 persons at 800 different sites. Most had chronic back problems (average, 8 years), but remained relatively functional, as judged by the apparently high rate of continued employment. At the end of the 6-week program, 80.7% reported improvement in pain. However, there was no control group, and placebo effects plus natural history certainly could account for much of the improvement.

We have reported a randomized trial of a program adapted from the YMCA's.[39] This trial used the three relaxation exercises described by Kraus,[24] but only nine additional stretching exercises, which were prescribed uniformly for all subjects. The control group was prescribed no exercise but received instruction in back care, application of local heat, and equally frequent follow-up (twice weekly for 2 weeks). Of 125 subjects who completed the trial, all with chronic back problems, the exercise group reported significantly greater improvement in pain severity, pain frequency, and self-assessed level of activity. Unfortunately, most subjects did not continue exercising after the 4-week intervention, and group differences were lost 2 months later. Thus, the trial suggested at least modest subjective improvements, but it appeared that continuing efforts would be necessary to maintain patient compliance with the exercise regimen.

FLEXION EXERCISES

At least three randomized trials of isometric flexion exercise regimens have been reported, with conflicting results. Although the apparent contradictions could be a result of different study populations, this remans uncertain. The first trial was reported in 1968 by Kendall and Jenkins,[40] from a physical therapy clinic. The 47 subjects were randomly allocated to one of three exercise regimens: mobilizing exercises, isometric flexion exercises, or extension exercises. The patient sample was not described, except to say that the subjects had "long-standing backache" and no evidence of systemic disease or spondylolisthesis. "The majority" had suffered from symptoms for over 1 year. After 3 months of therapy, there was significantly greater improvement in symptoms among the subjects in the flexion group than in either of the other regimens. In the extension group, 5 of 14 were said to be worse, as were 2 of 14 in the mobilizing group, and none in the flexion group.

A decade later, Davies and colleagues[41] sought to replicate several aspects of the Kendall and Jenkins study. Their trial included 47 subjects with subacute back pain (greater than 3 weeks' duration but less than 6 months), who were randomly allocated to isometric flexion exercises, extension exercises, or no exercise. All three groups received short-wave diathermy. The subjects were young adults (mean age, 25 years); only 21% were unable to work at entry, and all resumed their normal work during the trial. No significant differences were observed among the groups in outcomes (pain relief, time to resume work, or time to resume sporting activities). Nonetheless, both exercise regimens resulted in a larger percentage of improved subjects than the nonexercise regimen (93% for extension, 86% for flexion, and 66% for nonexercise), and low statistical power may have prevented the results from achieving significance. Three patients were initially worse with flexion exercises (only one withdrew), and none were made worse by extension exercises.

The most recent trial[9] was conducted in a primary care setting (Canadian family physician practices) with a somewhat older patient sample (mean age, 41 years). These subjects (n = 252) had acute pain, with most episodes less than 6 days in duration. Patients were randomized to follow an isometric flexion exercise regimen (not further described) or no exercises. Those in the exercise group reported stopping drug therapy significantly sooner than the nonexercise group, but also had a significantly slower recovery of activities of daily living. There was a trend against the exercise regimen for range of motion and pain severity. By 6 weeks of follow-up, no differences in pain or activity reports were observed. Little information regarding exercise compliance was available.

In summary, these data suggest a potential benefit for flexion exercises among persons with chronic or subacute pain, but no benefit in primary care patients with acute back pain.

EXTENSION EXERCISES

The previous section on flexion exercise described two trials that compared flexion and extension regimens with somewhat differing results, one reporting a significant advantage for flexion exercise and one reporting no significant difference between regimens, but with a trend favoring extension exercises.

A recent study[42] of extension principles used an intensive regimen for 105 subjects with chronic low back pain. These patients had a median age of 45 years, and median pain duration of 15 years, yet 78% were still employed. They were randomized to receive one of three regimens: (1) a combination of isometric extension and flexion exercises with moderate intensity, taught in eight sessions over 1 month, (2) an intensive extension exercise regimen given in 30 sessions over 3 months, and (3) a mild version of the group 2 regimen with one-fifth the number of repetitions. The intensive extension regimen consisted of three exercises. Trunk lifting was performed with the patient lying prone on a couch and the trunk hanging free over the edge, supported by hands against the floor. With hands on forehead, the trunk was lifted to the greatest possible extent. Leg lifting was performed standing at the edge of the couch with the trunk leaning prone on the couch. The legs were then lifted bilaterally to the greatest possible extension of hips and spine. The pull to neck required sitting on a stool, grasping a weighted pulley device overhead, and pulling the weight down behind the neck and shoulders. Each exercise was performed 50 times, in series of 10 attempts with 1-minute rests in between.

Outcomes of the intensive exercise regimen were superior to the other regimens with regard to pain relief, activity limitation, and physiologic measures (muscle endurance and spine mobility). The authors emphasized that improvement was only apparent after about 2 months of treatment, as many patients noted increased discomfort from muscle fatigue and tenderness in the first month. The authors also noted the need for close supervision by a physical therapist during the first few months of this intensive regimen.

More recently, the McKenzie method has been evaluated in a randomized trial.[43] This study compared the McKenzie method (average, 5.5 treatment sessions) with a single-session educational program on low-back pain.[43] An advantage was reported for the McKenzie method in speed of return to work, recurrence rate, and total work absenteeism. However, the authors pointed out that some of the benefit may simply have resulted from nonspecific benefits of increased contact and attention in the McKenzie group.

OTHER IMPORTANT STUDIES

Some additional randomized trials of exercises for low back pain have been reported. Unfortunately, the studies of Coxhead and colleagues[44] and White[45] did not describe the exercise regimens tested and both were negative trials (exercises not superior to alternative treatments). The study of Lidstrom and Zachrisson[46] included two regimens with a combination of exercise types. Neither regimen was clearly superior to a nonexercise treatment group. None of these three trials discussed the potential problem of insufficient statistical power (too few subjects) to detect a clinically meaningful difference.

In 1987, a task force was commissioned by the province of Quebec to assess the literature on treatment of back pain and make recommendations for the management of occupational back problems.[47] After applying a set of methodologic criteria to the existing published literature, the task force provided a summary conclusion about current knowledge on the efficacy of various treatments, including strengthening exercises and stretching exercises. The task force members concluded that stretching exercises were commonly prescribed, but that no scientific evidence supported their use (prior to a more recent supportive trial).[39] Although they concluded that strengthening exercises were supported for certain subgroups by nonrandomized trials but not by convincing randomized studies, this conclusion preceded a recent well-designed trial.[42] The value of strengthening exercise was judged to be best demonstrated for persons with pain of greater than 7 weeks' duration, for postoperative patients, and for those with chronic pain syndromes. Unfortunately, no distinction was made between flexion and extension exercises.

A formal literature synthesis[48] detailed methodologic flaws in the existing literature and reached a similar conclusion. While the authors concluded that the efficacy of exercise for low back pain remains unclear, they also noted that the positive clinical trials tended to be better designed than the negative trials. They further observed that little evidence favors any particular exercise regimen.

Nonrandomized cohort studies[49,50] have suggested that intensive mixed exercise programs may be useful for patients with chronic back pain and work disability. These programs typically combine fitness, stretching, and strengthening exercises under frequent supervision. Randomized trials are not yet available.

Clinical Recommendations

GENERAL APPROACH TO BACK PAIN THERAPY

Those who are at greater risk to develop back pain share certain risk factors, including both obesity and cigarette smoking.[12,13,51,52] Evidence suggests that smoking cessation can reduce the risk of back pain.[12,52] Also, weight reduction (in overweight persons) may reduce the frequency and severity of back pain. In general, the emphasis in back pain therapy has shifted from prolonged bed rest to more active therapy.

Back pain can be subdivided into acute, subacute, and chronic conditions, each with prognostic implications, and this can influence therapeutic decisions. Exercise typically is used as one component of acute and subacute back pain therapy, with other common aspects, including brief bed rest and administration of nonsteroidal anti-inflammatory drugs (NSAIDs) and occasionally muscle relaxants.[34,47] Treatment for chronic low-back pain is usually complex, including multidisciplinary approaches to physical therapy, behavioral therapy, and drug therapy, in addition to exercise.[53]

Patients need to be reassured that most back problems are not disabling and that the prognosis for returning to regular activities is excellent. Increased activity that causes mild to moderate pain will not cause permanent harm and does not require activity limitation. When patients are advised to "let pain be your guide," the outcomes may be worse than when patients are given specific activity goals regardless of discomfort.[10] It is important to remember that compliance with any exercise regimen is problematic. While it may be true that sedentary persons benefit most, they also are least likely to follow an exercise program. Compliance will be enhanced by providing both verbal and written instructions[54] and by close supervision (more frequent follow-up).[55]

ACUTE BACK PAIN (LESS THAN 6 WEEKS' DURATION)

Bed rest may provide temporary symptomatic relief for individuals with acute mechanical low back pain, but probably does not alter the course of recovery. Bed rest recommendations (if any) should therefore be brief, with 2 to 3 days sufficient for most. Some ambulation can be permitted during this time, to limit muscular and cardiovascular deconditioning. Since standing results in smaller loads on the intervertebral disk than sitting, patients can be encouraged to begin walking regularly after bed rest is complete. After the acute episode has subsided (usually within 2 weeks), more rigorous aerobic conditioning should be recommended for most, as a means of preventing recurrence. The rationale is to improve muscle endurance, making subsequent strain less likely. A beneficial strengthening effect for the abdominal and lower-extremity muscles also will result.

When initiating an aerobic fitness program, the clinician should consider the patient's current level of fitness and comorbid conditions (such as cardiovascular disease or musculoskeletal limitation).[11] Recommendations for beginning this type of conditioning are provided in Chapter 1. The goals should be directed at achieving the functional level necessary for vocational or recreational pursuits, which should be a level achieved by the patient in the recent past.[11]

The specific aerobic mode is probably unimportant. Swimming, walking, jogging, and bicycling are all appropriate and can be prescribed according to patient preference. However, exercises that result in major twisting or bending forces on the spine (e.g., rowing, certain types of aerobic dance) need to be individually evaluated. Exercise sessions typically require at least 30 to 40 minutes, including warm-up and cool-down periods, with the aerobic component occupying at least 20 minutes. A minimum of three weekly exercise sessions (preferably five) are recommended. The warm-up and cool-down sessions should include muscle stretching, such as the exercises used by the YMCA.[24,26,27]

Patients with a neurologic deficit require different recommendations. These patients are likely to have a true herniated disk, and initial bed rest may need to be stricter and longer (about 1 week). Intermittent ambulation still may be advised to prevent the complications of prolonged rest. The management is highly individualized and is based on progression or improvement in the neurologic deficit. *If deficits persist for 6 weeks, surgical intervention is a reasonable consideration.* Even for surgical candidates, mild exercise such as walking may be advisable, since deconditioned patients may not tolerate surgery and later rehabilitation well.

SUBACUTE BACK PAIN (6 TO 12 WEEKS' DURATION)

This is an important clinical group, for whom optimal management may prevent the emergence of chronic pain syndromes. As most patients with acute back pain have improved by 6 weeks, this also is a group that has already demonstrated a worse-than-average clinical course. For these patients, referral to a physical therapist, back school, or YMCA program is appropriate. Although aerobic conditioning and stretching exercises can be helpful, the activities require supervision and greater adherence.

> **CASE:** R.P., a 42-year-old man, presented to the occupational health clinic in the hospital where he worked. He had a history of moderately severe back pain of nearly 4 months' duration, with two previous acute episodes. He had no symptoms of sciatica. He reported 3 days of overall activity limitation and 60 days of limited household activities in the 3 previous months.
>
> On physical examination, he was 180 cm (6') tall and weighed 99 kg (220 lb). Results of the neurologic examination were normal. Measured body composition was 27% fat.
>
> The patient entered a worksite exercise program that included both stretching and spinal extension exercises, as well as aerobic conditioning, three times weekly. After 6 months, he weighed 94 kg (210 lb), and body composition had fallen to 22% fat. Aerobic capacity, spinal flexion and abdominal and back strength were substantially increased. He reported that the pain was "much better" and that he had not limited his activities at all in the preceding 3 months.
>
> **COMMENT:** Like most persons with low back pain, this patient did not have a specific pathoanatomic diagnosis, and there was no neurologic impairment. He experienced weight loss, strength gains, and improved fitness, all of which may have helped to reduce the pain and enhance his overall activity level. This case illustrates the potential benefits of an exercise regimen that combines several physiologic goals.

An extension exercise program such as that described by McKenzie[29] probably should be added for individuals with subacute back pain. Those with radiating pain (to the leg) that centralizes on extension are certainly candidates, as well as those with simple back pain. This regimen should be avoided if pain is aggravated by extension, or if the patient clearly has spinal stenosis, spondylolisthesis, or moderate scoliosis. Supervision by a physical therapist is optimal, although the exercise in Figure 7–5 can be used with instructions to perform 10 repetitions, along with other extension exercises, in a single daily session.

CHRONIC BACK PAIN (MORE THAN 3 MONTHS' DURATION)

This group has a less favorable prognosis for recovery than those with pain of shorter duration, and there may be barriers to improvement, such as job dissatisfaction, substance abuse, psychological problems, symptom amplification, and financial disincentives.[53] Treatment of those with chronic low back pain should not be prescribed solely based on the reported association of pain with specific activities, as these individuals' symptoms do not generally correlate with measured physical performance.[56] Such patients can benefit from a formal, structured pain management program. Many such programs now advocate functional restoration, emphasizing a combination of aerobic and strengthening exercises.[53] Based on the work of Manniche and colleagues,[42] these patients can improve with extension exercises. Because these are quite strenuous, require specialized equipment, and demand supervision by a trained therapist, referral is usually necessary. In general, the focus of formal pain treatment programs has become the resumption of function.

> **CASE:** E.D., a 38-year-old woman, had a 4½-year history of back pain, with constant pain at the time of presentation. A computed tomography scan done 3 years previously showed a herniated disk at L5-S1, but she had been treated conservatively, without surgery. She was receiving NSAIDs, and in the past had been treated with corsets, chiropractic manipulation, and acupuncture. At the present time she had no symptoms of sciatica.
>
> Physical examination revealed normal findings on neurologic examination but limited spinal flexion. Plain spine films revealed a narrowed L5-S1 interspace.
>
> The patient began a stretching exercise regimen adapted from the program of Kraus and the YMCA. After 1 month, she reported that her pain was 95% better and occurred only occasionally. Spinal flexion was slightly increased.
>
> **COMMENT:** This patient showed a dramatic subjective improvement with a relatively nonintensive intervention. Despite the chronicity of pain, some of the improvement may have been due to placebo effects and the natural history of the disease. Nonetheless the stretching exercise regimen does appear to be associated with reduced frequency and severity of pain, and is readily available at many YMCAs.

While many persons enrolled in the treatment studies described here have apparently done well, they represent a highly selected and highly motivated subset of all persons with chronic low back pain. The challenge for primary care physicians in many cases will be to motivate and elicit the active participation of patients in such programs.

Summary

Low back pain is a common problem, and most is due to uncomplicated mechanical problems. Although few scientifically rigorous studies have documented the effectiveness of exercise as a treatment or prevention for low back pain, most reports support the view that a carefully chosen exercise regimen is likely to be more effective than bed rest in improving the patient's functioning, particularly if there is no neurologic deficit. A program of aerobic conditioning is helpful to many and appears to reduce the likelihood of recurrence of the pain. Patients with subacute or chronic pain frequently benefit from the addition of a specialized exercise regimen involving stretching, extension, or flexion. Although long-term compliance is often a problem, this can be overcome with written instructions, supervision, and close follow-up.

REFERENCES

1. Cyriax J: *Textbook of Orthopaedic Medicine*, ed 6. Williams & Wilkins: Baltimore, 1975, p 513.
2. Framer JW: Back pain and sciatica. *N Engl J Med* 1988; 318:291–300.
3. Cypress BK: Characteristics of physician visits for back symptoms: A national perspective. *Am J Public Health* 1983; 73:389–395.
4. Salkever DS: *Morbidity Costs: National Esti-*

mates and Economic Determinants. Washington DC: NCHSR Summary Series; October 1985. US Dept of Health and Human Services publication (PHS) 86-3393, pp 1-13.

5. Deyo RA: Early diagnostic evaluation of low back pain. *J Gen Intern Med* 1986; 1: 328-338.

6. White AA 3d, Gordon SL: Synopsis: Workshop on idiopathic low-back pain. *Spine* 1982; 7:141-149.

7. Waddell G: A new clinical model for the treatment of low back pain. *Spine* 1987; 12:632-644.

8. Deyo RA, Diehl AK, Rosenthal M: How many days of bed rest for acute low back pain? A randomized clinical trial. *N Engl J Med* 1986; 315:1064-1070.

9. Gilbert JR, et al.: Clinical trial of common treatments for low back pain in family practice. *BMJ* 1985; 291:791-794.

10. Fordyce WE, et al.: Acute back pain: A control-group comparison of behavioral vs traditional management methods. *J Behav Med* 1986; 9:127-140.

11. Nutter P: Aerobic exercise in the treatment and prevention of low back pain. *Occup Med* 1988; 3:137-145.

12. Deyo RA, Bass JE: Lifestyle and low-back pain: The influence of smoking and obesity. *Spine* 1989; 14:501-506.

13. Heliovaara M: Body height, obesity, and risk of herniated lumbar intervertebral disc. *Spine* 1987; 12:469-472.

14. Colt EW, Wardlaw SL, Frantz AG: The effect of running on plasma β-endorphin. *Life Sci* 1981; 28:1637-1640.

15. Fraioli F, et al.: Physical exercise stimulates marked concomitant release of β-endorphin and adrenocorticotropic hormone (ACTH) in peripheral blood in man. *Experientia* 1980; 36:987-989.

16. Rahkila P, et al.: Beta-endorphin and corticotropin release is dependent on a threshold intensity of running exercise in male endurance athletes. *Life Sci* 1988; 43:551-558.

17. Romano JM, Turner JA: Chronic pain and depression: Does the evidence support a relationship? *Psychol Bull* 1985; 97:18-34.

18. Blumenthal JA, et al.: Psychological changes accompany aerobic exercise in healthy middle-aged adults. *Psychosom Med* 1982; 44:529-536.

19. Dishman RK: Medical psychology in exercise and sport. *Med Clin North Am* 1985; 69:123-143.

20. Sinyor D, et al.: Aerobic fitness level and reactivity to psychosocial stress: Physiological, biochemical, and subjective measures. *Psychosom Med* 1983; 45:205-217.

21. Jackson CP, Brown MD: Analysis of current approaches and a practical guide to prescription of exercise. *Clin Orthop* 1983; 179:46-54.

22. Bigos SJ, Battié MC: Acute care to prevent back disability: Ten years of progress. *Clin Orthop* 1987; 221:121-130.

23. Nachemson A: The lumbar spine: An orthopedic challenge. *Spine* 1976; 1:59-71.

24. Kraus H: *Backache, Stress and Tension: Cause, Prevention and Treatment.* Simon and Schuster: New York, 1965.

25. Tollison CD, Kriegel ML: Physical exercise in the treatment of low back pain, II: A practical regimen of stretching exercise. *Orthop Rev* 1988; 17:913-923.

26. Kraus H, Nagler W, Melleby A: Evaluation of an exercise program for back pain. *Am Fam Physician* 1983; 28:153-158.

27. Kraus H, Melleby A, Gaston SR: Back pain correction and prevention: National voluntary organizational approach. *NY State J Med* 1977; 77:1335-1338.

28. Williams PC: *The Lumbosacral Spine, Emphasizing Conservative Management.* McGraw-Hill: New York, 1965, pp 80-93.

29. McKenzie RA: Prophylaxis in recurrent low back pain. *N Z Med J* 1979; 89:22-23.

30. Kopp JR, et al.: The use of lumbar extension in the evaluation and treatment of patients with acute herniated nucleus pulposus: A preliminary report. *Clin Orthop* 1986; 202:211-218.

31. Donelson R: The McKenzie approach to evaluating and treating low back pain. *Orthop Rev* 1990; 19:681-686.

32. Roland M, Morris R: A study of the natural history of low-back pain, II: Development of guidelines for trials of treatment in primary care. *Spine* 1983; 8:145-150.

33. Dillane JB, Fry J, Kalton G: Acute back syndrome: A study from general practice. *BMJ* 1966; 2:82.

34. Deyo RA: Conservative therapy for low back pain: Distinguishing useful from useless therapy. *JAMA* 1983; 250:1057-1062.

35. Department of Clinical Epidemiology and Biostatistics, McMaster University Health Sciences Center: How to read clinical journals, V: To distinguish useful from useless or even harmful therapy. *Can Med Assoc J* 1981; 124:1156-1162.

36. Cady LD Jr, Thomas PC, Karwasky RJ: Program for increasing health and physical fitness of fire fighters. *J Occup Med* 1985; 27:110-114.

37. Cady L, et al.: Strength and fitness and subsequent back injuries in firefighters. *J Occup Med* 1979; 21:269-272.

38. Monmaney T: Bouncing back from bad backs. *Newsweek* 1988; October 24.

39. Deyo RA, et al.: A controlled trial of transcutaneous electrical nerve stimulation (TENS) and exercise for chronic low back pain. *N Engl J Med* 1990; 322:1627-1634.

40. Kendall PH, Jenkins JM: Exercise for backache: A double-blind controlled trial. *Physiotherapy* 1968; 54:154-157.

41. Davies JE, Gibson T, Tester L: The value of exercises in the treatment of low back pain. *Rheumatol Rehabil* 1979; 18:243-247.

42. Manniche C, et al.: Clinical trial of intensive muscle training for chronic low back pain. *Lancet* 1988; 2:1473-1476.

43. Stankovic R, Johnell O: Conservative treatment of acute low back pain: A prospective randomized trial: McKenzie method of treatment versus patient education in "mini back school." *Spine* 1990; 15:120–123.

44. Coxhead CE, et al.: Multicentre trial of physiotherapy in the management of sciatic symptoms. *Lancet* 1981; 1:1065–1068.

45. White AWM: Low back pain in men receiving workmen's compensation. *Can Med Assoc J* 1966; 95:50–56.

46. Lidstrom A, Zachrisson M: Physical therapy on low back pain and sciatica: An attempt at evaluation. *Scand J Rehabil Med* 1970; 2:37–42.

47. Quebec Task Force on Spinal Disorders: Scientific approach to the assessment and management of activity-related spinal disorders: A monograph for clinicians. *Spine* 1987; 12(7:Suppl): S1–S59.

48. Koes BW, et al.: Physiotherapy exercises and back pain: A blinded review. *BMJ* 1991; 302:1572–1576.

49. Mitchell RI, Carmen GM: Results of a multicenter trial using an intensive active exercise program for the treatment of acute soft tissue and back injuries. *Spine* 1990; 15: 514–521.

50. Mayer TG, et al.: A prospective two-year study of functional restoration in industrial low back injury: An objective assessment procedure. *JAMA* 1987; 258:1763–1767.

51. Frymoyer JW, et al.: Epidemiologic studies of low-back pain. *Spine* 1980; 5:419–423.

52. Kelsey JL, et al.: Acute prolapsed lumbar intervertebral disc: An epidemiologic study with special reference to driving automobiles and cigarette smoking. *Spine* 1984; 9:608–613.

53. Mayer TG, Gatchel RJ: *Functional Restoration for Spinal Disorders: The Sports Medicine Approach.* Lea & Febiger: Philadelphia, 1988.

54. Glossop ES, et al.: Patient compliance in back and neck pain. *Physiotherapy* 1982; 68:225–226.

55. Sackett DL, Haynes RB, Tugwell P: *Clinical Epidemiology: A Basic Science for Clinical Medicine.* Little, Brown: Boston, 1985, pp 199–222.

56. Rainville J, et al.: The association of pain with physical activities in chronic low back pain. *Spine* 1992; 17:1060–1064.

PART IV

Metabolic Disorders

CHAPTER **8**

EXERCISE IN THE MANAGEMENT OF DIABETES MELLITUS

BARBARA N. CAMPAIGNE, PhD

EXERCISE, GLUCOSE,
   AND INSULIN
EFFECTS OF PHYSICAL TRAINING
   Type I Diabetes
   Type II Diabetes
   Insulin Sensitivity
   Lipids and Lipoproteins

CLINICAL RECOMMENDATIONS
   Screening

Management of the
   Complications of Diabetes
Glycemic Control
Insulin Absorption
Food Intake for Exercise
Timing of Exercise
Competition for the
   Individual with Diabetes

Exercise long has been known to benefit individuals with diabetes mellitus. Around 600 B.C., Indian physicians noted that the urine glucose was lowered when patients walked.[1] Prior to the discovery of insulin, exercise and diet were the sole means of treating diabetes mellitus. In 1916, Allen and colleagues[2] published the initial studies on the effects of exercise, concluding that physical activity complemented dietary management of diabetes. Despite these historical notes, only recently have researchers examined the glucose homeostasis adaptations to physical training. This chapter reviews the effects of exercise on diabetes and its complications, and the use of physical activity in managing diabetic patients.

Exercise, Glucose, and Insulin

Among normal individuals, physical activity affects both hepatic glucose output and glucose uptake by exercising muscle.[3] As shown in Table 8–1, during exercise, hepatic glucose output rises in both normal controls[4] (Situa-

Acknowledgments:
The author would like to gratefully acknowledge Margie DeHo for the careful typing of the manuscript.

Table 8–1 **THE EFFECTS OF THE STATE OF INSULINIZATION ON BLOOD GLUCOSE DURING EXERCISE**

Situation	Plasma Insulin	Hepatic Production	Muscle Uptake	Blood Glucose
1*	Normal	Increased	Increased	Maintained
2†	Acutely deficient	Increased	Reduced	High
3‡	Chronically deficient	Reduced	Reduced	Low

*Normal controls.
†Nonketotic diabetic individuals.
‡Newly diagnosed diabetic patient with long-standing insulin deficiency.

tion 1) and in nonketotic diabetic individuals (Situation 2). Situation 3 shows the effects of exercise in a newly diagnosed patient with diabetes and long-standing insulin deficiency. In that situation, hepatic glycogen is depleted, resulting in inadequate liver glucose production during exertion.[5,6] Because of reduced glycogen stores, exercise-induced hypoglycemia can occur in these individuals.

Soon after the discovery of insulin, it was noted that insulin requirements diminished immediately following exercise,[7] but it was not until the early 1980s that exercise effects were systematically investigated. An early study[8] quantified the effects of exercise on meal-induced glycemic changes. Subjects were undergoing standard insulin treatment by multiple subcutaneous injections (MSI). For the majority, 45 minutes of moderate exercise after breakfast prevented hyperglycemia induced by both breakfast and lunch. Individual responses varied in this investigation, however, and not all patients demonstrated the effect. Another study of 10 MSI-treated subjects measured the 12-hour plasma insulin and glucose response to moderate (60% of maximal oxygen uptake [VO_{2max}]) exercise.[9] This trial confirmed the variability of the response to physical activity, underscoring the need to individualize recommendations for exercise in patients with diabetes. Recommendations will depend on both the activity (intensity and duration) and the pre-exercise blood glucose level.

Continuous subcutaneous insulin infusion (CSII) is used to manage diabetes for some patients. When studied, these individuals generally did not develop hypoglycemia after exercising in the postabsorptive state (after meals).[10] A group of such individuals showed no differences in plasma glucose or insulin levels 2 hours after breakfast on days when they exercised, as compared with a control, nonexercise day.[11] The researchers concluded that tightly controlled patients treated with CSII who performed 30 minutes of mild (30% to 40% VO_{2max}) or moderate (50% to 60% VO_{2max}) exercise 2 to 3 hours after a meal were not at an increased risk of developing hypoglycemia. However, some CSII patients may require changes in insulin infusion to prevent hypoglycemia (Table 8–2).

The immediate effects of exercise on blood glucose appear to be unaffected by training. Prior to training, the reduction in blood glucose following a bout of exercise was similar to that which occurred after both 6 and 12 weeks of regular aerobic conditioning.[12] Although there was no change in insulin dose, caloric intake was significantly increased on exercise days. This study supports

Table 8–2 **GUIDELINES FOR AVOIDING HYPOGLYCEMIA DURING AND AFTER EXERCISE**

Blood Glucose Monitoring
1. Monitor blood glucose immediately before, during (every 30 minutes), and 15 minutes after exercise.
2. Delay exercise if blood glucose level is 250 mg/dL or greater or if ketones are present.
3. Consume carbohydrates if blood glucose level is less than 90 mg/dL.
4. Learn individual glucose response to different types of exercise.
5. Avoid exercising late at night.

Insulin Therapy
1. Decrease the insulin dose.
   a. Intermediate-acting insulin: Decrease by 30%–35% on the day of exercise.
   b. Intermediate-acting and short-acting insulin: Omit dose of short-acting insulin that precedes exercise.
   c. Multiple doses of short-acting insulin: Reduce the dose prior to exercise by 30%–35% and supplement with carbohydrates.
   d. Continuous subcutaneous infusion: Eliminate mealtime bolus or increment that precedes or immediately follows exercise.
2. Avoid exercising muscle underlying injections of short-acting insulin for 1 hour after injection.
3. Do not exercise at the time of peak insulin action.

Adapted from Vitug et al.[19]

the observation that initiating regular exercise in diabetic individuals may require close monitoring of diet to maintain metabolic control. Reducing the insulin dose or increasing dietary intake can prevent exercise-induced hypoglycemia during the 12-hour period after exertion. Suggestions for food adjustments are listed in Table 8–3.

Effects of Physical Training

Only limited information is available on the long-term effects of exercise on mortality among diabetic individuals. Data from the Joslin Clinic [14] concerning 48 patients with 25 years of follow-up indicated that men who developed complications reported a lower frequency of physical activity, when compared with those who were complication-free. More recently, insulin-dependent diabetic patients were found to have a lower mortality and incidence of macrovascular disease when they had engaged in team sports in high school and college than did their sedentary counterparts.[13]

Exercise also may be effective in protecting against the development of noninsulin-dependent diabetes mellitus (NIDDM). A longitudinal epidemiologic study of adult men found that physical activity reduced the risk for developing diabetes, even when adjusted for obesity, hypertension, and parental history of diabetes.[15]

Several reviews[16–20] have been published concerning physical training and diabetes. Table 8–4 summarizes recent reports on the adaptation to physical training in patients with type I diabetes, or insulin-dependent diabetes mellitus (IDDM).

TYPE I DIABETES

Regular exercise has not consistently improved indices of glucose control among patients with IDDM. One of the first investigations[21] described the effects of regular activity among six adolescent diabetic boys during 6 months

Table 8-3 **GUIDELINES FOR FOOD ADJUSTMENTS TO PREVENT EXERCISE-INDUCED HYPOGLYCEMIA**

Type of Exercise	Blood Glucose	Adjustments to Food Intake or Insulin	Food Suggestions
Low to moderate intensity, short duration (e.g., walking ½ mile, leisurely bicycling <30 minutes)	<90 mg/dL	10–15 g carbohydrate per hour	One fruit or one bread exchange
Moderate intensity (e.g., tennis, swimming, jogging, leisurely bicycling, gardening, golfing, vacuuming for 1 hour)	≥90 mg/dL	Not necessary to increase food	
	<90 mg/dL	25–50 mg carbohydrate before exercise, then 10–15 g/hr of exercise	Half a meat sandwich with a milk or fruit exchange
	90–240 mg/dL	10–15 g carbohydrate per hour of exercise; not necessary to increase food	One fruit or one bread exchange
	≥250 mg/dL	Check for ketones; if ketotic, take supplemental insulin, do not begin exercise until blood glucose is under better control and ketones are negative	
Strenuous exercise (e.g., football, hockey, racquetball, soccer, running, strenuous bicycling or swimming, shoveling heavy snow)	<90 mg/dL	50 g carbohydrate; monitor blood glucose carefully	One meat sandwich (two slices bread) with a milk and fruit exchange
	90–170 mg/dL	25–50 mg carbohydrate, depending on intensity and duration	Half meat sandwich with a milk or fruit exchange
	180–250 mg/dL	10–15 g carbohydrate per hour of exercise	One fruit or one bread exchange

Modified from Etzwiler DD, et al.: *Learning to Live Well with Diabetes*. D.C.I.: Minnetonka, MN, 1987.

of a gymnastics program. Exercise was conducted for 1 hour, once a week. No change in mean glucose levels was seen after the 6-month program. However, other researchers have shown significant decreases in glycosylated hemoglobin levels (HbA$_1$) after physical training among children.[22,23] In one of these studies,[23] no additional interventions (such as advice on glucose monitoring, diet, or insulin dose) were undertaken. The children in both investigations had diabetes for approximately 5 years, and their glycosylated hemoglobin levels indicated relatively poor control (HbA$_1$ = 13%) prior to exercise.

Because HbA$_1$ has a long half-life, it may not accurately reflect recent blood glucose levels. Glycosylated albumin, a measure of the glucose-bound protein, has a shorter half-life (3 weeks) than HbA$_1$. Investigators have examined the effects of physical training on glycosylated albumin levels among adolescents.[24] A significant decrease in glycosylated albumin levels occurred after only 8 weeks of training.

However, some studies[25,26] have not reported these favorable changes.

Table 8–4 REPORTS OF THE EFFECTS OF PHYSICAL TRAINING AMONG INDIVIDUALS WITH INSULIN-DEPENDENT DIABETES

Author	Subjects	Mean Age (yr)	Diabetes Duration (yr)	Training Protocol	Training Effect	Effect on Blood Glucose	Comments
Children and Adolescents							
Larsson et al, 1964[21]	6 m 6 nondiabetic controls	16.3 16.5	7.3	6 months of 1h, 1×/wk gymnastics	VO_{2max} ↑ 35%	No change in glycosuria	
Dahl-Jorgensen et al, 1980[22]	14 8 diabetic controls	11.0	5.0	5 months of 1h, 2×/wk	No change in VO_{2max}	HbA$_1$ ↓ 8%, no change in 24h glycosuria	
Campaigne et al, 1984[23]	9 (4m, 5f) 10 diabetic controls (2m, 8f)	9.0 8.5	5.0 3.9	12 wk of 25 min, 3×/wk at 80% VO_{2max}	VO_{2max} ↑ 7%	HbA$_1$ ↓ 10%, FBG ↓ 16%	
Rowland et al, 1985[26]	13 (7m, 6f)	9.0 to 14.0	4.2	12 wk of 1h, 3×/wk at 60% HR reserve	VO_{2max} ↑ 9%	No change in HbA$_1$, 24h glycosuria, or FBG	
Landt et al, 1985[25]	9 (3m, 6f) 5 diabetic controls (2m, 3f)	16.1	6.7	12 wk of 45 min, 3×/wk at HR 160 bpm	VO_{2max} ↑ 9%	No change in HbA$_1$, or FBG	Increased insulin sensitivity
Stratton et al, 1987[24]	8 adolescents (4m, 4f) 8 diabetic controls (4m, 4f)	15.1 15.5	3.7 5.5	8 wk of 30-45 min, 3×/wk aerobic activities	Treadmill exercise time ↑ 12%	Glycosylated serum albumin ↓ 6%, no change in HbA$_1$, or FBG	
Adults							
Costill et al, 1979[34]	12 m 13 nondiabetic controls	21.1 23.2	3 mo 11.0	10 wk of 30 min, 5×/wk running at 60%-70% VO_{2max}	VO_{2max} ↑ 11% VO_{2max} ↑ 13%	FBG ↓ 17%	Increased oxidative enzyme activity
Peterson et al, 1980[31]	9 (3m, 6f)	26.0	10.0	8-10 months of 35 min 3×/wk at 70% maximum HR	Not documented	HbA$_1$ ↓ 30%	Split-dose insulin treatment and glucose monitoring also initiated with exercise

Continued

177

Table 8–4 **REPORTS OF THE EFFECTS OF PHYSICAL TRAINING AMONG INDIVIDUALS WITH INSULIN-DEPENDENT DIABETES**—*Continued*

Author	Subjects	Mean Age (yr)	Diabetes Duration (yr)	Training Protocol	Training Effect	Effect on Blood Glucose	Comments
Wallberg-Henriksson et al, 1982[27]	9 m	35.0	12.0	16 wk of 1 h 2-3X/wk at 60%-80% maximum HR	VO_{2max} ↑ 8%	No change in HbA_1 or 24h glycosuria	Increased insulin sensitivity, increased oxidative enzyme activity
Wallberg-Henriksson et al, 1984[28]	10 m 10 nondiabetic controls	32.0 30.0	14.0	8 wk of 45 min, 3X/wk at 60%-80% max HR	VO_{2max} ↑ 13% VO_{2max} ↑ 13%	No change in HbA_1 or mean blood glucose	Muscle capillarization changes influenced by duration of diabetes
Zinman et al, 1984[12]	13 (7m, 6f) 7 nondiabetic controls (2m, 5f)	30.0 30.0	14.0	12 wk of 45 min, 3X/wk at 60%-85% VO_{2max}	VO_{2max} ↑ 28% VO_{2max} ↑ 20%	No change in HbA_1 or FBG	Significant increase caloric intake on exercise days
Yki-Jarvinen et al, 1984[29]	7 (6m 1f) 6 diabetic controls (4m, 2f) 19 nondiabetic controls	26.0 24.0 27.0	7.0 9.0	6 wk of 30 min, 4X/wk at 70% VO_{2max}	VO_{2max} ↑ 8%	No change HbA_1, mean blood glucose, or 24h glycosuria	Increased insulin sensitivity; no change in insulin binding to erythrocytes
Baevre et al, 1985[46]	6 (2m, 4f)	16.9	7.0	6 mo of 30 min, 2X/wk at HR 130 bpm	VO_{2max} ↑ 19%	No change HbA_1 or FBG	Increased insulin binding to erythrocytes
Bak et al, 1989[30]	7 (4m, 3f) 7 nondiabetic controls (4m, 3f)	27.9 28.0	9.5	6 wk of 60 min, 3X/wk jogging	VO_{2max} ↑ 7%	HbA_1 ↓ 3%	Glycogen synthase activity ↑ 15%

Key: m = male, VO_{2max} = maximal oxygen uptake, ↑ = increased, HbA_1 = glycosylated hemoglobin, ↓ = decreased. f = female, FBG = fasting blood glucose, HR = heart rate.

Improvement in fitness, as determined by VO_{2max}, may be independent of changes in HbA_1, and younger patients can achieve an increase in oxygen uptake without improved blood glucose control.

Likewise, several investigations[12,27-29] of adults with IDDM have not shown improvements in glucose control (assessed by HbA_1, home-monitored blood glucose, or glycosuria) after physical training. Although a statistically significant decrease in HbA_1 levels (7.9% ± 0.4 to 7.7% ± 1.5) was found after 6 weeks of physical training in a more recent study,[30] the clinical significance of this small decrement is uncertain. Another investigative team found improved blood glucose control after regular exercise, but physical activity was initiated in conjunction with a split-dose insulin regimen and institution of glucose self-monitoring.[31]

Thus, the beneficial effect of regular exercise for long-term blood glucose control is unclear among patients with IDDM. The apparent discrepancy between studies of children and adults may, in part, reflect differences in training response, diabetes duration, and the potential for residual endogenous insulin production among younger subjects. The last aspect, if occurring in conjunction with increased insulin sensitivity, might result in greater metabolic improvement in younger individuals or in those with recent-onset IDDM.

TYPE II DIABETES

Unlike the equivocal results seen with type I diabetic patients, regular physical activity has led to consistent improvement in long-term indicators of glycemic control among patients with type II diabetes, or NIDDM.[32,33] Studies have documented significant decreases in HbA_1 after as little as 6 weeks of training among patients with NIDDM.[32,33]

Since obesity often is associated with hypertension, hyperlipidemia, and NIDDM, weight reduction (specifically fat loss) is a primary means of therapy in overweight type II diabetic patients. As discussed in Chapter 10, exercise alone does not always significantly lower body weight. Therefore, when fat loss is a goal, exercise should be combined with caloric restriction in the treatment of these patients.

INSULIN SENSITIVITY

Type I diabetes is characterized by an absolute insulin deficiency; type II diabetes is typified by insulin resistance and impaired insulin secretion. Physical training may alter glucose homeostasis by increasing insulin sensitivity. Although some studies describe stable insulin requirements associated with physical activity, others report a significant decrease in the insulin dose required during training.[30,34] The former finding may relate to reports that patients often increase caloric intake to compensate for the heightened insulin sensitivity (without decreasing the insulin dose).[12]

The glucose clamp technique uses an insulin infusion to measure skeletal muscle sensitivity to insulin.[35] Studies using this methodology[25,27,29] have documented significant increases in insulin sensitivity following exercise conditioning, and type II diabetic patients have been observed to have a 30% to 35% increase in insulin-stimulated glucose disposal after physical training.[32,36] This increase likely is due to augmented muscle glucose uptake, since the hepatic production rate appears unchanged. In addition to calories burned with exercise, conditioning and caloric restriction in type II diabetic patients result in enhanced peripheral glucose use due to increased glycogen synthesis.[37,38]

The mechanism of increased insulin sensitivity is not understood completely. The glycogen storage capacity of skeletal muscle is decreased in those with IDDM.[30,39,40] Regular exercise counteracts this effect by increasing skeletal muscle enzyme activity,[30,40] which will augment glucose uptake and resynthesis of muscle glycogen stores.[41,42] Physical activity also may alter insulin binding,[43,44] a physiologic alteration that can be assessed by studying erythrocytes and monocytes.[38,45] In those with diabetes, insulin binding to erythrocytes has been reported to be unchanged[29] or increased after training. The increase appeared attributable to an elevated receptor number, but not increased affinity.[46] More recently, data suggest that muscular activity may directly relate to increased glucose transport as an additional factor leading to increased insulin sensitivity.[47]

Lipids and Lipoproteins

After 10 to 15 years of diabetes, individuals manifest accelerated atherosclerosis,[48] and abnormal lipid levels may contribute to this problem.[49] As discussed in Chapter 9, physical training may affect lipid profiles by increasing high-density lipoprotein (HDL) cholesterol, decreasing triglycerides, and possibly lowering low-density lipoprotein (LDL) cholesterol, especially if body fat is reduced. However, interpreting training effects on lipid and lipoprotein levels is difficult owing to the interactions among body composition, diet, and glycemic control on these variables.

In a cross-sectional study of women with type I diabetes, those with the best glycemic control had lower triglyceride levels and higher total HDL and HDL_2 cholesterol concentrations.[50] Also, those with greater aerobic capacity had higher HDL cholesterol and lower LDL cholesterol and triglyceride levels. Among diabetic patients, serum triglyceride and total cholesterol levels have been reported to decrease after training, and the HDL cholesterol to total cholesterol ratio has increased.[27,29] LDL cholesterol was decreased significantly after 12 weeks of physical training among a group of adolescent diabetics.[51] However, other investigations have not found these favorable changes.[46,50]

In summary, among insulin-dependent subjects, physical training may lower total cholesterol, triglycerides, and LDL cholesterol. However, these metabolic adaptations have not been demonstrated in type II patients without simultaneous weight loss. The major lipoprotein effect for those with type II diabetes appears related to triglyceride lowering, with a concomitant increase in HDL cholesterol.[52]

Clinical Recommendations

SCREENING

The clinician seeing an individual with diabetes for the first time must assess glucose control, disease complications, cardiovascular risk factors, and general health.[53] Relevant clinical information that should be obtained is outlined in Table 8–5.

Table 8–5 **RECOMMENDED SCREENING PRIOR TO BEGINNING EXERCISE**

1. History and Physical Examination
   (For those newly diagnosed or without up-to-date records)
   a. Review all systems
   b. Identify other medical problems (e.g., asthma, arthritis)
2. Diabetes Evaluation
   a. Glycosylated hemoglobin (HbA$_1$)
   b. Ophthalmoscopic exam (retinopathy)
   c. Neurologic exam (neuropathy)
   d. Nephrologic evaluation (microproteinuria)
   e. Nutritional status (underweight or overweight)
3. Cardiovascular Evaluation
   a. Blood pressure
   b. Peripheral pulses, bruits
   c. 12-lead electrocardiogram
   d. Serum lipid profile (total cholesterol, triglycerides, high-density lipoprotein and low-density lipoprotein cholesterol)
   e. Graded exercise test* (those older than age 35 with history of documented coronary artery disease or multiple risk factors)

*According to the guidelines of the American College of Sports Medicine.

Patients who have had diabetes for more than 5 years, those older than age 35, and individuals with renal disease are at increased risk for coronary artery disease. In addition to diabetic patients' increased prevalence of atherosclerotic disease, exertional chest pain is less reliably associated with ischemia among these individuals.[54] These patients should undergo a careful examination for cardiovascular disease, including a graded exercise test, before exercise recommendations are made for them. Table 8–6 lists contraindications to exercise.

MANAGEMENT OF THE COMPLICATIONS OF DIABETES

Unique concerns for the diabetic patient include retinopathy, autonomic and peripheral (sensory) neuropathy, peripheral vascular disease, and renal dysfunction.

Renal insufficiency is a complication of diabetes that leads to increased morbidity and mortality.[5] Early detection of renal damage might allow selective management to offset disease progression. An exercise stress test to detect the early presence of albuminuria in diabetic adults has been proposed.[56]

Table 8–6 **CONTRAINDICATIONS TO EXERCISE**

Poor metabolic control
Any of the following conditions that have not been evaluated and managed: retinopathy, hypertension, neuropathy (autonomic or peripheral), nephropathy
Proliferative retinopathy with recent photocoagulation or surgery
Dehydration
Extreme environmental temperatures

Several studies have assessed the utility of exercise in identifying those at increased risk for developing nephropathy. Although data conflict, it appears that physical exertion can increase urinary albumin excretion in many patients.[57] Exercise-induced proteinuria is more common among patients with longer disease duration and is directly related to the level of systolic blood pressure elevation during exercise. The precise implications of the albuminuria, as well as the sensitivity and specificity of this analysis, are not known, which limits its utility as a screen for nephropathy.

Patients with proliferative retinopathy are at risk for vitreous hemorrhage, and exercise is contraindicated for these individuals until properly treated. Exercise resulting in large increases in systolic pressure (i.e., intense weight lifting, head stands, and high-intensity aerobic activity) also can cause retinal hemorrhage if proliferative retinopathy is present. In patients with background retinopathy, exercise is not prohibited, but low-impact activities that do not increase blood pressure excessively (e.g., moderate-intensity aerobic activities) are most suitable.

Patients with neuropathy are at risk for developing complications during exercise. If an autonomic neuropathy is present, individuals are more likely to develop hypotension after vigorous exercise, particularly when initiating an exercise program.[19] Although these individuals may have an elevated resting heart rate, their maximal heart rate can be lower than predicted. Because of potential chronotropic insufficiency during exercise, perceived exertion may be the most appropriate measure for exercise intensity recommendations (see Chapter 1). In addition, caution is warranted during exercise in hot and humid environments, because difficulty in thermoregulation and dehydration are increased. Finally, those with autonomic neuropathy may have reduced ability to detect hypoglycemia, requiring even more careful glucose monitoring, especially when initiating an exercise program.

Problems associated with foot injury and reduced peripheral circulation are important considerations, especially when the patient has a peripheral neuropathy. Close inspection of the feet and properly fitted footwear with optimal cushioning should be emphasized. Exercise that may lead to chronic foot trauma (prolonged hiking, jogging, or walking on uneven surfaces) should be avoided in this group. The feet should be inspected regularly, with careful note of blisters and calluses. Feet and toes should be kept clean and dry. Dry socks always should be used, and application of lubricating lotion to these areas is advisable before bed and after bathing.

GLYCEMIC CONTROL

Close glucose monitoring is recommended for patients with diabetes beginning an exercise program, because adjustments in management require individualization. These alterations can be accomplished most easily with careful recording of diet, activity, and insulin treatment. With the first several exercise sessions, blood glucose levels should be checked before the session, as often as every 15 minutes during the activity, immediately afterward, and 4 to 5 hours later. These records allow therapy changes to maintain near-normal blood glucose levels. When exercise is consistent in timing and duration, a routine can be developed to prevent hypoglycemia or hyperglycemia. Based on these blood glucose records, appropriate modifications in diet and oral hypoglycemic and insulin dosage can be recommended (see Tables 8–2 and 8–3).

CASE: A.V., a 55-year-old woman with type II diabetes, wanted to begin an exercise program. Physical examination revealed that she had nonproliferative retinopathy, as well as hypertension (blood pressure of 150/100 mm Hg), a weight of 67.5 kg (150 lb), and a height of 160 cm (5'4"). She underwent an evaluation, including a graded exercise test, which did not disclose electrocardiographic or hemodynamic evidence of ischemia. Her blood pressure response at maximal exercise was 260/90 mm Hg.

It was recommended that she engage in moderate-intensity, dynamic (60% maximal heart rate) activities with minimal impact (i.e., walking, swimming, cycling), as well as a stretching program. The heart rate and perceived exertion levels were chosen to coincide with training that maintained a systolic pressure at or below 180 mm Hg. After choosing stationary cycling, she came into the clinic three times per week for 1 month, so that her training level and blood pressure response could be monitored. Blood glucose was assessed before cycling, as well as 5 minutes and 15 minutes after exercise. She became hyperglycemic 5 minutes following exercise, but by 15 minutes she returned to near pre-exercise levels. After the initial month, she began a home program, monitoring her heart rate and perceived exertion, with clinic visits to assess progress every 6 weeks.

COMMENT: Exercise-induced hyperglycemia can be related to two situations. First, transient hyperglycemia occurring 5 minutes after exercise may be related to the normal increase in hepatic glucose output, which in part supplies muscle glucose during endurance activities. Thus, when exercise concludes, glucose production continues while its use is diminished, resulting in transient hyperglycemia. Second, exercise that is too intense causes a counter-regulatory increase in catecholamines and a further rise in hepatic glucose output, resulting in more prolonged hyperglycemia after exercise. Hyperglycemia persisting longer than 15 minutes after exercise suggests that the training intensity should be lowered. For this individual, glucose levels had returned to normal within 15 minutes after exercise. Thus, it was concluded that the exercise intensity was appropriate. After a month of monitored training, she was knowledgeable about glucose control and could appropriately regulate her own program.

INSULIN ABSORPTION

Under resting conditions, human insulin is absorbed more rapidly than porcine insulin. During exercise, they are both absorbed more rapidly and in a similar manner. Absorption is most enhanced when insulin is given immediately before exercise. This increase is not associated with greater cutaneous blood flow, but appears more related to mechanical stimulation of the injection site.[58] Absorption rates differ from various injection sites (i.e., thigh, abdomen, arm), and the site may be the most important variable on absorption rate, even greater than the mechanical stimulation of exercise.[32,59] The longer the interval between injection and exercise, the less important the injection site. Exercise should be avoided for 60 to 90 minutes after insulin injections to minimize potential effects of enhanced insulin absorption.

FOOD INTAKE FOR EXERCISE

Patients often ask how much carbohydrate they should consume during exercise. Although it is difficult to provide precise information because of large individual variation, useful estimates of energy requirements can be based on the intensity and duration of activity. Table 8–3 provides general guidelines for dietary modifications. Patients may increase their caloric intake to compensate for increased energy expenditure, but reductions in insulin dose prior to exercise may be more appropriate.[60] As discussed in Chapter 2, higher insulin levels may relate to increased cardiovascular risk, and thus reducing the amount of insulin may be beneficial. Patients using oral hypoglycemic agents may require a lower dosage.

TIMING OF EXERCISE

In general, the patient with diabetes should exercise at times when the insulin effects are lowest and blood glucose is on the rise. To minimize the risk of hypoglycemia, it is best to avoid exercising for 60 to 90 minutes after insulin injection and coincident with peak insulin action. To prevent hypoglycemia, a rapidly assimilated carbohydrate snack should be consumed prior to exercise. Exercising before insulin and breakfast may decrease the need for morning short-acting insulin. Once a physical activity schedule is established, insulin dose and caloric intake can be adjusted to optimize glycemic control.

COMPETITION FOR THE INDIVIDUAL WITH DIABETES

Diabetic athletes participating in competitions require further therapy adjustment. If an individual runs a 10-km race and usually runs 6 to 10 miles per day to train for the race, no change in insulin is necessary. For those using both long-acting and short-acting insulin, the short-acting insulin should be reduced in accordance with the distance and estimated time of the race. For example, if a race was to be held at 10:00 AM, with a light breakfast eaten 3 hours prior to competition and preceded by insulin injection 15 minutes before breakfast, a reduction in short-acting insulin would be indicated, because the peak action of insulin will be at race time. Also, the runner should begin an event with slightly elevated glucose levels, and should consume a rapidly assimilated carbohydrate every 15 to 20 minutes during competition. Since water is needed to maintain hydration and performance, a dilute glucose solution is recommended (such as some of the commercially available drinks, e.g., Exceed, Max). These solutions will help prevent hypoglycemia during exercise.

CASE: W.T., a 28-year-old man with IDDM diagnosed at age 11, sought treatment for frequent hypoglycemia. He had a 2-year history of exercise-induced hypoglycemia, which had responded well to a decrease in insulin dosage. Over the past year, however, he had experienced an increase in hypoglycemic episodes. He had been in good health and active all his life. More recently, he had become a competitive runner, training for and running in several races.

His physical examination revealed a height of 175 cm (5'10"), weight 77.4 kg (172 lb), blood pressure of 110/70 mm Hg, and HbA$_1$ of 9%. He was on a regimen of regular and lente (intermediate-acting) insulin in the morning and evening.

Because he was planning on running a 10-km race at the end of the week, he decreased his exercise. It was advised that he increase his caloric intake to ensure optimal glycogen storage, while maintaining his previous insulin dose. He began to monitor his blood glucose closely to maintain near-normal blood glucose levels (90 to 120 mg/dL).

After recovering from the race and resuming training, he began a program of careful self-monitoring of blood glucose throughout the day. He gradually reduced the evening lente insulin dose by 25%, after charting his blood glucose levels for several weeks and noting a consistent pattern of hypoglycemia during the night. The increase in exercise resulted in a lower insulin need. After 1 week, the frequency and severity of hypoglycemic occurrences was reduced. After 2 weeks, he experienced only one such episode, due to missing his evening snack.

COMMENT: Long-distance running is common today. When advising the diabetic runner, proper glycemic control is the most important consideration. Without appropriate control, muscle fuel utilization is affected, compromising training and performance. Hyperglycemia reduces the availability of free fatty acids, which are a major energy source for prolonged exercise. Hypoglycemia makes glucose unavailable as muscle fuel, hindering the intensity and duration of exercise, and if ketosis is present, both ketones and acidemia decrease exercise ability. Assessing the blood glucose is important before each exercise session. If severe hyperglycemia (blood glucose of 250 mg/dL or more) or ketones are present, exercise should not be undertaken until a more normoglycemic state is achieved.

For the diabetic individual who plans to race more than 10 miles, several unique situations may arise. Several days prior to long-distance competition, most athletes reduce their mileage and increase caloric intake to improve glycogen storage. For the diabetic runner, both of these measures increase blood glucose. It probably is advisable to increase both insulin dose and carbohydrate intake, thus permitting suitable glycogen storage while maintaining near-normal blood glucose levels. The typical carbohydrate-loading regimen practiced by competitive runners begins with a depletion phase of heavy exercise with reduced carbohydrate intake, followed by several days of light exercise and higher carbohydrate intake. However, this practice increases the risk of hypoglycemia and hyperglycemia, respectively, and is not recommended for diabetic individuals. Thus, the depletion phase should be omitted.

The anxiety of race day may produce symptoms simulating an insulin reaction, such as muscle weakness, nervousness, and irritability. Following prolonged physical activity, diabetic individuals can experience delayed hypoglycemia the following day. Some have reported hypoglycemic reactions occurring from 24 to 48 hours after exercise, which are probably related to depletion of glycogen or increased insulin sensitivity. Substantial amounts of liver and muscle glycogen are utilized during exercise of increased duration. Since replenishment of carbohydrate stores may take up to 24 to 48 hours, blood glucose may fall due to its preferential uptake for glycogen storage. To prevent hypoglycemia, foods high in carbohydrates (e.g., breads, pasta, juice) should be consumed soon after exercise. An increase in caloric intake is indicated, with the actual increases dependent on the intensity and duration of exercise (see

Table 8–3). Reducing the insulin dose also may be necessary, especially when snacking is not possible. Optimally, the depleted glycogen reserves should be replaced in the hours following exercise, but blood glucose may need monitoring for 48 hours after several hours of continuous exertion.

Summary

Exercise can be an important adjunctive therapy for those with diabetes. Liberalization of the diet, improved insulin sensitivity, reduced insulin requirements, modification of other cardiovascular risk factors, and weight loss are promoted by regular physical activity. Although exercise usually is safe, an exercise prescription necessitates careful review of metabolic control along with screening for consequences of diabetes. While general management recommendations can be provided, a unique regimen of diet and altered insulin will be required for optimal care of each individual.

REFERENCES

1. Sushruta SCS: *Vaidya Javavaji Trikamji Acharia.* Nirnyar Sagar Press: Bombay, India, 1938, p 11–13.
2. Allen FM, Stillman E, Fitz R: *Total Dietary Regulation in the Treatment of Diabetes.* Rockefeller Institute of Medical Research Monograph: New York, 1916, 11:486.
3. Wahren J: Glucose turnover during exercise in healthy man and in patients with diabetes mellitus. *Diabetes* 1979; 28(Suppl 1): 82–88.
4. Wahren J, Hagenfeldt L, Felig P: Splanchnic and leg exchange of glucose, amino acids, and free fatty acids during exercise in diabetes mellitus. *J Clin Invest* 1975; 55: 1301–1314.
5. VonMering A, Minkowski O: Diabetes mellitus nach pankreasexstirpation. Naunym Schmiedebergs. *Arch Parm* 1890; 26: 371–387.
6. Roch-Norlund AE: Muscle glycogen synthetase in patients with diabetes mellitus: Basal values, effects of glycogen depletion by exercise, and effects of treatment. *Scand J Clin Lab Invest* 1972; 29:237–242.
7. Lawrence RD: The effect of exercise on insulin action in diabetes. *BMJ* 1926; 1: 648–650.
8. Caron D, et al.: The effect of postprandial exercise on meal-related glucose intolerance in insulin-dependent diabetic individuals. *Diabetes Care* 1982; 5:364–369.
9. Campaigne BN, Wallberg-Henriksson H, Gunnarsson R: Glucose and insulin responses in relation to insulin dose and caloric intake 12h after acute physical exercise in men with IDDM. *Diabetes Care* 1987; 10:716–721.
10. Gooch BR, et al.: Exercise in insulin-dependent diabetes mellitus: The effect of continuous insulin infusion using the subcutaneous, intravenous and intraperitoneal sites. *Diabetes Care* 1983; 6:122–182.
11. Trovati M, et al.: Continuous subcutaneous insulin infusion and postprandial exercise in tightly controlled type I (insulin-dependent) diabetic patients. *Diabetes Care* 1984; 7:327–330.
12. Zinman B, Zuniga-Guajardo S, Kelly D: Comparison of the acute and long-term effects of exercise on glucose control in type I diabetes. *Diabetes Care* 1984; 7:515–519.
13. LaPorte RE, et al.: Pittsburgh Insulin-Dependent Diabetes Mellitus Morbidity and Mortality Study: Physical activity and diabetic complications. *Pediatrics* 1986; 78: 1027–1033.
14. Chazzan BI, et al.: Twenty-five to forty-five years of diabetes with and without vascular complications. *Diabetologia* 1970; 6: 565–569.
15. Helmrich SP, et al.: Physical activity and reduced occurrence of non–insulin-dependent diabetes mellitus. *N Engl J Med* 1991; 325:147–152.
16. Campaigne BN, Gunnarsson R: The effects of physical training in people with insulin-dependent diabetes. *Diabetic Med* 1988; 5:429–433.
17. Gunnarsson R, et al.: Exercise and physical training in Type I diabetes. Skandia International Symposia, *Recent Trends Diabetes Research* 1982; 101–111.
18. Richter EA, Ruderman NB, Schneider SH: Diabetes and exercise. *Am J Med* 1981; 70:201–209.
19. Vitug A, Schneider SH, Ruderman NB: Exercise and Type I diabetes mellitus. In KB Pardolf, ed: *Exercise and Sports Science Reviews.* Macmillan: New York, 1988, p 292.
20. Zinman B, Vranic M: Diabetes and exercise. *Med Clin North Am* 1985; 69:145–157.
21. Larsson Y, et al.: Functional adaptation to rigorous training and exercise in diabetic and non-diabetic adolescents. *J Appl Physiol* 1964; 19:629–635.

22. Dahl-Jorgensen K, et al.: The effect of exercise on diabetic control and hemoglobin A (HbA$_1$) in children. *Acta Paediatr Scand* 1980; 283(suppl):53–56.
23. Campaigne BN, et al.: Effects of a physical activity program on metabolic control and cardiovascular fitness in children with insulin-dependent diabetes mellitus. *Diabetes Care* 1984; 7:57–62.
24. Stratton R, et al.: Improved glycemic control after supervised eight-week exercise program in insulin-dependent diabetic adolescents. *Diabetes Care* 1987; 10:589–593.
25. Landt KW, et al.: Effects of exercise training on insulin sensitivity in adolescents with type I diabetes. *Diabetes Care* 1985; 8:461–465.
26. Rowland TW, et al.: Glycemic control with physical training in insulin-dependent diabetes mellitus. *Am J Dis Child* 1985; 139:307–310.
27. Wallberg-Henriksson H, et al.: Increased peripheral insulin sensitivity and muscle mitochondrial enzymes but unchanged blood glucose control in type I diabetics after physical training. *Diabetes* 1982; 31:1044–1050.
28. Wallberg-Henriksson H, et al.: Influence of physical training on formation of muscle capillaries in type I diabetes. *Diabetes* 1984; 33:851–857.
29. Yki-Jarvinen H, DeFronzo RA, Koivisto VA: Normalization of insulin sensitivity in type I diabetic subjects by physical training during insulin pump therapy. *Diabetes Care* 1984; 7:520–527.
30. Bak JF, et al.: Insulin receptor function and glycogen synthase activity in skeletal muscle biopsies from patients with insulin-dependent diabetes mellitus: Effects of physical training. *J Clin Endocrinol Metab* 1989; 69:158–164.
31. Peterson CM, et al.: Changes in basement membrane thickening and pulse volume concomitant with improved glucose control and exercise in patients with insulin-dependent diabetes mellitus. *Diabetes Care* 1980; 3:586–589.
32. Trovati M, et al.: Influence of physical training on blood glucose control, glucose tolerance, insulin secretion, and insulin action in non-insulin-dependent diabetic patients. *Diabetes Care* 1984; 7:416–420.
33. Schneider SH, et al.: Studies on the mechanism of improved glucose control during regular exercise in type II (non-insulin-dependent) diabetes. *Diabetologia* 1984; 26:355–360.
34. Costill DL, et al.: Training adaptations in skeletal muscle of juvenile diabetic. *Diabetes* 1979; 28:818–822.
35. DeFronzo A, Tobin JD, Andres R: Glucose clamp technique: A method for quantifying insulin secretion and resistance. *Am J Physiol* 1979; 237:E214–E223.
36. DeFronzo RA, Ferrannini E, Koivisto V: New concepts in the pathogenesis and

treatment of noninsulin-dependent diabetes mellitus. *Am J Med* 1983; 74:52–81.
37. Devlin JT, et al.: Enhanced peripheral and splanchnic insulin sensitivity in NIDDM men after single bout of exercise. *Diabetes* 1987; 36:434–439.
38. Burstein R, et al.: Acute reversal of the enhanced insulin action in trained athletes: Association with insulin receptor changes. *Diabetes* 1985; 34:756–760.
39. Saltin B, et al.: Muscle fiber characteristics in healthy men and patients with juvenile diabetes. *Diabetes* 1979; 28:93–98.
40. Wallberg-Henriksson H, et al.: Increased peripheral insulin sensitivity and muscle mitochondrial enzymes but unchanged blood glucose control in Type I diabetics after physical training. *Diabetes* 1982; 31:1022–1050.
41. Bogardus C, et al.: Effect of muscle glycogen depletion on in vivo insulin action in man. *J Clin Invest* 1983; 72:1605–1610.
42. Devlin JT, Horton ES: Effects of prior high-intensity exercise on glucose metabolism in normal and insulin-resistant men. *Diabetes* 1985; 34:973–979.
43. Soman VR, et al.: Increased insulin binding to monocytes after acute exercise in normal man. *J Clin Endocrinol Metab* 1978; 47:216–219.
44. Pederson O, Beck-Nielsen H, Hedig L: Increased insulin receptors after exercise in patients with insulin dependent diabetes mellitus. *N Engl J Med* 1980; 302:886–892.
45. Heath GW, et al.: Effects of exercise and lack of exercise on glucose tolerance and insulin sensitivity. *J Appl Physiol* 1983; 55:512–517.
46. Baevre H, et al.: Metabolic responses to physical training in young insulin-dependent diabetics. *Scand J Clin Lab Invest* 1985; 45:109–114.
47. Wallberg-Henriksson H: Repeated exercise regulates glucose transport capacity in skeletal muscle. *Acta Physiol Scand* 1986; 127:39–43.
48. Ganda OP: Pathogenesis of macrovascular disease in the human diabetic. *Diabetes* 1980; 29:931–942.
49. Goldberg RB: Lipid disorders in diabetes. *Diabetes Care* 1981; 4:561–572.
50. Gunnarsson R, et al.: Serum lipid and lipoprotein levels in female Type I diabetics: Relationships to aerobic capacity and glycemic control. *Diabetes Metab* 1987; 13:417–421.
51. Campaigne BN, et al.: The effects of physical training on blood lipid profiles in adolescents with insulin dependent diabetes mellitus. *Phys Sports Med* 1985; 13:83–89.
52. Lampman RM, et al.: The influence of physical training on glucose tolerance, insulin sensitivity, and lipid and lipoprotein concentrations in middle-aged hypertriglyceridemic, carbohydrate intolerant men. *Diabetologia* 1987; 30:380–385.
53. Campaigne BN: Evaluation and testing of

the diabetic patient prior to exercise prescription. In Hall LK, Meyer GC, eds: *Epidemiology, Behavior Change and Intervention in Chronic Disease*. Life Enhancement Publications: Champaign, Ill., 1988, pp 167–177.

54. Nesto RW, et al.: Angina and exertional myocardial ischemia in diabetic and nondiabetic patients: Assessment by exercise thallium scintigraphy. *Ann Intern Med* 1988; 108:170–175.

55. Balodimos NC: Diabetic nephropathy. In *Joslin's Diabetes Mellitus*. Lea & Febiger: Philadelphia, 1971, p 526.

56. Mogensen CE, Vittinghus E: Urinary albumin excretion during exercise in juvenile diabetes: A provocation test for early abnormalities. *Scan J Clin Lab Invest* 1975; 35:295–300.

57. Poortmans J, Dorchy H, Toussiant D: Urinary excretion of total proteins, albumin, and beta 2-microglobulin during rest and exercise in diabetic adolescents with and without retinopathy. *Diabetes Care* 1982; 5:617–623.

58. Fernqvist E, et al.: Effects of physical exercise on insulin absorption in insulin-dependent diabetics: A comparison between human and porcine insulin. *Clin Physiol* 1986; 6:489–497.

59. Berger M, et al.: Absorption kinetics and biologic effects of subcutaneously injected insulin preparations. *Diabetes Care* 1982; 5:77–91.

60. Stout RW: Diabetes and atherosclerosis: The role of insulin. *Diabetologia* 1979; 16:141–150.

CHAPTER 9

THE USE OF EXERCISE TO IMPROVE LIPID AND LIPOPROTEIN LEVELS

LINN GOLDBERG, MD, and DIANE L. ELLIOT, MD

Cardiovascular disease, a major cause of adult morbidity and mortality, is strongly associated with lipoprotein abnormalities.[1-6] Total cholesterol, low-density lipoprotein cholesterol (LDL-C), and apolipoprotein B (apo B) plasma levels are associated directly with cardiovascular disease, whereas high-density lipoprotein cholesterol (HDL-C) and apolipoprotein A-I (apo A-I) levels are inversely related to coronary atherosclerosis.[5,7-12] Although the association between triglyceride concentration and coronary heart disease is not as evident,[13] epidemiologic evidence reveals a direct relationship between triglyceride levels and coronary risk,[14,15] especially among women.[16] Evidence from the Helsinki Heart Study[17] revealed that the ratio of LDL-C to HDL-C, in combination with the serum triglyceride level, improves the prognostic value for assessing coronary heart disease risk.

Cardiovascular disease can be reduced by altering risk factors by nonpharmacologic therapy,[18,19] drug treatment,[8,20-22] or surgical intervention.[23] Benefits are related to reducing LDL-C[20-25] or increasing HDL-C concentrations.[8,19] Angiographic trials have provided evidence that lowering LDL-C reduces progression or increases regression of coronary lesions and decreases the incidence of cardiovascular events.[24-27] Moreover, prospective studies have shown that favorably changing lipoprotein levels results in reduced coronary morbidity and mortality.[8,20,22,28] Improving lipoprotein abnormalities would have a large health promotion impact, as it is estimated that up to 60 million adult Americans have lipid levels requiring therapy.[29]

As discussed in Chapter 1, physical inactivity is a risk factor for the development of cardiovascular disease.[30-35] Exercise may protect against cardiovascular disease in part by improving lipid and lipoprotein levels.[36-38]

This chapter reviews lipoprotein classes and their metabolism, the effect of physical activity on plasma lipids and lipoproteins, and the potential mechanisms involved. We review the clinical application of exercise as a treatment of lipoprotein abnormalities and the use of complementary dietary strategies.

Lipoproteins

LIPOPROTEIN CLASSES

Lipoproteins are macromolecules of lipids (cholesterol, triglyceride, and phospholipid) combined with proteins (apoproteins). Cholesterol is the precursor for cellular membranes and steroid hormones, and triglycerides are primarily used as a fuel source.[39,40] Apoproteins, with their unique binding sites, are associated with specific lipids and assist in regulating the metabolism of protein–lipid (apolipoprotein) complexes.[41]

Chylomicrons

Dietary fat and cholesterol are absorbed from the intestine and transported into the blood as exogenously derived, triglyceride-rich chylomicrons. After absorption, they are metabolized by lipoprotein lipase in extrahepatic tissues, resulting in production of free-fatty-acids, with the final remnant particle degraded by the liver.[40]

Very-Low-Density Lipoproteins (VLDL)

Unlike chylomicrons, VLDL primarily contains endogenous triglyceride. After formation in the liver, VLDL is transported to adipose tissue or muscle for storage or use. The enzyme lipoprotein lipase (located in many tissues, including adipose tissue and muscle) hydrolyzes VLDL, producing free fatty acids for uptake, while the remaining portion is converted to LDL-C, which can be further degraded by the liver.[42,43] Triglycerides, in the form of both chylomicrons and VLDL, are inversely related to HDL-C levels,[44] probably because HDL-C and triglyceride macromolecules compete for sites on apoprotein C-II (apo C-II), a cofactor for lipoprotein lipase. Apo C-II also serves as a transporter for HDL-C.[45,46]

Low-Density Lipoprotein Cholesterol (LDL-C)

LDL-C is a lipoprotein end product of triglyceride metabolism and is a major risk factor for coronary atherosclerosis.[7,47–49] It is formed by the catabolism of VLDL by lipoprotein lipase after degradation to intermediate-density lipoprotein.[50] The LDL particles are catabolized further by both receptor and nonreceptor mechanisms.[39]

High-Density Lipoprotein Cholesterol (HDL-C)

HDL-C is a family of heterogeneous lipoproteins and mainly consists of HDL_2 and HDL_3 subfractions. HDL has a protective effect against coronary artery disease.[6–10,47,51] It contains approximately equivalent amounts of lipid and protein, and usually represents 20% to 30% of the total plasma cholesterol.[46,50,51–53] The HDL_2 subfraction is lighter and contains more lipid; HDL_3 is heavier and is relatively lipid-poor.[44,52]

Newly formed HDL particles, secreted from the liver and ileum, contain both apo A-I and apoprotein E (apo E). These particles pick up free cholesterol from cells after esterification by the enzyme lecithin:cholesterol acyltransferase (see below). HDL-C transports cholesterol from extrahepatic tissues to cells requiring cholesterol or to the liver for elimination.[46,54] The HDL molecule enlarges as cholesterol is acquired, forming HDL_2. HDL_2 is thought to be converted to HDL_3 by the enzyme hepatic lipase. The function referred to as *reverse cholesterol transport* relates to the ability of HDL-C to augment cholesterol removal from atherogenic sites, supporting one potential mechanism of protection from coronary atherosclerosis.[55] In addition, HDL-C may inhibit cellular LDL-C uptake by its effect on the LDL-C receptor site.[56]

APOPROTEINS

Apoproteins are the protein components of plasma lipoproteins. Of 13 human apoproteins, 7 are considered major types.[43] Apoproteins have a role in lipid synthesis, transport, and catabolism. They serve as cofactors or enzymes in lipoprotein metabolism, facilitating lipid exchange among the various lipoprotein particles.[6,41,57–60] These substances also have been shown to mediate lipoprotein binding to cell receptors for enzyme activation.[58]

LIPOPROTEIN METABOLISM

LDL Cholesterol and VLDL

In general, changes in lipoprotein levels are due to an alteration in the rate of synthesis or catabolism. For example, certain drugs (lovastatin, simvastatin, pravastatin) inhibit the synthesis of LDL, while specific hormones (e.g., estrogens) can increase plasma LDL clearance by increasing LDL receptors in the liver.[61] LDL receptors are responsible for most LDL catabolism. A reduction in receptors increases plasma LDL-C, a condition found in familial hypercholesterolemia.[39,57]

Specific lipoprotein enzymes directly influence lipid concentrations. Lipoprotein lipase (LPL), present in muscle and adipose tissue, breaks down triglycerides (chylomicrons and VLDL) to produce fatty acids.[40,53] Free fatty acids can be used for energy production by the muscle or stored as fat. Lipoprotein lipase also converts VLDL to form LDL-C.[50] If LPL activity is reduced, inadequate metabolism of triglycerides will result in type I hyperlipoproteinemia.

HDL Cholesterol

The metabolism of HDL-C is under the control of enzymatic influences. Lecithin:cholesterol acyltransferase (LCAT) originates in the liver and circulates with HDL. This enzyme changes nascent HDL to a more mature HDL-C by esterifying free cholesterol, resulting in greater cholesterol accumulation within HDL-C.[42,62] In addition, this reaction results in the transfer of cholesteryl ester to other lipoproteins, including VLDL. Lipoprotein lipase, which metabolizes triglycerides,[40,53] can indirectly increase HDL-C concentrations[44-46] by lowering VLDL levels. The enzyme hepatic lipase breaks down HDL-C.[62] Either high hepatic lipase or low LCAT activity, or both, will reduce HDL-C concentrations.

CONFOUNDING VARIABLES IN ASSESSING LIPOPROTEINS

Assessing the effects of exercise on lipid metabolism requires accurate and reliable biochemical determinations of lipids, lipoproteins, and apoproteins. In the United States, a standardization program for lipid, cholesterol, and triglycerides is available through the Centers for Disease Control and Prevention and the National Heart, Lung, and Blood Institute.[63] However, not all laboratories use this methodology. Certain automated instruments report significantly higher cholesterol levels than the standardized procedures,[64] and HDL-C determinations have been shown to vary by as much as 15% to 38%.[65,66] Differences in storage and transport of samples also can alter HDL-C concentrations.[58] Apoprotein measurements have similar problems, because some apoproteins are stable for only a short time in a cooled environment,[67] and levels can be altered by various transport conditions.[68]

A related issue is the accuracy of the procedure for determining LDL-C. Some studies report a measured LDL-C, whereas most others use a formula advanced by Friedewald and colleagues,[69] based on total cholesterol, HDL-C, and triglyceride levels [LDL (mg/dL) = total cholesterol − HDL-C − (triglycerides/5)]. This calculation is used because specialized equipment is needed for the direct measurement of LDL-C, but it is less accurate than the Lipid Research Clinics' ultracentrifugation procedure. The derived method also may not estimate LDL-C levels as well as another formula based on data from over 10,000 subjects.[70] Friedewald's formula[69] is especially inaccurate when triglyceride levels are greater than 400 mg/dL.[70]

A number of competing influences alter both lipoprotein levels and lipid–exercise relationships. Dietary intake can obscure the ability of exercise to alter lipid and lipoproteins. For instance, ingestion of saturated fat unfavorably changes plasma lipoprotein levels.[71,72] There is wide individual variation in the effect of both dietary cholesterol and saturated fat on plasma lipid and lipoprotein levels.[73-75] Also, an increase in carbohydrate intake may elevate triglyceride levels[73] while reducing HDL-C.[76] Ingestion of n-6 polyunsaturated fat lowers levels of plasma cholesterol, LDL-C, HDL-C, triglycerides, and VLDL, while marine polyunsaturated fat (n-3) reduces triglycerides without affecting LDL-C.[74,75,77]

Other factors can change an individual's plasma lipid and lipoprotein levels. These include drug use, seasonal fluctuations, age, body composition (percentage of body fat), and the distribution of adiposity.[71,72,78-81] For example, higher levels of HDL-C have been associated with intake of ethanol, nicotinic acid, gemfibrozil, estrogen, phenytoin, and terbutaline.[8,82-84] HDL-C levels are reduced with use of anabolic steroids, zinc supplements, beta-adrenoreceptor antagonists, benzodiazepines, and cigarettes.[81,84-86] Triglyceride concentrations can be increased by alcohol ingestion, intake of saturated dietary fat, an increase in the percentage of body fat, and estrogen use.[87-89]

Effects of Exercise on Lipids, Lipoproteins, and Apoproteins

EFFECTS OF EXERCISE ON LIPIDS

Total Cholesterol

Evidence that exercise affects total cholesterol concentration is inconclusive.[37,38] However, assessing only total cholesterol can overlook changes in cholesterol subclasses and so not accurately reflect lipoprotein risk. For example, when an HDL-C increase is accompanied by a decrease in LDL-C, total cholesterol may not change, although the ratio of cholesterol to HDL-C or of LDL-C to HDL-C would indicate an improved lipoprotein risk profile.[7,20,47]

Observational studies[90-92] have documented a modest difference (4%–6%) in mean plasma cholesterol for endurance-trained athletes when compared with less active controls. Likewise, total cholesterol levels were found to be significantly lower among those in high fitness categories, determined by maximal treadmill time, when compared to those in low fitness categories.[93] However, assessment of aerobic fitness by maximal oxygen uptake has not shown a consistent correlation between fitness and total cholesterol concentration when age and body composition effects were removed.[94,95] Some studies of endurance-trained runners,[96] tennis players,[97] speed skaters,[98] and soccer players[99] have not observed a difference for total cholesterol when compared with sedentary controls. One study[100] actually found an increase in total cholesterol concentration among runners. Similar variability has been documented among those trained for speed or strength.[83,98,101] Most of these studies have been small, however, and were limited in assessment of confounding variables that could affect cholesterol levels.

Tran and colleagues[36] assessed the relationship between endurance exercise and change in plasma lipids and lipoproteins, using meta-analysis. The authors observed the interactions of exercise with age, initial lipid profile, percent body fat, body weight, and maximal oxygen consumption. This review involved interventions conducted over 26 years and represented 2,926 subjects (including controls). The findings suggested that exercisers had an average 10 mg/dL decrease in total cholesterol.

Prospective short-term (several weeks) training studies have observed lowering of cholesterol levels among healthy men[102,103] and those with type II diabetes mellitus.[104] Others, however, have not found a change in total cholesterol levels.[105,106]

Changes in body weight and composition may contribute to the lipid and lipoprotein response to physical training.[38] After running an average of 12 miles per week, formerly sedentary middle-aged men significantly lowered their mean total cholesterol level by 6% and increased their HDL-C levels by 8%.[107] At the conclusion of the 2-year intervention period, subjects had significantly decreased their body fat from 22% to 18%, a change in body composition that would contribute to these improvements.

Dietary habits have been found to alter the relationship between exercise and total cholesterol in prospective studies. Potential cholesterol-lowering effects of regular exercise are impeded by a moderately high-cholesterol diet. When normolipidemic healthy men exercised regularly and had their dietary daily intake of cholesterol increased from 200 mg to 600 mg, LDL-C and apo B plasma levels increased by averages of 10% and 13%, respectively.[108] The dietary change may have inhibited the LDL receptors and thus reduced LDL-C degradation.[39]

In general, the effect of small, short-term exercise trials on total cholesterol level is inconsistent or slightly beneficial. Conflicting results may be attributed to both the magnitude of response and confounding variables that affect plasma cholesterol. Importantly, changes in cholesterol subclasses can occur without changing the total cholesterol concentration.

Triglycerides

Athletes and others engaged in regular physical activity often have low plasma triglyceride levels. Several cross-sectional studies have documented lower triglyceride concentrations among highly active individuals, including male marathoners[109] and female and middle-aged male long-distance runners.[110,111] A potential contributing cofactor to low triglyceride levels is the observation that these subjects are often lean.[81,91,96,112,113] Greater leanness is not a necessary precondition for improved triglycerides, however. Of two groups of factory workers designated as physically active and sedentary, the physically active group had significantly lower triglyceride concentrations despite comparable age and body mass index.[114] Even when matched for age, weight, height, and body fat, a group of male long-distance runners had significantly lower triglyceride concentrations than controls.[115]

Intervention studies have demonstrated that exercise of moderate intensity among sedentary, hypertriglyceridemic individuals can produce a significant reduction (up to 45%) in plasma triglycerides.[116,117] The capacity of physical activity to lower triglyceride levels appears to have both an acute and chronic phase. Acute exercise assists reduction of postprandial triglyceride-rich lipoproteins, in part owing to utilization of substrate for muscle energy production.[116,118–121] As exercise continues, a further reduction of triglycerides occurs.[122,123]

Physically active individuals also have lower triglyceride levels independent of the previous exercise session and the acute response. Fit athletes are better able to metabolize serum triglycerides.[116–124] Trained men clear serum triglycerides more rapidly after the ingestion of a high-fat meal than do sedentary men, even when diet composition and body weight are controlled.[121]

Triglyceride uptake from the circulation is highly related to muscle lipoprotein lipase activity, which increases with a prolonged exercise period.[122] This heightened enzyme activity probably assists in replenishing muscle triglyceride after its reduction during exercise.

EFFECTS OF EXERCISE ON LIPOPROTEINS

LDL Cholesterol

Studies of exercise effects on LDL-C are limited to individuals with polygenic hyperlipidemia. As yet, no research has assessed the effect of physical activity on LDL-C among those with familial hypercholesterolemia.

Although self-report of exercise was strongly related to HDL-C and inversely associated with triglyceride levels in the Lipid Research Clinics' Coronary Primary Prevention Trial,[125] LDL-C was not related to activity levels. Similarly, others have reported that physical activity level appears independent of LDL-C concentrations.[107] However, one comparative study found that older and younger runners had lower LDL-C levels than sedentary controls.[126]

Meta-analysis of endurance exercise training studies found a significant reduction in LDL-C,[36] while others have found lower LDL-C levels following strength training.[127,128] The reported reductions are a 5% to 10% decrease in LDL-C concentration with daily aerobic exercise of moderate intensity in studies ranging from just 11 days to 16 weeks duration.[129,130] In an attempt to assess the effect of exercise intensity on lipoproteins, a group of 49 men were divided into four groups and evaluated before and after 12 weeks of stationary cycling.[131] Only those engaged in the intermediate training intensity (75% maximum heart rate) were found to lower their LDL-C level. Subjects exercising at higher (85% maximum) and lower (65% maximum) levels of training did not acquire beneficial changes. It is unclear whether this effect reflects a true relationship to training intensity, as the low number of participants reduces the statistical power to detect changes among the other groups.

Many prospective investigations have not reported lowering LDL-C concentrations, despite gains in strength or maximal oxygen uptake after weight lifting or endurance training.[106,132-134] However, these studies generally were performed on individuals who had normal lipid levels prior to enrollment, and lowering LDL-C may not have been clinically significant because initial levels were so low prior to engaging in exercise.

LDL-C is directly related to age, amount of dietary cholesterol and saturated fat, and percentage of body fat.[62,71,78,79] Thus, the effects of exercise on LDL-C concentration may depend on other variables, such as diet or body composition. Concentrations of LDL-C are not uniformly changed by weight loss produced either by diet alone or with an exercise program. In a 1-year randomized controlled trial, Wood and associates[135] analyzed lipids and lipoproteins after weight loss produced by diet as compared with weight loss produced by exercise. The exercisers were provided with a supervised program and individual prescriptions, based on estimates of the amount of energy necessary to progressively decrease body fat. Loss of approximately 5 kg of body fat over 1 year, whether by dieting or exercise, did not alter LDL-C levels. Despite this, both groups significantly increased HDL-C as compared to controls.

As with total cholesterol, aerobic exercise does not appear to lower LDL-C levels among those who do not undergo body composition changes. However, most studies have evaluated subjects with "normal" LDL-C levels, and few have assessed those at higher risk (LDL-C over 160 mg/dL).

Lipoprotein (Lp[a])

This lipoprotein is structurally related to LDL but has an additional glycoprotein [Apo(a)].[136,137] Increased plasma Lp(a) concentration may be an independent risk factor for coronary disease and myocardial infarction.[136,138] Preliminary research has found that exercise may influence the levels of Lp[a]. In physically fit, mostly normolipidemic, nonsmoking men, an 8-day skiing tour with daily trips of 12 to 25 km lowered Lp(a) concentrations.[139]

HDL Cholesterol

A reduced concentration of HDL-C is a strong predictor of coronary artery disease.[1,6-10,140] Both epidemiologic and prospective studies confirm the inverse relationship between plasma HDL-C and coronary atherosclerosis. Although it initially appeared that the protective effect was mainly due to HDL_2 fraction, more recent data have found that both HDL_2 and HDL_3 levels are associated with cardioprotection.[60]

Most studies indicate that exercise raises HDL-C. Laporte and associates[35] examined the relationship between HDL-C and activity levels. The lowest HDL-C levels occurred among patients confined to bed rest, and endurance athletes had the highest HDL-C. In a cross-sectional investigation[141] controlled for many variables known to alter HDL-C, higher levels were present among joggers than among those who were sedentary. HDL-C has been found to be directly related to parameters of physical fitness.[142] Various active men and women, including marathon runners, joggers, lumberjacks, swimmers, and ballet dancers, have been found to have higher levels of total HDL-C than their sedentary counterparts.[91,92,98,125,143-146] The differences in HDL-C levels between active and sedentary subjects have been as much as 15 to 20 mg/dL. However, most cross-sectional studies only have observed the effects of exercise among subjects with relatively normal lipid patterns, and comparisons did not always include considerations of body composition.

Prospective training studies generally have demonstrated that endurance exercise increases HDL-C concentrations. These studies have included healthy subjects,[103,146] obese individuals,[117,135] elderly men,[126] and dyslipidemic patients.[116,117]

Some investigations[106,147-149] have failed to detect significant changes in HDL-C after conditioning. However, these findings may be explained by other variables that counteract the favorable effect of exercise on HDL-C levels, including relatively normal initial HDL-C concentrations[150] and short duration of the exercise intervention.[149] The beneficial HDL-C response to exercise may require months of conditioning rather than the usual 4- to 12-week exercise-study time frame.[107,151] In addition, many investigations are limited by small subject numbers, which could have led to inadequate statistical power to detect significant differences.

HDL subfractions

As previously noted, HDL-C concentrations consist of two major components, HDL_2 and HDL_3. Myocardial infarction survivors show lower HDL_2 levels than do controls,[152,153] and some have also found this relationship for HDL_3.[153] The independent contributions of both HDL_2 and HDL_3 subfractions were found in a 5-year prospective study of 14,916 men, aged 40 to 84 years, matched for age and smoking status.[51] Both subfractions were associated with cardioprotection. However, the total HDL-C level probably is as potent a discriminator as either or both HDL-C subfractions.[51,154]

Higher physical fitness levels and exercise training have been primarily associated with increased HDL_2,[155] although one cross-sectional study[156] found exercise to be directly related to HDL_3. After 1 year of diet and training, HDL_2 cholesterol levels were higher for men who exercised and dieted than for males who only dieted.[157] However, the former group also had greater fat loss. A more consistent change in HDL_2 has been observed in prospective studies, but exercise has not had a major impact on the HDL_3 subfraction. Exercise may result in higher HDL_2 owing to reduced conversion of HDL_2 to HDL_3 in the liver.[158,159] Also, during lipoprotein lipase hydrolysis of triglyceride-rich lipoproteins (which occurs during exercise), lipids can be transferred to HDL_3, resulting in HDL_2-like particles.[52] These changes could improve HDL_2 levels and overall coronary risk without altering total HDL-C concentrations.

EFFECTS OF EXERCISE ON APOPROTEINS

Most studies relating apo A-I levels to coronary heart disease have found that, as with HDL-C, affected individuals have significantly lower levels of apo A-I than controls.[10,51] Apoprotein A-I and apo A-II are the major proteins of HDL_2 and HDL_3, respectively, while apo B is associated with LDL-C. A reduction in serum apo-A-I levels increases coronary heart disease risk, while apo B concentrations are directly related to coronary atherosclerosis; a high apo B-to-apo A-I ratio (>.98) is most strongly associated with disease severity.[160]

Exercise may alter apoprotein levels. Four days of intense training has lowered apo-B levels while also increasing the apo A-I-to-apo A-II ratio.[161] Physical training has been observed to increase apo A-I levels in young males, middle-aged men, and elderly exercisers.[125,162] Wood and colleagues[157] observed a significant increase in apo A-I among male dieters who also exercised, compared to controls and those who only dieted. However, not all studies have found beneficial changes. Sedentary men had no increase in apo A-I levels after 4 months of bicycling or running,[163] and similar negative results have been noted by other investigators.[164,165] The mixed results may reflect design problems similar to those of other exercise–lipid studies, including few study subjects and short duration of training, both of which limit the ability of these investigations to find significant differences in apolipoproteins after training.[164-166] In general, exercise appears either to result in no change in apolipoprotein concentrations or to increase apo A-I levels.

Potential Mechanisms of Action of Exercise in Lipid and Lipoprotein Metabolism

The beneficial relationship between exercise and lipoprotein levels may be explained by the effect of training on enzymes involved in lipoprotein metabolism. Investigators have studied the relationship of training and LPL,[43,45,46,53,167–172] LCAT,[166,173,174] and hepatic lipase.[175,176]

INCREASED LPL ACTIVITY

Lipoprotein lipase resides on the capillary wall of most tissues, where it is activated to hydrolyze chylomicrons and VLDL particles.[43,55] Reduced plasma LPL activity has been correlated with increased cardiovascular disease.[177] An increase in LPL activity is associated with lower triglyceride levels[167] and higher HDL-C concentrations.[44–46] LPL facilitates metabolism of triglycerides by hydrolysis,[178] often resulting in higher HDL-C levels. When LPL activity is increased by exercise, favorable effects on lipids and lipoproteins occur.

Endurance-trained individuals have high concentrations of LPL in both adipose and lean tissue.[142,168–170] Higher LPL levels among conditioned individuals result in plasma clearance of VLDL and triglyceride reduction.[123] Prospective evidence suggests that LPL activity increases with vigorous exertion.[129,130,142,170–172] Increased LPL activity has been observed soon after exercise and persists after prolonged bouts of exercise. After a 42-km race, LPL activity increased among trained men,[171] along with a reduction in triglycerides and an elevation in HDL-C levels. An increased rate of triglyceride catabolism after physical training also occurs for those with type IV hyperlipoproteinemia.[119] These studies are consistent with the observation that exercise increases catabolism of triglycerides rather than diminishing their synthesis.

Presumably, triglyceride and HDL-C changes that occur with exercise are due to changes in enzyme activity, but they also can result from alteration of regulatory apoproteins.[40] The triglyceride changes that accompany one bout of physical activity also may be augmented by the need to replenish muscle triglyceride reduced by the previous exercise period.[179] The more chronic effects of exercise on LPL activity could be the result of body composition changes, as adipose-tissue LPL activity is increased after weight loss alone, without exercise.[180]

LOWER HEPATIC LIPASE ACTIVITY

Other enzymes of lipoprotein metabolism have been investigated after exercise. Hepatic triglyceride lipase promotes clearance of HDL-C in the plasma by promoting its catabolism.[43,62] Endurance training may reduce HDL-C clearance because aerobically conditioned subjects have lower hepatic lipase activity.[145,181] However, lower body fat among exercisers reduces the significance of these findings. Hepatic lipase activity also is inversely correlated with HDL_2 levels and is directly associated with HDL_3 concentration.[45] This relationship has been observed after 15 weeks of exercise training in previously sedentary, middle-aged men[139] and in active military academy students.[142]

INCREASED LCAT ACTIVITY

Some of the effects of exercise on cholesterol metabolism may be explained by changes in the activity of LCAT, an enzyme activated by apo A-I.[182] This enzyme affects newly formed HDL-C, which, after being secreted from the liver or ileum, enhances acquisition of cholesterol from the periphery (e.g., arterial walls). LCAT esterifies free cholesterol and converts HDL_3 to HDL_2.[173,183] A single exercise session was shown to increase LCAT activity, and 7 weeks of training increased LCAT in an uncontrolled study.[103,184] However, another investigation found that LCAT did not increase after 13 weeks of training,[166] and no significant relationship between the change in LCAT concentration and HDL-C levels was apparent after 1 year of exercise.[91] Differences in the findings could be due to a number of factors affecting LCAT, including initial enzyme levels, as well as the substrate and end products that regulate LCAT concentrations.[185]

Clinical Applications of Exercise in Dyslipidemia

GENERAL CLASSIFICATION OF DYSLIPIDEMIA

When fasting elevated cholesterol or triglycerides are detected (i.e., a total cholesterol of 200 mg/dL or more or a triglyceride level of 150 mg/dL or greater), follow-up should include a repeat determination and measurement of HDL-C.[82,186,187] Based on the lipid profiles obtained from these measurements, dyslipidemia can be divided into several categories of risk (Table 9–1). Guidelines from the National Cholesterol Educational Program suggest that individuals with levels of LDL-C of 130 mg/dL or higher and individuals with LDL-C concentrations above 160 mg/dL who have two other coronary risk factors (male sex is considered a risk factor) require therapy.[82,187] Likewise, those with LDL-C of >100 mg/dL who have definite coronary heart disease should have a complete clinical evaluation and begin treatment to lower LDL-C.[187] Because a

Table 9–1 **RISK PROFILE OF LIPID AND LIPOPROTEIN CONCENTRATIONS WITHOUT OTHER RISK FACTORS PRESENT**

	Total Cholesterol* (mg/dL)	LDL Cholesterol (mg/dL)	HDL Cholesterol (mg/dL)	Triglycerides† (mg/dL)
High risk	≥245	≥190‡	≤35§	≥1,000**
Moderate risk	221–244	160–189‡††	36–44¶	500–999
Mild risk	201–220	130–159‡	45–54¶	250–499
Average risk	182–200	<100–129‡	55–65¶	151–249
Low risk	<182	<100	≥65¶	≤150

*Kannel WB, et al: Overall and CHD mortality rates in relation to major risk factors in 325,348 men screened for the MRFIT. *Am Heart J* 1986; 112:825–836.
†1992 NIH Consensus Conference on Treatment of Hypertriglyceridemia.[189]
‡National Cholesterol Education Program (NCEP) Expert Panel.[187]
§Helsinki Heart Study.[8]
¶Framingham Heart Study.[7]
**Hypertriglyceridemia of this magnitude increases the risk for pancreatitis and abdominal pain.
††NCEP Expert Panel (II), 1993, suggests >160 mg/dL is high risk, but recommends initiation of drug therapy at 190 mg/dL.

low level of HDL-C (below 35 mg/dL) is a significant coronary risk[10,20,140] and improving HDL-C concentration can reduce the myocardial infarction rate,[140] therapy should be initiated for individuals with low HDL-C levels. The patient's total atherosclerotic risk profile and present clinical status should be considered in a lipid-altering treatment program.[82,186–189]

After clinical assessment, it is necessary to exclude correctable secondary causes of dyslipidemia, such as hypothyroidism, nephrotic syndrome, diabetes mellitus, obstructive liver disease, and use of alcohol or medication that can influence lipid levels. If no secondary causes are present, patients should be advised to have other family members screened for lipid abnormalities.[82,186,188]

CLINICAL USE OF EXERCISE

Changes in lipid and lipoprotein levels occur with exercise. The major alterations induced by endurance exercise are a decrease in triglyceride level (mostly VLDL) and an increase in HDL-C concentration (Table 9–2). In planning an exercise program to improve the lipid profile, the factors listed on Table 9–3 need to be considered. Even if exercise does not enhance lipid and lipoprotein levels, however, it can alter other cardiovascular risk factors, as discussed in Chapters 2, 8, and 10 (i.e., hypertension, type II diabetes, obesity) and has the potential to reduce all-cause mortality.[32]

NUTRITIONAL THERAPY

Goals of dietary therapy are to reduce LDL-C and triglyceride levels. Nutritional interventions can complement regular physical activity and en-

Table 9–2 **EFFECT OF EXERCISE ON LIPIDS AND LIPOPROTEINS**

Plasma Constituent	Acute Changes	Chronic Changes	Comment
Triglycerides	$\downarrow\downarrow$	$\downarrow\downarrow$	Consistently found, even among those with hypertriglyceridemia (most studies are endurance exercise).
Total cholesterol	$\leftrightarrow$	$\leftrightarrow$ or $\downarrow$	Fat loss will contribute to decrease.
LDL-C	$\leftrightarrow$	$\leftrightarrow$	Some studies have observed a decrease with weight training; exercise-induced fat loss may reduce LDL-C.
HDL-C	$\uparrow\leftrightarrow$	$\uparrow$	A mild increase can be observed after an acute bout of exercise, possibly related to LPL activity and triglyceride utilization. The degree of change is somewhat dependent on pre-exercise levels. Lower levels have more potential to change (mainly endurance exercise).
HDL$_2$	*	$\uparrow$	Changes may be secondary to $\downarrow$ HL or $\uparrow$ LPL activity; few studies address this finding.
HDL$_3$	*	$\leftrightarrow$	Only a few studies are available.
Apoprotein A-I	*	$\leftrightarrow$ or $\uparrow$	Only a few studies are available.
Apoprotein B	*	$\leftrightarrow$	Only a few studies are available.

Key: $\downarrow$ = small or mild decrease, $\downarrow\downarrow$ = substantial decrease, $\uparrow$ = small or mild increase, $\leftrightarrow$ = no change, LDL-C = low-density lipoprotein cholesterol, HDL-C = high-density lipoprotein cholesterol, LPL = lipoprotein lipase, * = inadequate number of studies to justify trends or conclusion, HL = hepatic lipase.

Table 9–3 **CONDITIONS THAT WILL ENHANCE THE EFFECTS OF EXERCISE**

- Patients are sedentary
- Lipoprotein levels are abnormal (especially elevated triglycerides or depressed HDL cholesterol)
- Exercise training is long-term (>6 months)
- Body composition changes occur (↑ lean body mass, ↓ body fat)
- Diet is modified (e.g., ↓ saturated fat, ↑ omega-3 or omega-6 fatty acids)

hance changes in lipid and lipoprotein concentrations. In general, all animal fats are highly saturated (having few double bonds). Highly saturated fats will increase LDL-C concentration by suppressing liver LDL-receptor activity and thus decreasing breakdown of LDL-C.[189–191] Animal studies have shown that cholesterol ingestion also reduces hepatic LDL-receptor activity.[192] Limiting saturated fat and cholesterol intake can produce a decrease in LDL-C.[191]

Polyunsaturated fats, which are constituents of cellular membranes that are necessary for prostaglandin production, are not synthesized by the body and are considered essential.[193] High intake of polyunsaturated fatty acids (either omega-3 or omega-6 structures) can reduce LDL-C levels,[190,194,195] and the omega-3 fatty acids, found in high concentrations in fish, can lower plasma triglycerides.[196] Although the adult treatment panel of the 1993 Joint National Committee report[187] for high cholesterol recommended that patients initially (during phase 1) reduce total daily calories from fat to below 30% (< 10% saturated and less than 300 mg cholesterol), others have suggested lower intake of fat and cholesterol. The diet recommended for phase 2 is less than 25% of calories from fat, with less than 200 mg of cholesterol each day. Connor and Connor[196] recommend reducing total fat intake to 20% while limiting cholesterol consumption to 100 mg/d, with saturated fat comprising only 5% to 6% of daily calories.

Case Studies

CASE: M.T., a 26-year-old woman, managed a local exercise facility. She regularly exercised in a vigorous fashion, mainly by lifting weights, and competed in local and regional bodybuilding contests. Her family history was negative for premature cardiovascular disease or known cardiovascular risk factors. Although she had no complaints, a physical examination was requested along with body composition analysis and a cholesterol profile. The examination revealed a 173-cm (5'9"), 79-kg (175-lb) muscular woman, with low body fat (6% by hydrodensitometry). Results of her physical examination were normal, and no signs of virilization were present other than prominent muscle size.

Laboratory data revealed a total cholesterol of 160 mg/dL, HDL-C of 7 mg/dL, LDL-C of 128 mg/dL, and a 125 mg/dL triglyceride concentration. Further questioning revealed that she was using anabolic androgenic steroids prior to bodybuilding contests. She routinely took high doses of these drugs for 8 weeks while reducing her caloric intake.

COMMENT: Weight lifting, also known as resistive exercise, has gained popularity, and a number of health benefits can accrue from this form of training.[197] In several studies,[37,101,127,128] weight lifting has been found to impact favorably on lipid levels, mainly by lowering LDL-C or decreasing total cholesterol-to-HDL cholesterol ratios. Whether this is due to reduction in body fat, changes that follow an exercise program, or alteration of lipolytic enzymes is unclear. However, use of anabolic androgenic hormones in pharmacologic doses as a muscle-enhancing stimulus is associated with a number of adverse risks, including elevation of LDL-C and large reductions in HDL-C.[83] Although no long-term studies have been performed, the severe alterations associated with these drugs, especially if continued for prolonged periods, could lead to early coronary atherosclerosis. The potential benefits of training, especially for favorable lipid changes, are negated by the use of these drugs.

CASE: F.A., a 45-year-old white man, had a 15-year history of elevated blood pressure. Although he had been treated with various antihypertensive agents for several years, he complained of untoward effects with each attempted pharmacologic therapy. His diet was low in saturated fat, low in salt and, he reported, "very low in taste quality." Because a previous chemistry panel revealed a cholesterol of 270 mg/dL, his cholesterol was fractionated. His repeat total cholesterol was 268 mg/dL, with an HDL-C of 54 mg/dL, LDL-C of 162 mg/dL, and triglycerides of 260 mg/dL. His physical examination revealed a resting, seated blood pressure of 168/98 mm Hg. Results of thyroid function tests, blood urea nitrogen, glucose, urinalysis, and electrocardiogram (ECG) were normal. A 3-day dietary analysis confirmed a low intake of total fat (below 20%) and saturated fat (below 7%) and the avoidance of alcohol.

He enrolled in a 3 day/wk exercise class at the university hospital's Human Performance Laboratory, and complemented this with additional training on weekends. After 12 weeks of regular exercise, 5 days each week (30–45 minutes every session), his weight decreased 7 kg (15 lb) and blood pressure decreased to 130/84 mm Hg without pharmacologic intervention. A repeat lipoprotein panel revealed a total cholesterol of 240 mg/dL, HDL-C of 68 mg/dL, LDL-C of 138 mg/dL, and triglyceride level of 170 mg/dL. He continued to exercise, and after 3 years, his lipoprotein profile and blood pressure remain controlled.

COMMENT: This patient has three risks for coronary artery disease: (1) an elevated LDL-C, (2) hypertension, and (3) male sex. Therapy to reduce LDL-C should be initiated because of elevated LDL-C and two other risk factors. Although he adopted a diet that was low in saturated fat and cholesterol, it did not reduce his LDL-C to a reasonable level. Hypertension and dyslipidemia are often found in the same individual, as this patient demonstrates. Data from the National Health and Nutrition Survey II,[198] by staff of the National Heart, Lung and Blood Institute, suggest that 40% of persons who have a blood pressure of 140/90 mm Hg or more have total blood cholesterol levels of 240 mg/dL or greater.

Weight loss achieved by physical activity, even without reduced caloric intake, can decrease plasma triglycerides and elevate HDL-C, similar to weight loss induced by diet alone.[135] In this case, two major risk factors were favorably modified by nonpharmacologic measures. These patients should be followed closely, however, as these risk factors usually return to preintervention levels when lifestyle changes are discontinued.

CASE: M.R., a 36-year-old man, complained of right upper quadrant tenderness, which increased with sitting and standing and was reduced with the supine position. He denied any change in this discomfort with exertion and noted tenderness when he pressed on his right lower ribs anteriorly. He had had these symptoms in the past, but despite a medical work-up, no diagnosis was rendered. M.R. reported that he had gained approximately 7 kg (15 lb) over the past 8 months and had begun consuming 3 ounces of bourbon each night as a way to reduce stress from work. There was no history of early coronary disease, although his mother had "trouble with her pancreas" in the past. He had been an "athlete" in high school, but had not exercised regularly for at least 5 years.

The physical examination revealed a well-developed, mildly overweight man in no distress. Findings were remarkable for a 13-cm liver span only, while the rest of the physical examination was normal. His plasma glucose, amylase, liver function tests (aspartate aminotransferase, SGOT, prothrombin time, alkaline phosphate, and lactic dehydrogenase), renal function, and thyroid function were normal. Likewise, his electrocardiogram was without significant abnormality. The lipoprotein levels were cholesterol of 210 mg/dL, triglycerides of 1040 mg/dL, and an HDL-C of 34 mg/dL. An abdominal computerized tomographic scan revealed a normal pancreas and gallbladder, and the common bile duct was not dilated. The liver was reported to be near "water density."

COMMENT: M.R. has hypertriglyceridemia with an associated low HDL-C. It is important to avoid bile acid resins when treating this disorder, as these agents increase the triglyceride concentrations. Hypertriglyceridemia in this case has resulted in an enlarged, fatty liver. His alcohol intake could also promote hypertriglyceridemia. A diet rich in omega-3 fatty acids (fish oil), abstinence from alcohol, and regular exercise were recommended. He began exercising at his local health club, training on a stationary cycle for 30 minutes, four times a week. After 8 weeks of this nonpharmacologic intervention, along with alcohol abstinence, his triglycerides decreased to 360 mg/dL while HDL-C levels increased to 42 mg/dL. M.R.'s right upper quadrant pain, which was likely due to hepatomegaly, resolved after 3 weeks. Overall, his risk from pancreatitis was reduced and his HDL-C improved.

Summary

Exercise should be prescribed as a component of the initial therapy for lipid and lipoprotein disorders, especially among those with hypertriglyceridemia and low HDL-C. Regular physical activity can help to decrease body fat and will complement a diet that is low in saturated fat to favorably alter LDL-C levels. Adopting and maintaining an exercise program is of particular benefit to those with dyslipidemia who have other associated coronary risk factors, including obesity, non–insulin-dependent diabetes mellitus, and hypertension.

Like pharmacologic therapy, regular physical activity may not be effective for all forms of dyslipidemia. Further research should help delineate specific clinical conditions wherein lipoprotein responsiveness to exercise is most likely to occur.

REFERENCES

1. Miller ME, et al.: Relation of angiographically defined coronary artery disease to plasma lipoprotein subfractions and apolipoproteins. *BMJ* 1981; 282:1741–1744.
2. Naito HK: The association of serum lipids, lipoproteins, and apolipoproteins with coronary artery disease assessed by coronary arteriography. *Ann NY Acad Sci* 1985; 454:230–238.
3. Wallace RB, Anderson RA: Blood lipids, lipid-related measures, and risk of atherosclerotic cardiovascular disease. *Epidemiol Rev* 1987; 9:95–119.
4. Kannel WB, Castelli WP, Gordon T: Cholesterol in the prediction of atherosclerotic disease: New perspectives based on the Framingham Study. *Ann Intern Med* 1979; 90:85–91.
5. Brunzell JD, et al.: Apoproteins B and A-I and coronary artery disease in humans. *Arteriosclerosis* 1984; 4:79–83.
6. Whayne TF, et al.: Plasma apolipoprotein B and VLDL, LDL, and HDL cholesterol as risk factors in the development of coronary artery disease in male patients examined by angiography. *Atherosclerosis* 1981; 39:411–424.
7. Gordon T, et al.: High-density lipoprotein as a protective factor against coronary heart disease: The Framingham Study. *Am J Med* 1977; 62:707–714.
8. Manninen V, et al.: Lipid alterations and decline in the incidence of coronary heart disease in the Helsinki Heart Study. *JAMA* 1988; 260:641–651.
9. Gordon DJ, Rifkind BM: High-density lipoprotein: The clinical implications of recent studies. *N Engl J Med* 1989; 321:1311–1316.
10. Miller NE: Associations of high-density lipoprotein subclasses and apolipoproteins wth ischemic heart disease and coronary atherosclerosis. *Am Heart J* 1987; 113:589–597.
11. Maciejko JJ, et al.: Apolipoprotein A-I as a marker of angiographically assessed coronary artery disease. *N Engl J Med* 1983; 309:385–389.
12. Ordovas JM, et al.: Apolipoprotein A-I gene polymorphism associated with premature coronary heart disease and familial hypoalphalipoproteinemia. *N Engl J Med* 1986; 314:671–677.
13. Hulley SB, et al.: Epidemiology as a guide to clinical decisions: The association between triglyceride and coronary heart disease. *N Engl J Med* 1980; 302:1383–1389.
14. Austin M: Plasma triglycerides as a risk factor for coronary heart disease: The epidemiologic evidence and beyond. *Am J Epidemiol* 1989; 129:249–259.
15. Heyden S, et al.: Fasting triglyceride as predictors of total and CHD mortality in Evans County, Georgia. *J Chron Dis* 1980; 33:275–282.
16. Carlson LA, Bottiger LE: Serum triglycerides, to be or not to be a risk factor for ischemic heart disease? *Atherosclerosis* 1981; 39:287–291.
17. Manninen V, et al.: Joint effects of serum triglyceride and LDL-cholesterol and HDL-cholesterol concentrations on coronary heart disease risk in the Helsinki Heart Study: Implication for treatment. *Circulation* 1992; 85:37–45.
18. Hjerman I, et al.: Effect of diet and smoking intervention on the incidence of coronary heart disease: Report from the Oslo Study Group of a randomized trial in healthy men. *Lancet* 1981; 2:1303–1310.
19. Arntzenius AC, et al.: Diet, lipoprotein, and the progression of coronary atherosclerosis: The Leiden Intervention Trial. *N Engl J Med* 1985; 312:805–811.
20. Lipid Research Clinics Program: The Lipid Research Clinics Coronary Primary Prevention Trial results, I: Reduction in incidence of coronary disease. *JAMA* 1984; 251:351–364.
21. Lipid Research Clinics Program: The Lipid Research Clinics Coronary Primary Prevention Trial results, II: The relationship of reduction in incidence of coronary heart disease to cholesterol lowering. *JAMA* 1984; 251:365–374.
22. Levy RI, et al.: The influence of changes in lipid values induced by cholestyramine and diet on progression of coronary artery disease: Results of the NHLBI Type II Coronary Intervention Study. *Circulation* 1984; 69:325–337.
23. Buchwald H, et al.: Effect of partial ileal bypass surgery on mortality and morbidity from coronary heart disease in patients with hypercholesterolemia. *N Engl J Med* 1990; 323:946–955.
24. Blankenhorn DH, Nessim SA, Johnson RL: Beneficial effects of combined colestipol-niacin therapy on coronary atherosclerosis and coronary venous bypass grafts. *JAMA* 1987; 257:3233–3240.
25. Brown G, et al.: Regression of coronary artery disease as a result of intensive lipid-lowering therapy in men with high levels of apolipoprotein B. *N Engl J Med* 1990; 323:1289–1298.
26. Ornish D: Can lifestyle changes reverse coronary heart disease? Report of the Lifestyle Heart Trial. *Lancet* 1990; 336:129–133.
27. Loscalzo J: Regression of coronary atherosclerosis. *N Engl J Med* 1990; 323:1337–1339.
28. Canner PL, et al.: Fifteen-year mortality in Coronary Drug Project patients: Long-term benefit with niacin. *J Am Coll Cardiol* 1986; 8:1245–1255.
29. Sempos C, et al.: The prevalence of high blood cholesterol levels among adults in the United States. *JAMA* 1989; 262:45–52.
30. Ekelund LG, et al.: Physical fitness as a

predictor of cardiovascular mortality in asymptomatic North American men: The Lipid Research Clinics mortality follow-up study. *N Engl J Med* 1988; 319:1379–1384.

31. Berlin JA, Colditz GA: A meta-analysis of physical activity in the prevention of coronary heart disease. *Am J Epidemiol* 1990; 132:612–628.

32. Blair SN, et al.: Physical fitness and all-cause mortality: A prospective study of healthy men and women. *JAMA* 1989; 262:2395–2401.

33. Paffenbarger RS Jr, et al.: Physical activity, all-cause mortality, and longevity of college alumni. *N Engl J Med* 1986; 314: 605–613.

34. Slattery ML, Jacobs DR Jr, Nichaman MZ. Leisure time physical activity and coronary heart disease death: The US Railroad Study. *Circulation* 1989; 79:304–311.

35. Laporte RE, et al.: The spectrum of physical activity, cardiovascular disease, and health: An epidemiologic perspective. *Am J Epidemiol* 1984; 120:507–517.

36. Tran ZV, et al.: The effects of exercise on blood lipids and lipoproteins: A meta-analysis of studies. *Med Sci Sports Exerc* 1983; 15:393–402.

37. Goldberg L, Elliot DL: The effect of exercise on lipid metabolism in men and women. *Sports Med* 1987; 4:307–321.

38. Marti B, et al.: Fifteen-year changes in exercise, aerobic power, abdominal fat, and serum lipids in runners and controls. *Med Sci Sports Exerc* 1991; 23:115–122.

39. Brown MS, Goldstein JL: A receptor-mediated pathway for cholesterol homeostasis. *Science* 1986; 232:34–47.

40. Hussain MM, et al.: Chylomicron metabolism: Chylomicron uptake by bone marrow in different animal species. *J Biol Chem* 1989; 264:17931–17938.

41. Gotto AM: The plasma apolipoproteins: Regulation of the structure and function of plasma lipoprotein. *Cardiovasc Rev Rep* 1982; 3:1032–1035.

42. Miller NE: HDL metabolism and its role in lipid transport in dyslipoproteinemia and coronary heart disease: The significance of HDL-cholesterol. *Symposium Proceedings.* AVMD: New York, 1987, pp 6–11.

43. Eisenberg S: Metabolism of apolipoproteins and lipoproteins. *Current Opinion in Lipidology* 1990; 1:205–215.

44. Nikkila EA, Takinen MR, Sane T: Plasma high-density lipoprotein concentration and subfraction distribution in relation to triglyceride metabolism. *Am Heart J* 1987; 113:543–548.

45. Taskinen MR, Nikkila EA: High-density lipoprotein subfractions in relation to lipoprotein lipase activity of tissues in man: Evidence for reciprocal regulation of HDL_2 and HDL_3 levels by lipoprotein lipase. *Clin Chem Acta* 1981; 112:325–332.

46. Nikkila EA, Kuusi T, Taskinen M-R: Role of lipoprotein lipase and hepatic endothelial lipase in the metabolism of high-density lipoproteins: A novel concept on cholesterol transport in HDL cycle. In Carlson LA, Pernow B, eds: *Metabolic Risk Factors in Ischemic Cardiovascular Disease.* Raven Press: New York, 1982.

47. Pekkanen J, et al.: Ten-year mortality from cardiovascular disease in relation to cholesterol level among men with and without pre-existing cardiovascular disease. *N Engl J Med* 1990; 322:1700–1707.

48. Krauss RM: Relationship of intermediate and low-density lipoprotein subspecies to risk of coronary artery disease. *Am Heart J* 1987; 113:578–582.

49. Aro A, et al.: Lipoprotein lipid levels as indicators of the severity of angiographically assessed coronary artery disease. *Atherosclerosis* 1986; 62:219–275.

50. Rudney H, Sexton RC: Regulation of cholesterol biosynthesis. *Annu Rev Nutr* 1986; 6:245–272.

51. Stampfer MJ, et al.: A prospective study of cholesterol, apolipoproteins, and the risk of myocardial infarction. *N Engl J Med* 1991; 325:373–381.

52. Krauss RM: Regulation of high-density lipoprotein levels. *Med Clin North Am* 1982; 66:403–430.

53. Eckel RH: Lipoprotein lipase: A multifunctional enzyme relevant to common metabolic diseases. *N Engl J Med* 1989; 320: 1060–1068.

54. Miller GJ, Miller NE: Plasma high-density lipoprotein concentration and development of ischemic heart disease. *Lancet* 1975; 1:16–19.

55. Phillips MC, Rothblat GH: Cholesterol flux between high-density lipoproteins and cells. In Catapano AL, Salvioli G, Veryani C, eds: *High-Density Lipoproteins: Physiopathological Aspects and Clinical Significance.* Raven Press: New York, 1987, pp 57–86.

56. Carew TE, et al.: A mechanism by which high-density lipoproteins may slow the atherogenic process. *Lancet* 1976; 1: 1315–1317.

57. Goldstein JL, Brown MS: The LDL-receptor defect in familial hypercholesterolemia. In Havel, RJ, ed: *The Medical Clinics of North America: Symposium on Lipid Disorders.* WB Saunders: Philadelphia, 1982, pp 469–484.

58. Alaupovic P, Curry MD, McConathy WJ: Quantitative determination of human plasma apolipoproteins by electroimmunoassays. In Carlson LA, Paoletti IR, Weber G, eds: *International Conference on Atherosclerosis.* Raven Press: New York, 1978, pp 109–115.

59. Goot AM: The plasma apolipoproteins: Regulation of the structure and function of plasma lipoproteins. *Cardiovasc Rev Rep* 1982; 3:1032–1035.

60. Stampfer MJ, et al.: A prospective study of cholesterol, apolipoproteins, and the risk of myocardial infarction. *N Engl J Med* 1991; 325:373–381.

61. Windler E, et al.: The estradiol-stimulated lipoprotein receptor of rat liver. *J Biol Chem* 1980; 255:10464–10471.

62. Eisenberg S: High-density lipoprotein metabolism. *J Lipid Res* 1984; 25:1017–1058.

63. Lipid Research Clinics Program: *Manual of Laboratory Operations, Lipid and Lipoprotein Analysis*, ed 2. Washington, DC: Dept of Health and Human Services, 1982.

64. Blank DW, et al.: The method of determination must be considered in interpreting blood cholesterol levels. *JAMA* 1986; 256: 2867–2870.

65. Superko HR, Bachorick PS, Wood PD: High-density lipoprotein measurements: A help or hindrance in practical clinical medicine? *JAMA* 1986; 256:2714–2717.

66. Warnick GR, Alberts JJ, Teng-Leary E: HDL-cholesterol: Results of interlaboratory proficiency tests. *Clin Chem* 1980; 26: 169–170.

67. Brown SA, et al.: Effects of blood collection and processing on radioimmunoassay results for apolipoprotein A-I in plasma. *Clin Chem* 1988; 34:920–924.

68. Hankinson SE, et al.: Effect of transport conditions on the stability of biochemical markers in blood. *Clin Chem* 1989; 35: 2313–2316.

69. Friedewald WT, Levy RI, Fredrickson DS: Estimation of the concentration of low-density lipoprotein cholesterol in plasma without use of preparative ultracentrifuge. *Clin Chem* 1972; 18:499–502.

70. DeLong DM, et al.: A comparison of methods for the estimation of plasma low- and very-low-density lipoprotein cholesterol. *JAMA* 1986; 256:2372–2377.

71. Quig DW, et al.: Effects of short-term aerobic conditioning and high-cholesterol feeding on plasma and total lipoprotein cholesterol levels in sedentary young men. *Am J Clin Nutr* 1983; 38:825–834.

72. Sacks FM, et al.: Effect of ingestion of meat on plasma cholesterol of vegetarians. *JAMA* 1981; 246:640–644.

73. Ullmann D, et al.: Will a high-carbohydrate, low-fat diet lower plasma lipids and lipoproteins without producing hypertriglyceridemia? *Arteriosclerosis Thrombosis* 1991; 11:1059–1067.

74. Caggiula AW: Optimum nutritional therapy in treatment of hyperlipoproteinemias. *Arteriosclerosis* 1989; 9:106–110.

75. Connor WE, Connor SJ: The dietary prevention and treatment of coronary heart disease. In Connor WE, Bristow JD, eds: *Coronary Heart Disease: Prevention, Complications and Treatment.* JB Lippincott: Philadelphia, 1985, pp 43–64.

76. Schonfeld G, et al.: Alterations in levels and interrelations of plasma apolipopro-teins induced by diet. *Metabolism* 1976; 25:261–275.

77. Illingworth DR, Ullmann D: The effects of omega-3 fatty acids on risk factors for cardiovascular disease. In Karel M, Lees RS, eds: *Omega-3 Fatty Acids in Health and Disease.* Marcel Dekker: New York, 1990, pp 39–70.

78. Avogaro P, et al.: HDL-cholesterol, apolipoprotein A and B, age, and index of body weight. *Atherosclerosis* 1978; 31:85–91.

79. Terry RB, et al.: Regional adiposity patterns in relation to lipids, lipoprotein cholesterol, and lipoprotein subfraction mass in men. *J Clin Endocrinol Metab* 1989; 68: 191–199.

80. Freedman DS, et al.: Body fat distribution and male/female differences in lipids and lipoproteins. *Circulation* 1990; 81: 1498–1506.

81. Hurley BF, et al.: High-density lipoprotein cholesterol in bodybuilders vs. power lifters: Negative effects of androgen use. *JAMA* 1984; 252:507–513.

82. Illingworth DR: Lipid-lowering drugs: An overview of indications and optimum therapeutic use. *Drugs* 1987; 33:259–279.

83. Ernst N, Fisher M, Smith W: The association of plasma high-density lipoprotein cholesterol with dietary intake and alcohol consumption: The Lipid Clinic Program Prevalence Study. *Circulation* 1980; 62 (suppl IV):51–52.

84. Wallace RB, et al.: Alterations of plasma high-density lipoprotein cholesterol levels associated with consumption of selected medications: The Lipid Research Clinics Program Prevalence Study. *Circulation* 1980; 62(suppl IV):77–82.

85. Lehtonen A, Marniemi J: Effect of atenolol on plasma HDL-cholesterol subfractions. *Atherosclerosis* 1984; 51:335–338.

86. Sasaki J, et al.: Decreased concentration of high-density lipoprotein cholesterol in schizophrenic patients treated with phenothiazines. *Atherosclerosis* 1984; 51: 163–169.

87. Nestel PJ, Hirsch EZ: Mechanism of alcohol-induced hypertriglyceridemia. *J Lab Clin Med* 1965; 66:357–365.

88. Molitch ME, Oill P, Odell WD: Massive hyperlipidemia during estrogen therapy. *JAMA* 1974; 227:522.

89. Grundy SM, et al.: Transport of very-low-density lipoprotein triglycerides in varying degrees of obesity and hypertriglyceridemia. *J Clin Invest* 1978; 63:1274–1283.

90. Wood PD, et al.: The distribution of plasma lipoproteins in middle-aged male runners. *Metabolism* 1976; 25:1249–1257.

91. Hartung GH, et al.: Relation of diet to high-density lipoprotein cholesterol in middle-aged marathon runners, joggers, and inactive men. *N Engl J Med* 1980; 302:357–361.

92. Wood PD, et al.: Plasma lipoprotein distri-

butions in male and female runners. *Ann NY Acad Sci* 1977; 301:748–763.

93. Cooper KH, et al.: Physical fitness levels vs. selected coronary risk factors: A cross-sectional study. *JAMA* 1976; 236:166–169.

94. Montoye HJ, Block WD, Gayle R: Maximal oxygen intake and blood lipids. *J Chron Dis* 1978; 31:111–118.

95. McDonough JR, Kusumi F, Bruce RA: Variations in maximal oxygen intake with physical activity in middle-aged men. *Circulation* 1970; 41:743–751.

96. Lehtonen A, Viikari J: Serum triglycerides and cholesterol and serum high-density lipoprotein cholesterol in highly physical active men. *Acta Med Scand* 1978; 204: 111–114.

97. Vodak PA, et al.: HDL-Cholesterol and other plasma lipid and lipoprotein concentrations in middle-aged male and female tennis players. *Metabolism* 1980; 29: 745–752.

98. Farrell PA, et al.: A comparison of plasma cholesterol, triglycerides, and high-density lipoprotein cholesterol in speed skaters, weight-lifters, and nonathletes. *Eur J Appl Physiol* 1982; 481:77–82.

99. Schnabel A, Kindermann W: Effect of maximal oxygen uptake and different forms of physical training on serum lipoproteins. *Eur J Appl Physiol* 1982; 48: 263–277.

100. Rotkis TC, et al.: Relationship between high-density lipoprotein cholesterol and weekly running mileage. *J Cardiac Rehabil* 1982; 2:109–112.

101. Elliot DL, et al.: Characteristics of anabolic-androgenic steroid-free competitive male and female bodybuilders. *Phys Sports Med* 1987; 15:169–179.

102. Altekruse EB, Wilmore JH: Changes in blood chemistries following a controlled exercise program. *J Occup Med* 1973; 15: 110–113.

103. Lopez SA, et al.: Effect of exercise and physical fitness on serum lipids and lipoproteins. *Atherosclerosis* 1974; 20:1–9.

104. Ruderman NB, Ganda OP, Johansen K: The effect of physical training on glucose tolerance and plasma lipids in maturity onset diabetes. *Diabetes* 1979; 28(suppl 1):89–92.

105. Leon AS, et al.: Effects of a vigorous walking program on body composition, carbohydrate and lipid metabolism of obese young men. *Am J Clin Nutr* 1979; 32: 1776–1787.

106. Allison PG, et al.: Failure of exercise to increase high-density lipoprotein cholesterol. *J Cardiac Rehabil* 1981; 1:257–262.

107. Haskell WL, et al.: Strenuous physical activity, treadmill exercise test response, and plasma high-density lipoprotein cholesterol: The Lipid Research Clinic Program Prevalence Study. *Circulation* 1980; 62: 53–61.

108. Griffin BA, Skinner ER, Maughan RJ: The acute effects of prolonged walking and dietary changes in plasma lipoprotein concentrations and high-density lipoprotein subfractions. *Metabolism* 1988; 37: 535–541.

109. Wood P, Haskell W: The effect of exercise on plasma high-density lipoproteins. *Lipids* 1979; 14:417–427.

110. Martin RP, Haskell WL, Wood PD: Blood chemistry and lipid profiles of elite distance runners. *Ann NY Acad Sci* 1977; 301:346–360.

111. Wood PD, et al.: Increased exercise level and plasma lipoprotein concentrations: A one-year randomized, controlled study in sedentary middle-aged men. *Metabolism* 1983; 32:31–39.

112. Krotkiewski M, et al.: Impact of obesity on metabolism in men and women: Importance of regional adipose tissue distribution. *J Clin Invest* 1983; 72:1150–1162.

113. Tran ZV, Weltman A: Differential effects of exercise on serum lipid and lipoprotein levels seen with changes in body weight: A meta-analysis. *JAMA* 1985; 254:919–924.

114. Hagan RD, Gettman LR: Maximal aerobic power, body fat and serum lipoproteins in male distance runners. *J Cardiac Rehabil* 1983; 3:331–337.

115. Zavaroni I, et al.: Habitual leisure-time physical activity is associated with differences in various risk factors for coronary artery disease. *J Gen Intern Med* 1989; 226: 417–421.

116. Gyntelberg F, et al.: Plasma triglyceride lowering by exercise despite increased food intake in patients with type IV hyperlipoproteinemia. *Am J Clin Nutr* 1977; 30:716–720.

117. Hanefeld M, et al.: Effects of exercise on hyperlipidemia in obesity. In Bjorntorp P, Jairella M, Howard AN, eds: *Recent Advances in Obesity Research: Third International Congress on Obesity*. John Liebe: London, 1981, pp 348–353.

118. Krotkiewski M, et al.: Effects of long-term physical training on body fat, metabolism, and blood pressure in obesity. *Metabolism* 1979; 28:650–658.

119. Hanefeld M, et al.: More exercise for the hyperlipidemic patient. *Ann Clin Res* 1988; 20:77–83.

120. Havei RJ, Pernon B, Jones NL: Uptake and release of free fatty acids and other metabolites in the legs of exercising men. *J Appl Physiol* 1967; 23:90–96.

121. Ahlborg G, et al.: Substrate turnover during prolonged exercise in men. *J Clin Invest* 1974; 53:1080–1090.

122. Cullinane E, et al.: Acute decrease in serum triglycerides with exercise: Is there a threshold for an exercise effect? *Metabolism* 1982; 31:844–847.

123. Sady SP, et al.: Prolonged exercise augments plasma triglyceride clearance. *JAMA* 1986; 256:2552–2555.

124. Hurley BF, et al.: Muscle triglyceride utilization during exercise: Effect of training. *J Appl Physiol* 1986; 60:562–567.

125. Gordon DJ, et al.: Habitual physical activity and high-density lipoprotein cholesterol in men with primary hypercholesterolemia: The Lipid Research Clinics Coronary Primary Prevention Trial. *Circulation* 1983; 67:512–520.

126. Tamai T, et al.: The effects of physical exercise on plasma lipoprotein and apoprotein metabolism in elderly men. *J Gerontol* 1988; 43:75–79.

127. Johnson CC, et al.: Diet and exercse in middle-aged men. *J Am Diet Assoc* 1982; 81:695–701.

128. Goldberg L, et al.: Changes in lipid and lipoprotein levels after weight training. *JAMA* 1984; 252:504–506.

129. Brownell KD, Bachorik PS, Ayerle RS: Changes in plasma lipid and lipoprotein levels in men and women after a program of moderate exercise. *Circulation* 1982; 65:477–484.

130. Peltonen P, et al.: Changes in serum lipids, lipoproteins, and heparin-releasable lipolytic enzymes during moderate physical training in man: A longitudinal study. *Metabolism* 1981; 30:518–526.

131. Stein RA, et al.: Effects of different exercise training intensities on lipoprotein cholesterol fractions in healthy middle-aged men. *Am Heart J* 1990; 119(2 pt 1):277–283.

132. Kokkinos PF, et al.: Effects of low- and high-repetition resistive training on lipoprotein-lipid profiles. *Med Sci Sports Exerc* 1988; 20:50–54.

133. Manning JM, et al.: Effects of a resistive training program on lipoprotein-lipid levels in obese women. *Med Sci Sports Exerc* 1991; 23:1222–1226.

134. Williams PT, et al.: The effects of running mileage and duration on plasma lipoprotein levels. *JAMA* 1982; 247:2674–2679.

135. Wood PD, et al.: Changes in plasma lipids and lipoproteins in overweight men during weight loss through dieting as compared with exercise. *N Engl J Med* 1988; 319:1173–1179.

136. Morrisett JD, et al.: Association of lipoprotein Lp(a), plasma lipids, and other lipoproteins with coronary artery disease documented by angiography. *Circulation* 1986; 74:758–765.

137. Gaubatz JW, et al.: Human plasma lipoprotein (a): Structural properties. *J Biol Chem* 1983; 258:4582–4589.

138. Rhoads GG, et al.: Lp(a) lipoprotein as a risk factor for myocardial infarction. *JAMA* 1986; 256:2540–2544.

139. Hellsten G, et al.: Lipids and endurance physical activity. *Atherosclerosis* 1989; 75:93–94.

140. Frick MH, et al.: The Helsinki Heart Study: Primary prevention trial with gemfibrozil in middle-aged men with dyslipidemia. *N Engl J Med* 1987; 317:1237–1245.

141. Nakamura N, et al.: Physical fitness: Its contribution to serum high-density lipoprotein. *Atherosclerosis* 1983; 48:173.

142. Kuusi T, et al.: Plasma high-density lipoproteins HDL_2, HDL_3, and postheparin plasma lipases in relation to parameters of physical fitness. *Atherosclerosis* 1982; 41: 209–219.

143. Masarei JRL, Pyke JE, Pyke FS: Physical fitness and plasma HDL-cholesterol concentrations in male business executives. *Arteriosclerosis* 1982; 42:77–83.

144. Lehtonen A, Viikari J: The effect of vigorous physical activity at work on serum lipids with special reference to serum high-density lipoprotein cholesterol. *Acta Physiol Scand* 1978; 104:117–121.

145. Herbert PN, et al.: High-density lipoprotein metabolism in runners and sedentary men. *JAMA* 1984; 252:1034–1037.

146. Kiens B, et al.: Increased plasma HDL-cholesterol and apo A-I in sedentary middle-aged men after physical conditioning. *Eur J Clin Invest* 1980; 10:203–209.

147. Savage MP, et al.: Exercise training effects on serum lipids of prepubescent boys and adult men. *Med Sci Sports Exerc* 1986; 18:197–204.

148. LaRosa JC, et al.: Effect of long-term moderate physical exercise in plasma lipoproteins. *Arch Intern Med* 1982; 142: 2269–2274.

149. Lipson LC, et al.: Effect of exercise conditioning on plasma high-density lipoproteins and other lipoproteins. *Atherosclerosis* 1980; 37:529–538.

150. Sutherland W, Woodhouse S: Physical activity and plasma lipid concentrations in men. *Atherosclerosis* 1980; 37:285–289.

151. Wood PD, et al.: Increased exercise level and plasma lipoprotein concentrations: A one-year, randomized, controlled study in sedentary middle-aged men. *Metabolism* 1983; 32:31–39.

152. Kauppinen-Makelin R, Nikkila EA: Serum lipoproteins in patients with myocardial infarction. *Atherosclerosis* 1988; 74:65–74.

153. Hamsten A, et al.: Serum lipoproteins and apolipoproteins in young male survivors of myocardial infarction. *Atherosclerosis* 1986; 59:223–235.

154. Cremer P, et al.: Incidence rates of fatal and nonfatal myocardial infarction in relation to the lipoprotein profile: First prospective results from the Gottingen risk, incidence and prevalence study (GRIPS). *Klin Wochenschr* 1988; suppl 11:42–49.

155. Sasaki J, et al.: Mild exercise therapy increases serum high-density lipoprotein 2 cholesterol levels in patients with essential hypertension. *Am J Med Sci* 1989; 197:220–223.

156. Manttari M, et al.: Lifestyle determinants of HDL_2 and HDL_3-cholesterol levels in a hypercholesterolemic male population. *Atherosclerosis* 1991; 87:1–8.

157. Wood PD, et al.: The effects on plasma li-

poproteins of a prudent weight-reducing diet, with and without exercise, in overweight men and women. *N Engl J Med* 1991; 325:461–466.

158. Rauramaa R, Salonen JT, Kukkonen-Harjula K: Effects of mild physical exercise on serum lipoproteins and metabolites of arachidonic acid: A controlled randomized trial in middle-aged men. *BMJ* 1984; 288: 603–606.

159. Haskell WL: The influence of exercise training on plasma lipids and lipoproteins in health and disease. *Acta Med Scand* 1986; 711(suppl):25–37.

160. Pan QX, et al.: The study of serum apoprotein levels as indicators for the severity of angiographically assessed coronary artery disease. *Am J Clin Pathol* 1991; 95: 597–600.

161. Magnus P, et al.: Increase in the ratio of serum levels of apoprotein A-I and A-II during prolonged physical strain and calorie deficiency. *Eur J Appl Physiol* 1984; 53:21–24.

162. Danner SA, et al.: Effect of physical exercise on blood lipids and adipose tissue composition in young healthy men. *Atherosclerosis* 1984; 53:83–90.

163. Hespel P, et al.: Changes in plasma lipids and apoproteins associated with physical training in middle-aged sedentary men. *Am Heart J* 1988; 115:786–792.

164. Huttunen JK, et al.: Effects of moderate physical exercise on serum lipoproteins. *Circulation* 1979; 60:1220–1229.

165. Freyman JF, et al.: Effects of 12 weeks of exercise training on plasma lipids and apoproteins in middle-aged men (Abstract). *Med Sci Sports Exerc* 1982; 14:103.

166. Iltis PW, et al.: Different running programs: Plasma lipids, apoproteins and lecithin: cholesterol acyltransferase in middle-aged men. *Ann Sports Med* 1984; 2:16–21.

167. Huttunen JK, et al.: Post-heparin plasma lipoprotein lipase in normal subjects and in patients with hypertriglyceridemia: Correlations to sex, age, and various parameters of triglyercide metabolism. *Clin Sci Mol Med* 1976; 50:249–260.

168. Lithell H, et al.: Changes in lipoprotein lipase activity and lipid stores in human skeletal muscle with prolonged heavy exercise. *Acta Physiol Scand* 1979; 107: 257–261.

169. Nikkila EA, et al.: Lipoprotein lipase activity in adipose tissue and skeletal muscle of runners: Relation to serum lipoproteins. *Metabolism* 1978; 27:1661–1671.

170. Marniemi J, et al.: Lipoprotein lipase of human postheparin plasma and adipose tissue in relation to physical training. *Acta Physiol Scand* 1980; 110:131–135.

171. Kantor MA, et al.: Acute increase in lipoprotein lipase following prolonged exercise. *Metabolism* 1984; 33:454–457.

172. Lithell H, et al.: Lipoproteins, lipoprotein lipase, and glycogen after prolonged physi-

cal activity. *J Appl Physiol* 1984; 57: 698–702.

173. Glomset JA: The plasma lecithin:cholesterol acyltransferase reaction. *J Lipid Res* 1968; 9:155.

174. Marniemi J, et al.: Dependence of serum lipid and lecithin:cholesterol acyltransferase levels on physical training of young men. *Eur J Appl Physiol* 1982; 49:25–35.

175. Grosser J, Scherecker O, Greten H: Function of hepatic triglyceride lipase in lipoprotein metabolism. *J Lipid Res* 1981; 22: 437–439.

176. Jansen H, Birkenhager JC: Liver lipase-like activity in human and hamster adrenocortical tissue. *Metabolism* 1981; 30:428–431.

177. Brier C, et al.: Essential role of post-heparin lipoprotein lipase activity and of plasma testosterone in coronary artery disease. *Lancet* 1985; 1:1242–1244.

178. Taskinen M-R: Lipoprotein lipase in hypertriglyceridemias. In Borensztajn J, ed: *Lipoprotein Lipase.* Evener: Chicago, 1987, pp 102–128.

179. Oscai LB, Essig DA, Palmer WK: Lipase regulation of muscle triglyceride hydrolysis. *J Appl Physiol* 1990; 69:1571–1577.

180. Schwartz RS, Brunzell JD: Increase of adipose tisue lipoprotein lipase activity with weight loss. *J Clin Invest* 1982; 67: 1425–1430.

181. Williams PT, et al.: Lipoprotein subfractions of runners and sedentary men. *Metabolism* 1986; 35:45–52.

182. Fielding CJ, Shore VG, Fielding PE: A protein cofactor of lecithin:cholesterol acyltranferase. *Biochem Biophys Res Commun* 1972; 46:1493–1498.

183. Glomset JA: High-density lipoproteins in human health and disease. *Adv Intern Med* 1980; 25:91–116.

184. Frey I, et al.: Influence of acute maximal exercise in lecithin:cholesterol acyltransferase activity in healthy adults of differing aerobic performance. *Eur J Appl Physiol* 1991; 62:31–35.

185. Williams PT, et al.: Associations of lecithin:cholesterol acyltransferase (LCAT) mass concentrations with exercise, weight loss, and plasma lipoprotein subfraction concentrations in men. *Atherosclerosis* 1990; 82:53–58.

186. Tyroler HA: Review of lipid-lowering clinical trials in relation to observational epidemiologic studies. *Circulation* 1987; 76: 515–522.

187. Summary of the Second Report of the National Cholesterol Education Program (NCEP) Expert Panel on detection, evaluation, and treatment of high blood cholesterol in adults. *JAMA* 1993; 269:3015–3023.

188. Avins AL, Haber RJ, Hulley SB: The status of hypertriglyceridemia as a risk factor for coronary heart disease. In Rifkind BM, Lippel K, eds: *Clin Lab Med* 1989; 9:153–168.

189. National Heart, Lung, and Blood Institute Consensus Development Panel: Treatment of hypertriglyceridemia. *JAMA* 1984; 251: 1196–1200.
190. Ahrens EJ, Hirsch J, Insull W: The influence of dietary fats on serum lipid levels in man. *Lancet* 1957; 1:943–953.
191. Connor WE, Connor SL: The dietary treatment of hyperlipidemia. *Med Clin North Am* 1982; 66:485–518.
192. Spady DK, Dietschy JM: Interaction of dietary cholesterol and triglycerides in the regulation of low-density lipoprotein transport in the hamster. *J Clin Invest* 1988; 81:300–309.
193. Goodnight SH Jr., et al.: Polyunsaturated fatty acids, hyperlipidemia, and thrombosis. *Arteriosclerosis* 1982; 2:87–113.
194. Becker N, et al.: Effects of saturated mono-unsaturated and omega-6 polyunsaturated fatty acids on plasma lipids, lipoproteins and apoproteins in humans. *Am J Clin Nutr* 1983; 37:355–360.
195. Connor WE, et al.: Cholesterol valance and fecal neutral steroid and bile acid excretion in normal men fed dietary fats of different fatty acid composition. *J Clin Invest* 1969; 48:1363–1375.
196. Connor WE, Connor SL: Diet, atherosclerosis and fish oil. *Adv Intern Med* 1990; 35:139–171.
197. Stone MH, Blessing D: Resistive training and selected effects. *Med Clin North Am* 1985; 69:109–122.
198. National Education Programs Working Group Report on the Management of Patients with Hypertension and High Blood Cholesterol. *Ann Intern Med* 1991; 114: 224–237.

CHAPTER 10

EXERCISE AND OBESITY

DIANE L. ELLIOT, MD, and LINN GOLDBERG, MD

Obesity is a condition characterized by excess body fat. It is associated with an increased prevalence of hypertension, hyperlipidemia, diabetes, degenerative arthritis, and certain cancers.[1,2] The usual indices of obesity include the Metropolitan Life Insurance height–weight charts, body mass index (weight [kg] / height[meters]^2), and the percentage of body fat. Obesity is defined as a body weight more than 20% above a desirable level, a body mass index greater than 30, or a percentage of body fat of more than 30% for women and 20% for men.[1,3]

Weight loss alters conditions associated with obesity. Elevated blood pressure may be reduced[4-6] with regression of left ventricular hypertrophy (see Chapter 2)[7]; total and high-density lipoprotein cholesterol[8-11] are favorably changed (see Chapter 9); and glucose tolerance improves among those with type II diabetes [12-14] (see Chapter 8).

Recent reviews[3,15,16] have outlined the pathogenesis of obesity and alternative treatments for it. Therapy confined to dietary measures alone has little success in sustaining weight loss,[17] and the addition of exercise to a comprehensive program of caloric reduction and behavior modification can improve results.[18,19] In this chapter, the components of energy balance and their relationship to obesity and physical exertion are reviewed. We present practical recommendations for using physical activity to achieve a reduction in body fat.

Exercise and Caloric Balance

INTAKE

Nonobese individuals can increase their physical activity with little body fat loss. In 1983, Wilmore[20] reviewed 58 studies that examined the effect of exercise training on body composition. The investigations generally involved nonobese subjects participating in training studies to assess effects other than weight loss. Combined data demonstrated an average 1% decrease in body fat. Although the changes were significant, their magnitude was small. Others have observed that aerobic exercise alone results in only minor changes in body weight and composition among normal-weight individuals.[21]

The effects of exercise on acute and chronic food consumption have been the topic of several reviews.[22,23] Among humans, physical exertion's long-term effects on caloric intake have been studied best in the controlled setting of a metabolic ward. In that way, activity can be altered while accurately monitoring spontaneous food consumption. Studies suggest that the impact of training on caloric intake differs between lean and obese individuals. The nonobese do not lose a clinically significant amount of weight with exercise, because calories are increased to compensate for energy expenditure and maintain a stable body weight.[24] However, when overweight women augmented caloric expenditure by means of physical activity, their food ingestion did not increase, resulting in a slow, steady weight loss.[25]

These results parallel other research on the regulation of appetite. Internal mechanisms may govern lean individuals' appetite and caloric intake, whereas external cues could be more important among obese individuals.[26] The results imply that, among the obese, the addition of exercise may be an effective method to achieve a negative caloric balance with resultant weight loss.

EXPENDITURE

Caloric expenditure involves three components: basal or resting metabolic rate (BMR), energy expended with exertion, and the thermic effect of food.[27] Physical activity can interact with each aspect of caloric use.

Basal Metabolic Rate

The BMR accounts for approximately 75% of daily caloric expenditure. BMR correlates with the fat-free or lean body mass. Obese individuals have an increase in both body fat and lean body mass. Because overweight individuals have greater lean mass for their height, BMR is increased when compared to that of nonobese individuals of similar age, gender, and height.[28] A lower BMR is not a major factor in maintenance of obesity, as the obese have normal BMRs (per kilogram of lean weight) when compared to lean individuals.[28]

The chronic effects of training on the BMR are not well-established. Some researchers[29-31] have found that endurance-trained men have higher BMRs per kilogram of lean weight, but others[32] have not found that fitness level affects this parameter. In a detraining study, BMR was found to decline among endurance athletes after 3 days without exercise.[33] Thus, even if trained individuals have an augmentation in BMR, that effect may relate to the last bout of exertion, rather than to a sustained effect of the conditioned state.

Although training appears to have minimal effects on the BMR when at a stable weight, regular exercise may affect the lowered BMR induced by reduced calorie consumption. A negative caloric balance can result in loss of lean tissue. Because BMR relates to the lean body mass, preserving lean mass will help maintain one's metabolic rate. Regular exercise accompanying caloric restriction reduces the loss of lean tissue,[10,34-37] an effect that helps maintain the total BMR, as well as optimizing body composition changes.

However, loss of lean body mass during weight reduction does not account for the total decrease in resting metabolic rate. Severe caloric restriction (<300 kcal/d) results in a lowering of BMR,[38,39] and even a moderate decrement (<800 kcal/d) can, over time, be associated with a decrease in BMR per kg of lean body mass.[36,40-43] The basis for this change is not understood, but it seems to relate to metabolic adaptations to the negative caloric intake.[44]

Not all investigators have observed a significant decrement in BMR during reduced food intake, perhaps because of the short durations of the studies[45] and the mild caloric restriction in them.[46] Longer protocols, with moderate reduction in caloric consumption (700 to 800 kcal/d), have generally demonstrated a BMR decrement. Whether regular physical activity can prevent this additional decrease is not clear. Several studies have examined the question, and results vary (Table 10–1).

Three studies[36,40,42] found no effect of exercise on BMR, even when training was of sufficient intensity to achieve an increase in aerobic capacity.[42] Three other investigators[41,43,47] reported that regular exertion (4 to 7 days per week) prevented the decrease in metabolic rate. Generally, the studies noting an exercise effect were of longer duration and had a greater number of subjects. Animal research on the interaction of caloric restriction and activity suggests that physical activity may attenuate the decrease in BMR, an effect that diminishes as caloric restriction becomes more severe.[48] Additional variables, such as intensity of exercise, net caloric restriction, and individual factors, need to be better defined to determine the impact of exercise on BMR in those with calorie-reduced diets.

Energy Use with Exercise

The calories expended with exercise represent the component of daily caloric consumption most amenable to alteration. In this context, the term "exercise" refers to both the activities of daily living (i.e., climbing stairs, walking) and regular physical conditioning.

Many studies have sought to determine whether obese individuals are less physically active than lean individuals. Measures of activity include self-report, records by observers, and activity monitors. In general, obese individuals' activity is either decreased or the same as their lean counterparts.[49,50] However, the studies are difficult to compare because of differences in activity indices, age, gender, and the degree and duration of obesity. When the evaluation was performed on a metabolic unit, lean and obese individuals had similar physical activity levels,[51] although the generalizability of that observation to the natural environment is in question. Only four studies[52-55] have assessed physical activity and the degree of obesity, and no relationship has been observed. Finally, it is unclear whether a reduction in physical activity is a cause or consequence of obesity, since lean individuals who gained weight through force-feeding on a metabolic ward also decreased their activity

Table 10–1 STUDIES OF THE EFFECT OF CALORIC RESTRICTION AND EXERCISE ON BASAL (RESTING) METABOLIC RATE

Author	Subjects	Study Duration	Groups	Exercise Frequency	Diet	Results
Hammer et al.[46]	26 F	16 wk	D, DE	5X/wk	800–1,400 kcal	No change in BMR per LBM in either group
Belko, Barbieri, and Wong[45]	11 F	6 wk	D, DE	6X/wk	1,000 kcal deficit each group	No change in BMR per LBM in either group
Hill et al.[36]	8 F	6 wk	D, DE	Daily	800 kcal	Both groups' BMR decreased approximately 20%
van Dale et al.[42]	12 F	12 wk	D, DE	4X/wk	700–800 kcal	19%–26% decrease in BMR per LBM; no change with exercise
Warwick and Garrow[40]	3 F	12 wk	3 wk D alternate 3 wk DE	Daily	800 kcal	Total BMR decreased; no change with exercise
Donahoe et al.[41]	12 F	12 wk	D, then DE	≥4X/wk	800 kcal	3%–7% decrease in BMR on diet, reversed with exercise
van Dale and Saris[43]	20 F	14 wk	D, DE	4X/wk	700–800 kcal	12% decrease in BMR per LBM reversed with exercise weeks 5–14
Mole et al.[47]	4 F 1 M	4 wk	2 wk D 2 wk DE	Daily	500 kcal	13% decrease in BMR with diet, reversed toward baseline with exercise

Key: F = female; D = diet only; DE = diet plus exercise; BMR = basal (resting) metabolic rate; LBM = lean body mass; M = male.

levels.[56] Obese individuals are not more efficient (calorie sparing) during exercise; that is, they expend calories normally with physical activity. Although those who are obese may be less physically active in their usual daily routine, when they exert themselves, caloric use is normal.[57-59]

The majority of additional caloric use induced by physical activity occurs during the period of exercise. However, a residual augmentation in metabolic rate persists after exertion. The extra calories expended during the recovery interval have been called recovery energy expenditure, or excess post-exercise oxygen consumption. Although initial studies[54,55] of metabolic rate following exertion suggested a sustained elevation, more recent evidence[60-62] indicates that the usual bout of aerobic training produces only a small, transient effect on the metabolic rate. More prolonged exertion or exercise of increased intensity may cause a more sustained effect on recovery energy expenditure.[63-65] As yet, no differences have been defined in this parameter between obese and lean individuals.

Thermic Effect of Food

The third component of energy expenditure occurs following ingestion of food. Eating results in an increase in metabolic rate, a phenomenon termed the thermic effect of food (TEF). The increased expenditure is a minor component of total daily caloric use, generally equivalent to 10% to 15% of the meal's total caloric value.

In 1967, Miller and Mumford[66] first suggested that exercise potentiated the thermic effect of food, a finding also observed by other investigators. Segal and Pi-Sunyer[67] reviewed the literature on the interaction of exercise and the TEF. Some studies of lean individuals have found augmentation of thermogenesis by exercise,[68-70] but others have not observed this effect.[71,72] An exercise-associated increase in the TEF has not been observed in obese individuals.[71] These discrepant findings may relate directly to obesity's pathogenesis or to the many variables affecting TEF, such as previous diet, meal composition, and glucose tolerance.[73]

Research on the effect of exercise training on TEF also has produced inconsistent results, with both an increase[74] and a decrease[29,30,75,76] reported. This finding may relate to the TEF being highest at an "optimal" fitness level and lower when the individual is untrained or overtrained. When fitness, as reflected by maximal oxygen consumption (Vo_{2max}), and the TEF were compared among nonobese men, those with intermediate fitness levels (mean Vo_{2max}, 53 mL / kg / min) had the highest TEF, while both more highly trained and untrained men had lower TEF levels.[31] There was considerable individual variability in the response, however, which was unaccounted for by aerobic capacity.

In summary, regular exercise favorably impacts caloric balance and aids weight loss (Table 10 – 2). Some obese individuals may be less physically active, and exercise (both with training and in activities of daily living) increases caloric expenditure for all people. The primary difference between obese and nonobese individuals may be less compensatory food ingestion among the latter when physical activity is increased. Importantly, training preserves lean tissue during weight loss, and in that way helps maintain the BMR. Also,

Table 10-2 **EXERCISE AND ENERGY BALANCE**

Energy Balance Component	Exercise Benefits among the Obese
Intake	Caloric intake may not match the additional caloric expenditure.
Expenditure Basal (resting) metabolic rate	Greatest component of total caloric expenditure. Exercise maintains BMR by preserving LBM. Exercise possibly prevents the BMR decrease associated with moderate or severe caloric restriction.
Exercise energy expenditure	Most modifiable component of total caloric expenditure. No difference in exercise efficiency, and calories are expended normally with exercise.

Key: BMR = basal (resting) metabolic rate; LBM = lean body mass.

regular physical activity may attenuate the BMR fall that can occur during moderate and severe caloric restriction.

Exercise as Therapy

STUDY OF EXERCISE FOR WEIGHT LOSS

Only recently has exercise been an explicit component of weight control recommendations. In a 1979 review,[77] exercise was evaluated in only 6% of programs studied. Controlled investigations among adults evaluating diet and diet plus exercise are outlined in Table 10-3. Results are difficult to compare, as training frequencies and caloric intakes differed. Research has been limited by the need to meet the dual requirements of many subjects and precise monitoring. The studies with power limited by few subjects were often conducted with careful monitoring of intake and exertion. Conversely, those investigations with many subjects had less ability to monitor diet and the amount of exertion. Lack of adherence to the intervention in larger studies may have confounded results, as investigators have noted that subjects who exercised did not restrict calories as well as the diet-only participants.[42]

Most research does not demonstrate greater weight loss with the addition of exercise to caloric restriction.* However, regular physical activity increases fat loss and preserves lean body mass, whereas weight loss produced by diet alone often reduces both muscle and fat mass.[10,34-37]

Investigators have speculated that low-intensity exertion, due to its preferential fat use, may be more effective for weight loss. However, total caloric expenditure, rather than intensity of exertion, appears to be the factor related to weight loss. Ballor and associates[81] compared caloric restriction with high- and low-intensity supervised exercise among 27 obese women. The training intensity did not affect weight loss, and both groups had similar fat loss and preservation of fat-free mass. Although low-intensity exercise theoretically

*References 10, 34-37, 42, 46, 78-80.

Table 10–3 STUDIES COMPARING THE EFFECTS OF DIET VS. DIET AND EXERCISE ON WEIGHT LOSS AND BODY COMPOSITION

Author	Subjects	Study Duration	Groups	Exercise Frequency	Diet	Results
Duddleston and Bennion[78]	12 F	6 wk	D, E, DE, C	4X/wk	1,200 kcal	Weight loss not different
Garrow et al.[79]	37 F	3 wk	D, DE	Daily; alternate weeks	800 kcal	Weight loss not different
Bogardus et al.[80]	15 F, 3 M	12 wk	D, DE	≥3X/wk	450 kcal/m²	Weight and fat loss not different
Hammer et al.[46]	26 F	16 wk	D, DE	5X/wk	800–1,400 kcal	Weight and fat loss not different
van Dale et al.[42]	2 F	12 wk	D, DE	4X/wk	700–800 kcal	Weight and fat loss not different
Belko, Barbieri, and Wong[45]	11 F	6 wk	D, DE	6X/wk	1,000 kcal/d deficit/grp	Weight loss greater D; fat loss not different DE & D
Zuti and Golding[34]	25 F	16 wk	D, E, DE	5X/wk	500 kcal deficit/grp	Weight loss not different; E preserved LBM
Weltman, Matter, and Stamford[10]	28 M	10 wk	D, E, DE, C	4X/wk (walk)	500 kcal < maintenance	Weight loss not different DE & D; DE lost less lean and more fat than D
Pavlou et al.[35]	72 M	8 wk	DE	3X/wk	400–1,110 kcal	Weight loss not different; E decreased loss of LBM and increased fat loss
Hill et al.[36]	8 F	6 wk	D, DE	Daily	800 kcal	Weight loss not different; E preserved LBM and increased fat loss
Ballor et al.[37]	40 F	8 wk	C, D, DE, E	3X/wk (resistance)	1,000 kcal < maintenance	Weight loss not different DE & D; E decreased loss of LBM
Hagen et al.[21]	48 F, 48 M	12 wk	D, E, DE, C	5X/wk	1,200 kcal	Weight and fat loss greater DE than D
van Dale and Saris[43]	20 F	14 wk	D, DE	4X/wk	700–800 kcal	No difference between groups at 5 wk; at 14 wk, E increased loss of weight and fat

Key: F = female; D = diet only; E = exercise only; DE = diet and exercise; C = control; M = male; LBM = lean body mass.

may preferentially utilize fat, in reality the total caloric output is the major factor affecting body composition change.

In addition, individuals using regular physical activity with their weight-loss program are more likely to maintain a weight loss. Among investigations with follow-up data,[82-85] subjects who lost weight with exercise better maintained their loss at 6 to 12 months than nonexercisers. Thus, regular exercise can both maximize body composition change and increase the probability of maintaining a weight loss.[86]

Recently, researchers have assessed the caloric expenditure due to movements during the usual daily routine. Individuals who lose weight have been noted to have a significant reduction in this aspect of caloric expenditure.[87] The researchers estimated that this reduction was approximately 500 kcal/d. Adding caloric use with exercise may compensate for this concealed decrement in caloric needs.

CASE: E.K., a 70-year-old woman, was self-referred for knee pain. She had a 2-year history of knee stiffness, which initially responded to nonsteroidal anti-inflammatory drugs (NSAIDs). However, her complaints increased such that she was unable to pull her golf cart without pain. She had been healthy all her life, but "always overweight." Although her clothes felt tighter during the past year, she did not weigh herself over this period.

Physical examination revealed a height of 165 cm (5'6"), weight of 95 kg (212 lb), and blood pressure of 190/100 mm Hg. Significant findings included arterial narrowing on funduscopic examination and an apical S_4 gallop noted during her cardiac examination. She had evidence of degenerative arthritis in both knees.

Because of upcoming travel plans, the patient did not want to begin a weight loss program. Her blood pressure was controlled with a diuretic, and joint symptoms were improved with various NSAIDs. After 6 months, her knees became more painful and she decided to begin a weight loss program. At that time her weight was 94 kg (208 lb), and her measured resting metabolic rate was 870 kcal/d.

Initially, a program of walking, swimming, behavior modification, and a low-fat, moderately calorie-restricted diet (800 to 900 kcal/d) was begun. She was successful at slowly losing weight. After 4 months, 12 kg (27 lb) had been lost. Her blood pressure was well controlled, despite reducing the diuretic dose. She was able to golf and bowl with only occasional use of NSAIDs, and her weight loss was maintained over a 2-year follow-up period.

COMMENT: For certain population subgroups, such as African Americans and the elderly, the morbidity associated with obesity is not as well established.[88] Although overweight hypertensive patients once were believed to have less morbidity associated with their high blood pressure, data suggest that the morbidity from hypertension is not reduced among obese individuals.[89] Conditions associated with obesity in any age-group can be improved with weight loss, and therapeutic success more often requires only a moderate weight loss (e.g., 10 to 15 lb) rather than a normalization of body composition.[4,5]

EXERCISE AND ABDOMINAL OBESITY

Abdominal obesity has been recognized as a greater cardiovascular risk than generalized (gluteofemoral or gynecoid) obesity.[90-92] Although abdominal obesity presents a greater risk, it also may be more amenable to treatment. Some researchers have attributed variability in body weight and composition to the number of fat cells.[93] Fat with an abdominal distribution is characterized by adipocyte hypertrophy (bigger fat cells), rather than the adipocyte hyperplasia (more fat cells) that may accompany gluteofemoral fat. Training studies suggest that exercise achieves weight loss by reducing fat cell size. Thus, android or hypertrophic obesity would be more susceptible to exercise effects.[94-96]

> **CASE:** W.M., a real estate salesman, was self-referred because he turned 40 and wanted to "get in better shape." He considered himself to be in good general health and had no medical problems. His weight had increased slowly since college, especially over the past 3 to 4 years.
>
> Physical examination revealed a weight of 103 kg (230 lb) and height of 183 cm (6'1"). Physical findings other than body weight were normal, and results of laboratory studies included a total cholesterol level of 255 mg/dL, with a high-density lipoprotein (HDL) cholesterol level of 39 mg/dL. A graded exercise test revealed no evidence of ischemic heart disease, and a below average Vo_{2max} of 27 mL/kg/min.
>
> The patient began a program of aerobic exercise four times each week, with additional upper- and lower-body strength training. He and his wife both participated, and they were able to arrive at a schedule wherein they worked out together at a health club each morning. Over the following year, the patient's weight slowly decreased without explicit attempts at caloric reduction. Approximately 1 year after entry, he weighed 14 kg (30 lb) less, and his body fat had decreased by 7%. His cholesterol level was 220 mg/dL with an HDL level of 40 mg/dL.
>
> **COMMENT:** Improvement in serum cholesterol and carbohydrate tolerance with weight reduction may be greatest in patients with abdominal obesity.[97] This patient's total cholesterol was reduced 35 mg/dL, his HDL cholesterol was stable and his risk ratio (total cholesterol-to-HDL cholesterol) was improved. Several training studies have demonstrated that aerobic conditioning alone can result in weight loss.[11,98,99] It is of interest that although most controlled studies of diet and exercise have used women subjects (see Table 10-3), reduction of body fat by physical training without dietary restriction has been demonstrated only among men.[11,98,99] Whether the apparent disparity in results relates to hormonal differences, hypertrophic versus hypoplastic obesity, or other physiologic variables is not known.

EXERCISE AND VERY-LOW-CALORIE DIETS

Exercise can assist in the management of weight loss even when caloric restriction is severe. Morbid obesity, defined as a body weight twice the desirable or being more than 100 lb overweight, has high associated morbidity and mortality.[100] Caloric restriction with a medically supervised very-low-calorie diet (VLCD) has been used to achieve weight loss among a small subset of individuals who are morbidly obese. These programs are often restricted to 300 to 500 kcal / d and include high-biologic-value protein, with additional vitamin and electrolyte supplements. Although development of gallstones and symptomatic cholecystitis are complications of VLCD and bariatric surgery,[101,102] when appropriately monitored, VLCD can be safe and effective.[103,104]

Despite the marked negative caloric balance associated with these diets, exercise capacity is preserved. Initially, muscle glycogen content is reduced, and endurance decreases (walking to exhaustion at 65% to 70% of VO_{2max}). After 6 weeks, however, the muscles' glycogen content increases toward normal levels, and endurance improves as muscles adapt to greater use of lipids as a fuel for aerobic exercise.[105]

> **CASE:** M.C., a 32-year-old nurse, was seen for obesity. She believed that her health was otherwise good. She had weighed 68 kg (150 lb) at high school graduation, and had steadily gained weight since that time. Many attempts to lose weight resulted in transient losses of 5 to 7 kg (10 to 15 lb).
>
> Physical examination revealed a height of 175 cm (5'10"), weight of 122 kg (270 lb), and 49% body fat. She began a very-low-calorie diet with close medical supervision. The program also provided behavior modification and advice on exercise. While on the diet, she maintained a program of slow-paced walking, gradually increasing exercise frequency and duration, up to 4 miles each day.
>
> The initial month's weight loss included equal amounts of lean mass and body fat, but subsequent weight reduction was essentially all fat loss. Over 4 months, her weight decreased 37 kg (83 lb) while her metabolic rate per kilogram of lean body mass decreased 19%. At that time she began a refeeding diet, stabilizing her body weight on an intake of 2,000 kcal/d, and reported that this program was "much harder than fasting." Even after 2 months after the refeeding diet, while her weight had been stable for a month, her BMR (per kilogram lean body mass) remained depressed to a level similar to that during the modified fast.

> **COMMENT:** Surprisingly, exercise in combination with a very-low-calorie diet has not uniformly increased weight loss, affected body composition changes,[106,107] or altered resting oxygen consumption.[108] In a study where weight loss was increased by exercise, the additional decrement was less than half that anticipated from the predicted caloric expenditure.[107] This reduced ability of exercise to increase total weight loss is difficult to explain in light of a recent study[47] of five subjects on very-low-calorie diets who trained for 30 minutes per day at 60% VO_{2max}. The authors observed that regular physical activity reversed the depressed metabolic rate that occurred with severe caloric restriction.

In 1963, Buskirk and colleagues[109] suggested that during severe caloric restriction, regular exercise may not cause additional weight loss. But the definition of severe calorie restriction may differ for each individual, depending on their BMR and other components of caloric expenditure. At present, it appears that exercise may be most useful when added to a program of mild to moderate caloric restriction.

Recommendations for Exercise in Obesity Management

There are no reliable predictors of success with a weight loss program.[110] Because limited evidence suggests that repeated unsuccessful dieting may impede subsequent attempts,[111] we recommend maximum therapy with a combined program (caloric restriction, exercise, and behavior modification) for all motivated individuals.[18,19]

CALORIC RESTRICTION

The degree of caloric restriction can be estimated from the individual's predicted or measured BMR. We recommend 500 kcal less than the individual's predicted caloric expenditure (BMR + 25%) or an intake of at least 800 kcal/d. BMR can be estimated as 850 kcal/m^2 for women and 900 kcal/m^2 for men, or if body composition is available, BMR in kcal is approximately 500 plus 20 times the lean body mass in kilograms.[112]

PRE-EXERCISE ASSESSMENT

Recommending physical training requires pre-exercise assessment and explicit advice about the mode, intensity, duration, and frequency of exertion. Since obesity often is associated with an increased prevalence of cardiovascular risk factors, graded exercise testing may be indicated prior to prescribing an exercise program.

Even morbidly obese patients may be evaluated on the treadmill, although those patients generally need alteration in the testing protocol. This is normally done by beginning with slow walking without treadmill elevation, followed by gradual increases in speed to achieve maximal exertion. This evaluation protocol enhances subjects' ability to complete testing.[113]

TRAINING RECOMMENDATIONS

Aerobic exercise is recommended for obesity management, because it provides the greatest caloric expenditure per minute of training. Epstein and Wing[114] performed a meta-analysis of studies on the effectiveness of exercise for weight loss. The number of exercise sessions per week is related to success, and data suggest that a frequency of four times a week is needed to produce significant weight loss.[115,116] Modes of aerobic training, including walking, running, and bicycling (each using similar training intensities) produced similar effects on body composition.[98] Although in one study,[117] swimming was found to result in less body-weight loss than walking and bicycling programs, patient preference and availability of training sites and equipment are greater influences on choosing a program than the theoretic advantage of a particular training regimen.

Exercise intensity requires individualization. Because compliance and caloric expenditure, rather than an immediate increase in aerobic endurance, are the objective, the prescription is aimed at achieving the exercise habit. Predicting compliance with training is difficult, and some studies have suggested that a lower-intensity program, such as walking or bicycling, achieves greater compliance.[118,119] Some overweight individuals prefer lower-intensity exercise, sustained over a long interval, to more intense exertion.[120] After a pattern of regular activity is established, training intensity can be increased. Over the long term, higher-intensity training will improve aerobic capacity and ultimately will allow more calories to be expended for exercise sessions of similar duration.

Most research on weight loss has concentrated on aerobic conditioning, with little attention directed toward weight training or resistive exercise. Weight lifting can be structured to produce aerobic gains (circuit style with low resistance, multiple repetitions, and short rests between sets) or maximize strength increase (priority style with moderate resistance, 5 to 10 repetitions, and longer rests between sets). For most individuals, caloric expenditure with traditional strength training techniques is not as great as with circuit lifting or aerobic conditioning,[120,121] but strength training does use calories and can increase lean body mass.[121] Ballor and colleagues[37] compared weight and body composition changes when diet was combined with resistance training in 40 women. Over 8 weeks, dieting weight trainers had total-weight and body-fat changes comparable to a diet-only group. However, weight lifting subjects demonstrated an increase in lean body mass, despite the loss in total weight. When studies of the effects of exercise on body mass and composition were assessed by meta-analysis, the authors[122] noted that weight training by men both facilitated fat loss and preserved or increased lean body mass. While aerobic exercise may maintain lean body mass, an increase is generally not observed.

Training considerations for morbidly obese individuals include their greater heat intolerance[123] and movement restriction.[124] Because of potential problems with musculoskeletal trauma and balance, stationary cycling (which reduces the influence of body weight on exertion and lower-extremity trauma) often is preferable. Alternatively, a slow walking program, aimed at eventually achieving a sustained 2-mile distance, also is an effective approach for morbidly obese individuals.[113]

We advise working toward an aerobic (e.g., walking, bicycling, swimming) conditioning program with sessions four to five times per week. Rather than emphasize achieving the intensity × duration recommendations for aerobic conditioning, the focus should be on achieving regular activity with its additional caloric expenditure. Exercise is structured to augment caloric use by approximately 2,000 kcal/wk. When feasible, a calisthenic or resistive training program, especially designed to exercise upper-body musculature, also is recommended two to three times per week. The caloric expenditure of typical exercise activities is listed in Table 10-4.

The principles of training progression outlined in chapter 1 also apply for obese individuals. Initial low-intensity exercise is recommended for those without prior experience with aerobic conditioning, as well as for moderate to morbidly overweight and severely deconditioned individuals. An increase in training intensity is prescribed as compliance and initial musculoskeletal fitness levels are achieved (usually in 4 to 6 weeks). Besides increasing energy expenditure through exercise, the benefits of burning calories during daily routine activities are emphasized as a component of the lifestyle changes required to maintain weight loss.

Exercise usually will be combined with dietary change and behavior modification, and the positive changes can be complementary. For example, the

Table 10-4 **APPROXIMATE ADDITIONAL CALORIC EXPENDITURE FOR 30 MINUTES' ACTIVITY***

Activity	Calories
Backpacking	250
Badminton	200
Baseball	160
Basketball	300
Bicycling at 5.5 mph	150
Bicycling at 7 mph	200
Bicycling at 12 mph	310
Bowling	150
Canoeing (4 mph)	220
Carpentry	135
Chopping wood	250
Dancing (moderate)	150
Dusting	90
Fencing	300
Football	300
Gardening	150
Golfing (using cart)	120
Golfing (carrying clubs)	200
Handball (social)	330
Handball (competitive)	350
Hiking	180
Horseback riding	200
Making beds	150
Mowing grass (power)	140
Racquetball	300
Running at 5.5 mph	375
Running at 7 mph	500
Sailing	150
Sitting, writing	50
Standing, light activity	80
Skiing (vigorous downhill)	350
Skiing (cross-country at 2.5 mph)	300
Soccer	300
Softball	150
Swimming (crawl)	180
Tennis (singles)	270
Volleyball (noncompetitive)	170
Walking at 2 mph	120
Walking at 4 mph	220
Walking at 5 mph	270
Washing floors	150

*Values are estimates and will vary with intensity of exertion.

enhanced self-efficacy that comes from being active may make the individual less likely to overeat, while the social support mobilized for calorie reduction also can be used to reinforce exercise. When interviewed, women who were successful at sustaining a weight loss were those who exercised and had developed their own strategies for maintaining their weight.[125] The practitioner's role is to collaborate with patients on designing, refining, and adhering to their programs of exercise and dietary change.

Summary

Obesity is a prevalent condition with significant morbidity and increased mortality. Its pathogenesis is not understood. Regular exercise and increased activity in daily routines will augment caloric use and maintain muscle mass during negative caloric balance. In addition, regular physical activity increases the chances of maintaining a weight loss. Both dietary change and the exercise prescription use analogous behavior-modification strategies. Prescribing exercise for obese individuals follows the principles used with healthy patients (Chapter 1). Additional considerations include modifying exercise for mechanical limitations and an emphasis on total caloric expenditure rather than on the intensity parameters usually followed for aerobic conditioning.

REFERENCES

1. Simopoulos AP, Van Itallie TB: Body weight, health, and longevity. *Ann Intern Med* 1984; 100:285–295.
2. Van Itallie TB: Health implications of overweight and obesity in the United States. *Ann Intern Med* 1985; 103(6 pt 2):983–988.
3. Bray GA, Gray DS: Obesity, I: Pathogenesis. *West J Med* 1988; 149:429–441.
4. Dornfeld LP, et al.: Obesity and hypertension: Long-term effects of weight reduction on blood pressure. *Int J Obesity* 1985; 9:381–389.
5. Fagenberg B, et al.: Blood pressure control during weight reduction in obese hypertensive men: Separate effects of sodium and energy restriction. *BMJ* 1984; 288: 11–14.
6. Schotte DE, Stunkard AJ: The effects of weight reduction on blood pressure in 301 obese patients. *Arch Intern Med* 1990; 150:1701–1704.
7. MacMahon SW, Wilcken DEL, MacDonald GJ: The effect of weight reduction on left ventricular mass. *N Engl J Med* 1986; 314: 334–339.
8. Brownell KD, Stunkard AJ: Differential changes in plasma high-density lipoprotein cholesterol in obese men and women during weight reduction. *Arch Intern Med* 1981; 141:1142–1146.
9. Follick MJ, et al.: Contrasting short- and long-term effects of weight loss on lipoprotein levels. *Arch Intern Med* 1984; 144:1571–1574.
10. Weltman A, Matter S, Stamford BA: Caloric restriction and / or mild exercise: Effects on serum lipids and body composition. *Am J Clin Nutr* 1980; 33:1002–1009.
11. Wood PD, et al.: Changes in plasma lipids and lipoproteins in overweight men during weight loss through diet as compared with exercise. *N Engl J Med* 1988; 319: 1173–1179.
12. Hughs TA, et al.: Effects of caloric restriction and weight loss on glycemic control, insulin release and resistance, and atherosclerotic risk in obese patients with type II diabetes mellitus. *Am J Med* 1984; 72:7–17.
13. Amatrida JM, Richeson JF, Welle SL: The safety and efficiency of a controlled low-energy (very-low-calorie) diet in the treatment of non-insulin-dependent diabetes and obesity. *Arch Intern Med* 1988; 148: 873–877.
14. Bauman WA, et al.: Early and long-term effects of acute caloric deprivation in obese diabetic patients. *Am J Med* 1988; 85:38–46.
15. Bray GA, Gray DS: Obesity, II: Treatment. *West J Med* 1988; 149:555–571.
16. Elliot DL, Goldberg L, Girard DE: Obesity: Pathophysiology and practical management. *J Gen Intern Med* 1987; 2:188–198.
17. Bennett W: Dietary treatments of obesity. *Ann NY Acad Sci* 1987; 499:250–263.
18. Council on Scientific Affairs: Treatment of obesity in adults. *JAMA* 1988; 260: 2547–2551.
19. Weinsier RL, et al.: Recommended therapeutic guidelines for professional weight control programs. *Am J Clin Nutr* 1984; 40:865–872.
20. Wilmore JH: Body composition in sports and exercise: Directions for future research. *Med Sci Sports Exerc* 1983; 15: 21–31.
21. Hagan RD, et al.: The effects of aerobic conditioning and / or caloric restriction in overweight men and women. *Med Sci Sports Exerc* 1986; 18:87–94.
22. Pi-Sunyer FX: Exercise effects on calorie intake. *Ann NY Acad Sci* 1987; 499: 94–103.
23. Porikos KP, Pi-Sunyer FX: Regulation of food intake in human obesity: Studies with caloric dilution and exercise. *Clin Endocrinol Metab* 1984; 13:547–561.
24. Woo R, Pi-Sunyer FX: Effect of increased physical activity on voluntary intake in lean women. *Metabolism* 1985; 34: 836–841.
25. Woo R, Garrow JS, Pi-Sunyer FX: Volun-

tary food intake during prolonged exercise in obese women. *Am J Clin Nutr* 1982; 36:478–484.

26. Schacter S: Obesity and eating. *Science* 1968; 161:751–756.
27. Horton ES: Introduction: An overview of the assessment and regulation of energy balance in humans. *Am J Clin Nutr* 1983; 38:972–977.
28. Ravussen E, et al.: Twenty-four-hour energy expenditure and resting metabolic rate in obese, moderately obese, and control subjects. *Am J Clin Nutr* 1982; 35:566–573.
29. LeBlanc J, et al.: Hormonal factors in reduced postprandial heat production of exercise-trained subjects. *J Appl Physiol* 1984; 56:772–776.
30. Poehlman ET, Melby CL, Badylak SF: Resting metabolic rate and postprandial thermogenesis in highly trained and untrained males. *Am J Clin Nutr* 1988; 47:793–798.
31. Poehlman E, et al.: Aerobic fitness and resting energy expenditure in young adult males. *Metabolism* 1989; 38:85–90.
32. Hill JO, et al.: Meal size and thermic response to food in male subjects as a function of maximum aerobic capacity. *Metabolism* 1984; 33:743–749.
33. Tremblay A, et al.: Effect of a three-day interruption of exercise training on resting metabolic rate and glucose-induced thermogenesis in trained individuals. *Int J Obesity* 1988; 12:163–168.
34. Zuti WB, Golding LA: Comparing diet and exercise as weight reduction tools. *Phys Sportsmed* 1976; 4(1):49–53.
35. Pavlou KN, et al.: Effects of dieting and exercise on lean body mass, oxygen uptake, and strength. *Med Sci Sports Exerc* 1985; 17:466–471.
36. Hill JO, et al.: Effects of exercise and food restriction on body composition and metabolic rate in obese women. *Am J Clin Nutr* 1987; 46:622–630.
37. Ballor DL, et al.: Resistance weight training during caloric restriction enhances lean body weight maintenance. *Am J Clin Nutr* 1988; 47:19–25.
38. Bray G: Effect of caloric restriction on energy expenditure in obese patients. *Lancet* 1969; 2:397–398.
39. Elliot DL, et al.: The sustained decrement in resting metabolic rates following massive weight loss. *Am J Clin Nutr* 1989; 49:93–96.
40. Warwick PM, Garrow JS: The effect of addition of exercise to a regimen of dietary restriction on weight loss, nitrogen balance, resting metabolic rate, and spontaneous physical activity in three obese women in a metabolic ward. *Int J Obesity* 1981; 5:25–32.
41. Donahoe CP Jr, et al.: Metabolic consequences of dieting and exercise in the treatment of obesity. *J Consult Clin Psychol* 1984; 52:827–836.
42. van Dale D, et al.: Does exercise give an additional effect in weight reduction regimens? *Int J Obesity* 1987; 11:367–375.
43. van Dale D, Saris WHM: Repetitive weight loss and weight regain: Effects on weight reduction, resting metabolic rate, lipolytic activity before and after exercise and/or diet treatment. *Am J Clin Nutr* 1989; 49:409–416.
44. Danforth E Jr: The role of thyroid hormones and insulin in the regulation of energy metabolism. *Am J Clin Nutr* 1983;
45. Belko AZ, Barbieri TF, Wong EC: Effect of energy and protein intake and exercise intensity on the thermic effect of food. *Am J Clin Nutr* 1986; 43:863–869.
46. Hammer RL, et al.: Caloric-restricted low-fat diet and exercise in obese women. *Am J Clin Nutr* 1989; 49:77–85.
47. Mole PA, et al.: Exercise reverses depressed metabolic rate produced by severe caloric restriction. *Med Sci Sports Exerc* 1989; 81:29–33.
48. Ballor DL, et al.: Exercise training attenuates diet-induced reduction in metabolic rate. *J Appl Physiol* 1990; 68:2612–2617.
49. Thompson KJ, et al.: Exercise and obesity: Etiology, physiology, and intervention. *Psychol Bull* 1982; 91:55–79.
50. Pacy PJ, Webster J, Garrow JS: Exercise and obesity. *Sports Med* 1986; 3:89–113.
51. Schutz Y, et al.: Spontaneous physical activity measured by radar in obese and control subjects studied in a respiratory chamber. *Int J Obesity* 1982; 6:23–28.
52. Chirico AM, Stunkard AJ: Physical activity and human obesity. *N Engl J Med* 1960; 263:935–940.
53. Dorris RJ, Stunkard AJ: Physical activity: Performance and attitudes of a group of obese women. *Am J Med Sci* 1957; 233 (6):622–628.
54. Stunkard A, Pestka J: The physical activity of obese girls. *Am J Dis Child* 1962; 103:812–817.
55. Tryon WW: Activity as a function of body weight. *Am J Clin Nutr* 1987; 46:451–455.
56. Simms EAH, et al.: Experimental obesity in man. *Trans Assoc Am Phys* 1968; 81:153–170.
57. Bray GA: The energetics of obesity. *Med Sci Sports Exerc* 1983; 15:32–40.
58. Passmore R, Johnson RE: Some metabolic changes following prolonged moderate exercise. *Metabolism* 1960; 9:452–456.
59. deVries HA, Gray DE: After effects of exercise upon resting metabolic rate. *Res Q* 1963; 34:314–321.
60. Freedman-Akabas S, et al.: Lack of sustained increase in V_{O_2} following exercise in fit and unfit subjects. *Am J Clin Nutr* 1985; 41:545–549.
61. Brehm BA, Gutin B: Recovery energy expenditure for steady state exercise in run-

ners and nonexercisers. *Med Sci Sports Exerc* 1986; 18:205–210.

62. Elliot DL, Goldberg L, Kuehl KS: Does aerobic conditioning cause a sustained increase in metabolic rate? *Am J Med Sci* 1988; 296:249–251.

63. Bielinski R, Schutz Y, Jequier E: Energy metabolism during the post-exercise recovery in man. *Am J Clin Nutr* 1985; 42:69–82.

64. Bahr E, et al.: Effect of duration of exercise on excess post-exercise O_2 consumption. *J Appl Physiol* 1987; 62:485–490.

65. Maehlum S, et al.: Magnitude and duration of excess post-exercise oxygen consumption in healthy young subjects. *Metabolism* 1986; 35:425–429.

66. Miller DS, Mumford P: Gluttony, I: An experimental study of overeating and low- and high-protein diets. *Am J Clin Nutr* 1967; 20:1223–1229.

67. Segal KR, Pi-Sunyer FX: Exercise and obesity. *Med Clin North Am* 1989; 73:217–236.

68. Young JC, et al.: Prior exercise potentiates the thermic effect of a carbohydrate load. *Metabolism* 1980; 35:1049–1053.

69. Samueloff S, Beer G, Blondheim SH: Influence of physical activity on the thermic effect of food in young men. *Isr J Med Sci* 1982; 18:193–196.

70. Zahorska-Murkiewicz B: Thermic effect of food and exercise in obesity. *Eur J Appl Physiol* 1980; 44:231–235.

71. Welle SL, Campbell RG: Normal thermic effect of glucose in obese women. *Am J Clin Nutr* 1983; 37:87–92.

72. Schutz Y, Bessard T, Jequier E: Exercise and postprandial thermogenesis in obese women before and after weight loss. *Am J Clin Nutr* 1987; 45:1424–1432.

73. Devlin JT, Horton ES: Potentiation of the thermic effect of insulin by exercise: Differences between lean, obese and non-insulin-dependent men. *Am J Clin Nutr* 1986; 43:884–890.

74. Davis JR, et al.: Variations in dietary-induced thermogenesis and body fatness with aerobic capacity. *Eur J Appl Physiol* 1983; 50:319–329.

75. Poehlman ET, et al.: Influence of caffeine on the resting metabolic rate of exercise-trained and inactive subjects. *Med Sci Sports Exerc* 1985; 17:689–694.

76. Tremblay A, Cote J, LeBlanc J: Diminished dietary thermogenesis in exercise-trained human subjects. *Eur J Appl Physiol* 1983; 52:1–4.

77. Wing RR, et al.: Intermittent low-calorie regimen and booster sessions in the treatment of obesity. *Behav Ther* 1984; 22:448–449.

78. Duddleston AK, Bennion M: Effect of diet and/or exercise on obese college women. *J Am Diet Assoc* 1970; 56:126–129.

79. Garrow JS, et al.: Factors determining weight loss in obese patient in a metabolic ward. *Int J Obesity* 1978; 2:441–447.

80. Bogardus C, et al.: Effects of physical train-

81. Ballor DL, McCarthy JP, Wilterdink EJ: Exercise intensity does not affect the composition of diet and exercise-induced body mass loss. *Am J Clin Nutr* 1990; 51:142–146.

82. Dahlkoetter J, Callahan EF, Linton J: Obesity and the unbalanced energy equation: Exercise versus eating habit change. *J Consult Clin Psychol* 1979; 47:898–905.

83. Harris MB, Hallbauer ES: Self-directed weight control through eating and exercise. *Behav Res Ther* 1973; 11:523–529.

84. Gormally J, Rardin D, Black S: Correlates of successful response to a behavioral weight control clinic. *J Counseling Psychol* 1980; 27:179–191.

85. Stalones PM, Johnson WG, Christ M: Behavior modification for obesity: The evaluation of exercise, contingency management and program adherence. *J Consult Clin Psychol* 1978; 46:463–469.

86. King AC, et al.: Diet vs. exercise in weight maintenance. *Arch Intern Med* 1989; 149:2741–2746.

87. Weigles DS, et al.: Weight loss leads to a marked decrease in nonresting energy expenditure in ambulatory human subjects. *Metabolism* 1988; 37:930–936.

88. Andres R, et al.: Impact of age on weight goals. *Ann Intern Med* 1985; 103:1030–1033.

89. Bloom E, et al.: Does obesity protect hypertensives against cardiovascular disease? *JAMA* 1986; 256:2972–2975.

90. Krotkiewski M, et al.: Impact of obesity on metabolism in men and women. *J Clin Invest* 1983; 72:1150–1162.

91. Bjorntorp P: Classification of obese patients and complications related to the distribution of surplus fat. *Am J Clin Nutr* 1987; 45:1120–1125.

92. Ostlund RE, et al.: The ratio of waist to hips circumference, plasma insulin level, and glucose intolerance as independent predictors of the HDL_2 cholesterol level in older adults. *N Engl J Med* 1990; 322:229–234.

93. Bjorntorp P, et al.: Effects of physical training on glucose tolerance, plasma insulin and lipids on body composition in men after myocardial infarction. *Acta Med Scand* 1972; 192:439–443.

94. Krotkiewski M, et al.: Effects of long-term physical training on body fat, metabolism, and blood pressure in obesity. *Metabolism* 1979; 28:650–658.

95. Bjorntorp P, et al.: Physical training in human obesity, III: Effects of long-term physical training on body composition. *Metabolism* 1973; 22:1467–1475.

96. Bjorntorp P, et al.: The effect of physical training on insulin production in obesity. *Metabolism* 1970; 19:631–638.

97. den Beston C, et al.: Resting metabolic rate

and diet-induced thermogenesis in abdominal and gluteal-femoral obese women before and after weight reduction. *Am J Clin Nutr* 1988; 47:840–847.

98. Pollack ML, et al.: Effects of mode of training on cardiovascular function and body composition of adult men. *Med Sci Sports Exerc* 1975; 7:139–145.

99. Leon AS, et al.: Effects of a vigorous walking program on body composition and carbohydrate and lipid metabolism of obese young men. *Am J Clin Nutr* 1979; 32:1776–1787.

100. Van Itallie TB: "Morbid" obesity: A hazardous disorder that resists conservative treatment. *Am J Clin Nutr* 1980; 33:358–363.

101. Liddle KA, Goldstein RB, Saxton J: Gallstone formation during weight-reduction dieting. *Arch Intern Med* 1989; 149:1750–1753.

102. Schmidt JH, et al.: The case for prophylactic cholecystectomy concomitant with gastric restriction for morbid obesity. *Ann Surg* 1988; 54:269–272.

103. Wadden TA, Stunkard AH, Brownell KD: Very-low-calorie diets: Their efficacy, safety and future. *Ann Intern Med* 1983; 99:675–684.

104. Lockwood DH, Amatrida JM: Very low calorie diets in the management of obesity. *Annu Rev Med* 1984; 35:373–381.

105. Phinney SD, et al.: Capacity for moderate exercise in obese subjects after adaptation to a hypocalorie, ketogenic diet. *J Clin Invest* 1980; 66:1152–1161.

106. Lampman RM, Schteingart DE, Foss MS: Exercise as a partial therapy for the extremely obese. *Med Sci Sports Exerc* 1985; 18:19–24.

107. Wirth A, et al.: Metabolic effects and body fat mass changes in obese subjects on a very-low-calorie diet with and without intensive physical training. *Ann Nutr Metabol* 1987; 31:378–386.

108. Krotkiewski M, et al.: The effect of a very-low-calorie diet with and without chronic exercise on thyroid and sex hormones, plasma proteins, oxygen uptake, insulin and c peptide concentrations in obese women. *Int J Obesity* 1981; 5:287–293.

109. Buskirk ER, et al.: Energy balance of obese patients during weight reduction: Influence of diet restriction and exercise. *Ann NY Acad Sci* 1963; 111:918–939.

110. Gilbert S, Garrow JS: A prospective controlled trial of outpatient treatment for obesity. *Human Nutr Clin Nutr* 1983; 370:4–9.

111. Brownell KD, et al.: The effects of repeated cycles of weight loss and regain in rats. *Physiol Behav* 1987; 38:459–464.

112. Cunningham JJ: A reanalysis of the factors influencing basal metabolic rate in normal adults. *Am J Clin Nutr* 1980; 33:2372–2374.

113. Foss ML, Lampman RM, Schteingart D: Physical training program for rehabilitating extremely obese patients. *Arch Phys Med Rehabil* 1976; 57:425–429.

114. Epstein LH, Wing RR: Aerobic exercise and weight. *Addict Behav* 1980; 5:371–388.

115. Pollack ML, Cureton TK, Greninger L: Effects of frequency of training on working capacity, cardiovascular function, and body composition of adult men. *Med Sci Sports Exerc* 1969; 1:70–74.

116. Pollack ML, et al.: Effects of training two days per week at different intensities on middle-aged men. *Med Sci Sports Exerc* 1972; 4:192–197.

117. Gwinup G: Weight loss without dietary restriction: Efficacy of different forms of aerobic exercise. *Am J Sports Med* 1987; 15:275–279.

118. Sallis JF, et al.: Predictors of adoption and maintenance of physical activity in a community sample. *Prev Med* 1986; 15:331–341.

119. Kriska AM, et al.: A randomized exercise trial in older women: Increased activity over two years and the factors associated with compliance. *Med Sci Sports Exerc* 1986; 18:557–572.

120. Geissler CA, Miller DS, Shah M: The daily metabolic rate of the post-obese and the lean. *Am J Clin Nutr* 1989; 45:914–920.

121. Kuehl K, Elliot DL, Goldberg L: Predicting caloric expenditure during multistation resistance exercise. *J Appl Sport Sci* 1990; 4:63–67.

122. Ballor DL, Keesey RE: A meta-analysis of the factors affecting exercise-induced changes in body mass, fat mass and fat-free mass in males and females. *Int J Obesity* 1991; 15:717–726.

123. Bar-Or O, Lundegren HM, Buskirk ER: Heat tolerance of exercising obese and lean women. *J Appl Physiol* 1969; 26:403–409.

124. Foss ML, et al.: Initial work tolerance of extremely obese patients. *Arch Phys Med Rehabil* 1975; 56:63–67.

125. Kayman S, Burold W, Stern JS: Maintenance and relapse after weight loss in women: Behavioral aspects. *Am J Clin Nutr* 1990; 52:800–807.

CHAPTER 11

THE INFLUENCE OF EXERCISE ON OSTEOPOROSIS AND SKELETAL HEALTH

ERIC S. ORWOLL, MD

PHYSICAL ACTIVITY AND BONE MASS
  Bone Cell Physiology
    Basic multicellular units
    The mechanostat
  Epidemiologic Studies
    Cross-sectional research
    Longitudinal investigations
    Confounding variables
    Studies of adverse effects

MANAGEMENT OF SKELETAL HEALTH
  Osteoporosis Detection
  Initial Evaluation and Management
  Exercise as Therapy

The skeleton is a dynamic and metabolically complex tissue that responds to a variety of stimuli. Mechanical forces long have been understood to be of major importance. In 1892 Wolff[1] published his monograph, *The Law of Bone Remodeling*, in which he proposed that mechanical loading led to changes in the bones' metabolic activity and subsequently to alterations in skeletal size and shape. Convincing evidence links the skeleton's mechanical environment to its morphology[2] and to its biochemical and cellular activity. This association led to the hypothesis that physical activity could prevent and treat metabolic bone disease, particularly osteoporosis. However, the relationship between physical activity and metabolic bone diseases, and the usefulness of exercise in osteoporosis prevention and therapy, are only gradually becoming clear. In this chapter, the skeletal response to exercise is reviewed, and therapeutic applications of physical training are discussed.

Physical Activity and Bone Mass

BONE CELL PHYSIOLOGY

Basic Multicellular Units

Understanding the potential influence of exercise requires knowledge of bone physiology. Changes in bone size and shape can result from longitudinal growth, bone modeling (shape change by addition or subtraction of cortical bone), or bone remodeling (bone turnover and replacement). During childhood, longitudinal bone growth and modeling are dominant forces; for adults, remodeling is of primary importance. All these processes are mediated by heterogeneous populations of cells organized into microanatomically distinct units (basic multicellular units; BMU) in bone.[3] Osteoclasts (bone resorption), osteoblasts (bone formation), and a variety of supporting cells make up the BMU, and work in a coordinated fashion to remove small packets of existing bone and replace them with newly formed bone. The number and activity of BMU determine the rate at which change occurs. Within this process, the potential exists to considerably alter the size and shape of existing bone, even in adults.

The rate at which new BMU arise, and their activity, are affected by a number of factors, including hormones (e.g., parathyroid hormone, $1,25\text{-}(OH)_2D$, glucocorticoids) and local substances (e.g., growth factors, cytokines), as well as the hematologic environment and growth. Mechanical force must, therefore, be viewed as a component of a complex regulatory environment, and bone remodeling activity reflects the sum of these interacting influences.

The relationship between mechanical use and bone mass is well established. Complete immobilization results in the rapid onset (within days) of accelerated bone resorption, as evidenced by an increase in urine calcium and hydroxyproline levels,[4-9] and heightened osteoclastic activity.[10,11] At the same time, osteoblastic activity and bone formation are reduced.[12] If immobilization is continued, loss can be as much as 50%.[13-17] Similar events occur in weightlessness.[18-22] Bone mass recovers when activity resumes, but whether bone loss is completely reversible is unknown.[23]

The Mechanostat

A physiologic process must exist that links mechanical activity to the functional status of bone remodeling cells. In conceptual terms, Frost[24] has referred to this linkage as the *mechanostat*, a useful framework for considering activity's effect on bone. This model proposes a classic feedback relationship between mechanical use and bone strength, such that mechanical stimulation incites accumulation or preservation of bone, and a reduction in stimulation results in the perception (by the mechanostat) of a positive bone balance, leading to bone loss. At stable levels of mechanical activity, bone balance would be maintained. In this way, the immobilization of a broken limb leads to demineralization,[25] and vigorous activity stimulates bone accumulation. Other humoral and cellular effectors of bone cell activity have been postulated to modulate the mechanostat's set point.[26,27] For example, a change in the endocrine milieu (hypogonadism or glucocorticoid excess) might alter the mechanostat's threshold and reduce its perception of mechanical signals, despite no change in actual levels of mechanical stimulation. The resulting perception of a positive bone balance would lead to an increase in osteoclastic activity and bone loss.

Although the mechanostat concept provides a model for understanding the skeletal effects of physical activity, many of its components are not understood. There is biochemical evidence that mechanical loading directly affects bone remodeling,[20,28-30] but the mechanism by which mechanical force is translated to cellular and molecular action remains elusive. Electromechanical events also may be involved. Bone cells are anatomically positioned to detect mechanical strain, and changes in the shape of cells likely lead to biochemical responses.[31] In particular, streaming potentials (generated by fluid movement in bone in response to the minute distortion created by mechanical stress) may affect cell function. It has been suggested[31] that mechanical forces result in the generation of prostaglandins (particularly PGE_2) and cytokines in bone cells, which then act in the BMU environment to alter modeling or remodeling activity.[32,33] Bell and colleagues[30] reported that weight lifting may be associated with changes in endocrine modulators of mineral metabolism, resulting in an increase in new bone formation. Similarly, several groups[34,35] have reported that levels of insulin-like growth factor I, a humoral substance with osteoblast-stimulating properties, were higher in subjects engaged in weight training than in control or aerobically exercising groups.

An activity must produce a certain magnitude of strain (minimum effective strain), representing an actuation in the skeleton's normal strain distribution, to positively influence modeling and remodeling.[2] When this threshold is reached, remodeling is activated; if this level of stimulation is sustained, the result is local bone hypertrophy.[36]

The amount of strain necessary to maintain or remodel existing skeletal mass is becoming understood. Rubin and Lanyon,[37,38] reporting on experiments performed on isolated tibia in vivo, noted a rapid response to small changes in mechanical loading. This finding suggests that the mechanostat is sensitive and maintains tight coupling between load and bone strength, even within the normal or physiologic range of activity. If bone responds quickly to modest changes in activity, the utility of exercise in the prevention and therapy of osteoporosis would be greatly enhanced. Alternatively, based on in vivo data gauging the relationship between strain and skeletal response, Carter[39,42-44] postulated that within the physiologic activity range, the mechanostat is relatively quiescent. Thus, the mechanostat may respond to large loads (which exceed the minimum effective strain) more than to constant or repeated small strains.[42] This is illustrated in Figure 11-1, where bone mass declines below a certain lower limit of activity, is relatively constant in the range of activity associated with daily living, and then increases with higher levels of activity.[43]

In summary, a variety of factors, including strain magnitude, distribution, and rate of application, as well as number of loading cycles, probably are involved in determining the remodeling response to activity.[2] The activity-dependent component of bone mass is determined by the sum of all loading events.[2,44,45] Using this information, it may be possible to maintain bone using either frequent small loads or infrequent larger loads.[37,38]

In an applied context, these issues become important when designing an exercise prescription. For instance, would an hour of daily walking (a repeti-

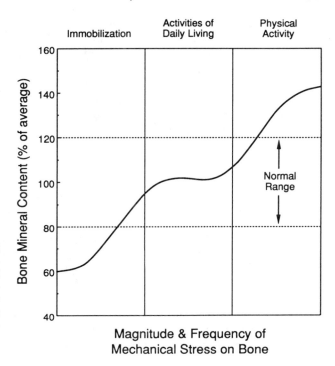

Figure 11–1 A proposed relationship between the history of mechanical strain and the induced change in skeletal mass. It may be at only very high or very low levels of strain that there is an important skeletal response. Adapted from Carter.[43]

tive low-strain activity) be as beneficial for skeletal health as a short burst of an activity producing higher strain levels (e.g., weight lifting)? The resolution of these differences will have important implications for the design of exercise programs for modulating bone mass. The development of these concepts is proceeding quickly[46] and promises to supply practical answers for those prescribing exercise.

EPIDEMIOLOGIC STUDIES

Cross-Sectional Research

Epidemiologic studies have related athletic populations to bone mineral density. Groups of accomplished athletes repeatedly have been shown to have greater skeletal mass than sedentary groups.[47-50] However, the skeletal changes associated with different physical activities have been the subject of debate. Weightbearing activity might be expected to produce greater skeletal strain, resulting in correspondingly larger bone mass. Most cross-sectional studies support this concept. Weight lifting and weightbearing exercises are associated with higher bone mineral density than nonweightbearing activities.[51,52] However, non-weightbearing exercise also seem to be associated with greater bone mass (e.g., tennis players' arm bones) than is found in sedentary groups.[53,54] Even swimming or water sports may confer skeletal benefits: swimmers have higher mineral densities than do sedentary control populations,[55-57] and swimming by animals produces a positive benefit.[58,59] Local muscle tension developed during these exercises may be of particular importance to stimulating bone density. However, in general, a trend suggests that more weightbearing activities (weight lifting, gymnastics) are associated with greater changes in bone remodeling and bone mass.[34]

The association between activity and bone mass is present in the general population. Researchers have observed that indices of physical fitness (VO_{2max}),[60-63] activity levels,[64-68] and muscle strength[60,62,69] correlate with higher bone mineral density.

In addition to one's aerobic ability, specific muscle group strength appears to be a predictor of bone mineral density, and may be the more proximate effector of the relationship between fitness and bone density.[60,62] Many studies suggest that exercise induces a localized skeletal response. For example, bone mass is greater in the dominant arm in tennis players and baseball pitchers. The strength in certain muscle groups correlates with bone mass in related regions (e.g., back extensor strength is associated with spine mineral density, and grip strength with forearm density).[60,62,69,70] Although the relationship between specific muscle strength and associated skeletal mineral density holds true, specific back strength also is related to femoral density, and grip strength to back density.[60,62,69] These correlations between activity or strength in one area and bone mass in another illustrate the complex nature of mechanical stimulation and skeletal physiology.

Most studies relating bone mass to muscle strength or activity level have been cross-sectional,[71] and are subject to many confounding variables (e.g., diet, other physical activities, the duration of exercise). The estimation of activity levels is difficult, because comparisons between athletes and sedentary subjects may have methodologic problems (selectional bias), and correlations between fitness or strength and bone mass are relatively weak and variable. Some studies are contradictory, indicating little benefit from exercise.[72] Thus, it remains unclear how much benefit may be gained from a given level or type of exercise. Certainly, the specifics of an exercise prescription (type, duration, intensity, frequency) are difficult to derive from these reports.

Longitudinal Investigations

Longitudinal studies would be the most powerful demonstration of physical activity's positive influence on bone strength. However, results are not yet clear. This may be due to several factors. Study groups have been heterogeneous, it has been difficult to achieve a high rate of sustained adherence to training, and varied types of training and bone-mass measurement techniques have been utilized.[71] Most commonly, training has involved moderate aerobic activities (walking, jogging, dancing), and some reports describe a reduction in the rate at which bone mass is lost. For instance, Smith and colleagues[73] reported a reduction in the rate of forearm bone loss in postmenopausal women engaging in regular aerobic exercise over a 3-year period. Others[74-78] have shown an apparent stabilization of bone mass in comparison to controls.

In several studies, an increase in bone mass was observed. Smith and coworkers[79] found that moderate exercise produced a gain in some (but not all) groups of elderly subjects. Margulis and associates[80] reported that intensive exercise in military recruits increased tibial bone mass; Williams and colleagues[81] observed an increase in bone mass in men training for a marathon. Dalsky and colleagues[82] found a 5% increase in spinal bone density among women engaged in weightbearing activity, and a group led by Chow[83] observed similar increases after either aerobic exercise or aerobic-plus-strength exercises. Although these positive findings are encouraging, at least two studies[82,84] have reported that exercise-accrued bone mass is lost rapidly when the activity level is reduced.

Not all studies have found a beneficial effect of exercise. Cavanaugh and Cann[85] found no effect of brisk walking in postmenopausal women in a 12-month study, and Sinaki and coworkers[86] were unable to demonstrate a beneficial effect of back-strengthening exercises on vertebral bone mass, despite increase in muscle strength. Gleeson and associates[87] reported that a moderate weight lifting program produced only a slight increase in bone mass in young women compared to controls, and they concluded that weight lifting was not an effective approach to increasing bone mass. However, half of the exercising subjects did not complete the study's exercise program. In a relatively short (9-month) study, Rockwell and colleagues[88] described more spinal bone loss in a group of premenopausal weight lifters than in a control group.

As with cross-sectional studies, longitudinal trials have methodologic difficulties. Most problematic is the absence of randomization (only two studies randomized subjects to exercise and control groups; one[77] was inconclusive and the other[83] showed a positive exercise effect. In other trials, the groups often have not been well-matched, and dropout rates have been high (up to 50%). Hence, the confidence with which exercise can be prescribed as a means to increase bone mass, or even to maintain skeletal health, is not great. Although some data and animal experiments are compelling, available studies with humans provide only limited support for increased activity in the prevention or treatment of osteoporosis.

Confounding Variables

Exercise regimens effective in some groups may be ineffective in others. Age is a particularly important variable, because bone may be less responsive to mechanical stimuli among older individuals.[89] In animal experiments, moderate, long-term treadmill exercise was successful in retarding trabecular bone loss when begun in youth, but when commenced after middle age, did not have a beneficial effect.[90-94] Permissive factors reduced or even lost with aging may result in a lack of an exercise response. For instance, it has been postulated that gonadal steroids are necessary for an anabolic effect of exercise on bone,[5,95] and some studies have reported that the benefits of training seen in premenopausal women are absent in postmenopausal subjects.[94] Similar findings have been noted in the castrated male.[96] Also, dietary calcium deficiency may blunt the ability of exercise to positively change bone metabolism.[95,97]

In addition to variables affecting the response to exercise, factors that correlate with physical activity (e.g., calcium intake or muscular coordination) may influence bone health. As with younger individuals, increased activity among the elderly may be associated with increased bone mass,[52,60,63-65] which in turn should have a positive effect on fracture risk. However, a reduced fracture rate may be a function of other factors also altered by exercise. Falls are a major risk factor for fracture.[98] Increased physical activity[99] and musculoskeletal function[100] are related to lower fracture rates in the elderly, potentially because falls are fewer in stronger, more active individuals.[101] Stronger bones may be a concomitant of a more vigorous, coordinated individual.

Studies of Adverse Effects

A certain level of mechanical stress is needed for maintenance of bone strength, but excessive physical activity can be detrimental. Overexercise actually may lead to reductions in bone mass.[102] Also, when increasing force is applied to any structure, failure (fracture) will occur. Although normal bone provides considerable resistance to fracture, at some intensity of mechanical usage (higher than the minimum effective strain but lower than that required for frank fracture), microdamage accumulates and can lead to failure.

> **CASE:** B.R., a 31-year-old healthy man, developed persistent right foot pain. He had jogged regularly for several years. However, over the past 3 months he had embarked on progressively more strenuous training in preparation for his first marathon. While running 40 miles per week, he noted foot pain that increased to severe discomfort. Examination revealed plantar tenderness, and a radiograph showed a typical stress fracture in the distal first metatarsal.

> **COMMENT:** Stress fractures (the march fracture of army recruits) are encountered when repeated mechanical stress leads to an accumulation of microfractures and ultimately to focal damage. Stress fractures frequently are encountered in those unaccustomed to physical activity.[80,103] Although microfractures are routinely noted in normal bones,[26,106] they usually are not sufficiently large to result in clinical disease. Under normal conditions (normal activity levels), a reparative response occurs after microfracture, consisting of (1) activation of new BMU, (2) formation of microcallus at the site of damage, and (3) adequate repair without symptoms.[107] When the balance is altered, however, so that damage is greater than repair, mechanical failure occurs. Hence, extreme mechanical use in healthy bone or, alternatively, more modest usage in bone less capable of repair (e.g., low-turnover osteoporosis, vitamin D deficiency) results in a clinically similar outcome.

In Figure 11–2, Heaney[108] has summarized a proposed relationship between the physical stress of activity, the mechanical strength of bone, and the likelihood of fracture. Fatigue (stress) fractures become more likely with con-

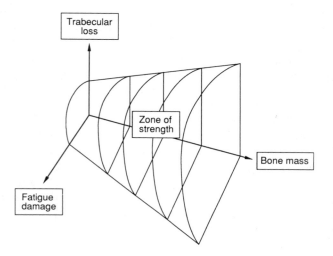

Figure 11–2 The interactions of bone mass, bone architecture, and mechanical fatigue. Whereas fracture may occur even in healthy bone with very high mechanical usage, reductions in bone mass or architectural integrity make fracture more likely at lower levels of mechanical stress. Adapted from Heaney,[108] with permission.

ditions that reduce bone strength or reparative potential. A study attempting to define the underlying cause of women athletes' stress fractures[109] found that those with stress fractures had lower bone mineral density than a control group (as well as several risk factors for osteopenia). This suggests that patients with stress fractures, whether athletic or sedentary, should be evaluated for the presence of metabolic bone disease. This evaluation should include a history and physical examination (with particular attention to risk factors such as menstrual dysfunction, dietary inadequacy, alcohol use, and concurrent endocrine disorder), multichemistry screening, and a measurement of bone mineral density using a precise and accurate technique (e.g., dual x-ray absorptiometry). Since the cause of stress fractures is focused mechanical force (possibly in the presence of an underlying metabolic disorder), a reduction in activity should allow healing via the formation of typical callus and bony union.

> **CASE:** M.S., an 18-year-old woman, sustained a proximal tibial fracture after a seemingly inconsequential trauma. She had been working toward a career in ballet, an effort requiring physical conditioning and the maintenance of strict weight limits. Although she began menstruating at age 12, menses ceased at age 16. There had been two previous metatarsal fractures at age 17, which healed with short periods of restricted activity.
>
> Bone mineral density was measured at vertebral and proximal femoral sites using dual energy x-ray absorptiometry and was found to be less than age- and sex-matched controls. The tibial fracture healed with appropriate therapy, and it was recommended that she liberalize her diet or decrease her exercise schedule. She refused, citing her intense desire to succeed in ballet.

> **COMMENT:** Physical activity can be excessive, especially when associated with deleterious alterations in the nutritional or metabolic environment (e.g., exercise-induced amenorrhea), and can result in bone loss and skeletal weakness. The relationship between vigorous physical activity and amenorrhea among women of reproductive age is well established.[109-118] Primary amenorrhea, or delayed menarche, has been repeatedly described in young women involved in demanding physical activities, including ballet, running, and gymnastics. In these situations, bone mass is frequently less than in age-matched, menstruating, sedentary control women.

Among women, secondary amenorrhea can be a sequela of sustained vigorous physical activity[119] and increases the risk of osteopenia and fractures.[119-127] Fractures in this setting frequently have the character of stress fractures[128] (illustrating the interaction between mechanical use, metabolic state, and bone strength) and also can include fractures typical of other osteopenic states (e.g., vertebral fractures, femoral fractures).

There is a relationship among body weight, adiposity, and the onset and maintenance of menstruation.[129-131] Among female athletes with amenorrhea, body weight is consistently less than among sedentary control populations, and prospective trials have implicated weight loss as a component of the etiology of exercise-induced amenorrhea.[120] Weight loss in these individuals results from the caloric demands of their activities and frequently is compounded by self-determined dietary restrictions meant to maintain body weight within desired limits.

Estimates of caloric intake among amenorrheic women athletes are sometimes surprisingly low,[121] and nutritional status correlates with risk of stress fracture in ballet dancers.[132] Several studies have documented the adverse effects of dietary restriction on bone mass.[133] In addition, eating disorders (anorexia, bulemia) may occur in the amenorrheic–osteopenic exerciser, and can contribute to the etiology of bone disease.[134-137] Stress itself may play a part in the menstrual dysfunction[114,116,138] and has been associated with alterations in other endocrine systems.[118] The similarity of exercise amenorrhea to hypothalamic amenorrhea and anorexia nervosa has been noted.[138,139] Interestingly, although similar effects of intense training on gonadal function have been reported among men,[140] no relationship between excessive exercise and osteopenia has been reported.

Hence, the pathophysiology of osteoporosis in this setting is multifactorial. First, exercise-induced amenorrhea is associated with low estrogen levels, a major risk factor for bone loss. Secondly, caloric restriction has in itself been associated with bone loss. (Low body weight also apparently confers some risk of osteopenia.) Specific nutrient inadequacies, particularly dietary calcium deficiency, may contribute to the risk. The confluence of these negative factors is sufficient to overcome any positive skeletal effects associated with exercise. In essence, the set point of the mechanostat is altered such that bone loss proceeds despite high mechanical usage. Interestingly, in a study[123] comparing exercising, amenorrheic women to amenorrheic but sedentary women, both groups exhibited osteopenia. However, the exercisers were not as severely affected as the sedentary subjects. Thus it would appear that exercise compensates for the bone loss induced by estrogen deficiency, but only partially. An increase in caloric intake or a reduction in exercise intensity will result in both the resumption of menses and greater bone mass.[141,142]

Whether the osteoporosis is completely reversible is uncertain. Drinkwater and colleagues[142] observed that women athletes with histories of prior irregular menstrual periods had lower spinal bone densities than did those with regular periods, suggesting some residual effect on bone mass.

A practical approach to the amenorrheic athlete would be to encourage adequate calcium intake, as well as adequate calories. If amenorrhea continues, a reduction in exercise levels is appropriate. If measures of bone mass reveal osteopenia, the patient should be strongly encouraged to reduce the level of exercise or consider estrogen replacement therapy. Women who do not choose to alter dietary and exercise habits risk further bone loss and skeletal fractures.

Management of Skeletal Health

CASE: B.D., a 60-year-old postmenopausal woman, was referred for the prevention of osteoporosis. She had a mastectomy for nonmetastatic breast carcinoma 10 years before and has never taken estrogen replacement therapy. She is otherwise healthy, although sedentary. She is concerned particularly because of her mother's history of vertebral fracture. A physical examination is unremarkable, and screening laboratory values are normal. Her vertebral and proximal femoral bone densities are found to be below the mean for her age, but still within the age-adjusted normal range (mean ± SD). The patient is told she does not have osteoporosis now, but that because of her relatively low bone mineral measurements, she should attempt to minimize any further bone loss.

The patient has several questions: How is osteoporosis detected? How can osteoporosis be prevented or treated? Can exercise help, and if so, what kinds of activity would be best?

COMMENT: The basic evaluation, prevention, and treatment of the osteoporotic patient have recently been reviewed,[143] and are summarized here in the context of a discussion of exercise and its utility.

OSTEOPOROSIS DETECTION

The diagnosis of osteoporosis should be based on either the presence of a fracture in the absence of important trauma (after excluding focal bone disorders such as cancer and infection) or an abnormally reduced bone mineral density. Reduced bone mineral density should be considered the precursor of fracture, in the same way that hypertension is considered a risk factor for cardiovascular events.

In the absence of fracture, the indications for measurement of bone mineral density are becoming more clear. It should not be used as a screening procedure, but rather applied when bone disease is suspected or when risk of osteoporosis is high (Table 11–1).[144,145] Bone mineral density can be measured with the use of several techniques, including single photon absorptiometry (radius or calcaneus), quantitative computed tomography (vertebrae), dual photon absorptiometry (vertebrae, proximal femur, whole body, radius), and dual-energy x-ray absorptometry (vertebrae, proximal femur, whole body radius). Data indicate that measures of bone mineral density are predictive of fracture risk.[146-150] None of these techniques is more useful than the others in this regard. Single photon absorptiometry is least expensive, and quantitative CT scan most costly. Bone mineral density measures may reflect only a compo-

Table 11–1 **RISK FACTORS FOR OSTEOPENIA**

Race (white or Asian)
Sex (female)
Age (>50)
Postmenopausal status
Excess glucocorticoid levels
Malabsorption
Alcoholism
Tobacco abuse
Anticonvulsant medications
Renal insufficiency
Hepatic insufficiency
Family history of osteoporosis
Hyperthyroidism
Hyperparathyroidism
Cancer
Chronic pulmonary diseases
Inadequate calcium nutrition

nent (albeit an important one) of fracture risk, however. Other issues that have been suggested to be of potential relevance include material properties of bone and its microarchitecture.[149]

INITIAL EVALUATION AND MANAGEMENT

Once osteoporosis is identified, an evaluation for potential etiologies is warranted. History and physical examination should focus on known risk factors for bone disease (e.g., dietary insufficiencies, endocrine disorders, gastrointestinal disease, use of certain drugs, alcohol abuse, menstrual dysfunction). The laboratory evaluation can be helpful, with particular attention to potential risks identified during the history and physical examination. Radiographs of the spine or other areas of interest can aid in the diagnosis and staging of bone disease. Although not helpful in quantitating bone mass, radiographs are helpful in excluding pathologic fractures (from cancer or infection) and determining the extent of current fractures (particularly in the spine).

The therapeutic approach is based on two basic principles: elimination (if possible) of risk factors for continued bone loss (see Table 11–1) and the prescription of measures to prevent further bone loss or to improve existing bone status. Frequently, therapy includes the treatment of endocrine disorders, ensuring adequacy of calcium and vitamin D in the diet, and discontinuing or reducing detrimental medications. In addition, specific therapies may include estrogen replacement, calcitonin, bisphosphonates, fluoride, and other agents.

After osteoporotic patients (or those at risk for development of osteoporosis) are provided specific recommendations, periodic follow-up is used to monitor clinical, biochemical, radiographic, or densitometric parameters and judge the effectiveness of therapy. Sequential bone mineral density measures may be used to assess stabilization or improvement in bone mass, which is an indicator of treatment success.

EXERCISE AS THERAPY

Osteoporosis prevention among susceptible individuals is the goal. Exercise may be an effective strategy, either by improving the peak bone mass attained in young adulthood or by reducing the rate of bone loss in later life. In 1984, the NIH Consensus Development Conference recommended moderate exercise as an approach to prevent bone loss, and exercise appears to be one of the mainstays of the osteoporosis prevention programs advocated by physicians.[150] Despite sophisticated means to measure exercise intensity and bone mass, however, the ability to prescribe an exercise program of documented effectiveness still does not exist. Nevertheless, although the type, duration, frequency, and intensity of exercise (the basics of an exercise prescription) for the prevention of osteoporosis are estimates from limited data, guidelines can be reasonably developed.

An individual who retains normal bone mineral content but is at risk for bone disease (e.g., a postmenopausal woman who cannot use estrogen replacement therapy, has a strong family history of osteoporosis, or needs glucocorticoid therapy) can use exercise as a mainstay for preventing osteoporosis. With normal bone mineral density, the risk of fracture is low, and relatively strenuous exercise, including weightbearing exercise, can be prescribed. For example, a program with components of aerobic activities and weight training could be tailored to the individual's abilities and predilections, using guidelines as outlined in Chapter 1. Other factors (nutrition, gonadal function) also should be optimized to maximize the exercise effect.

Developing an exercise prescription for those who have a reduced bone mineral content but who have not yet experienced fractures is more difficult. It is likely that weightbearing exercises are most effective in eliciting a positive skeletal response. However, with a reduction in bone mass, fractures from moderate or little trauma are more likely. In this situation, the type and intensity of exercise must be altered. Activities that involve a significant risk of falls or other trauma should be avoided. Aerobic activities (dance, bicycling, walking, calisthenics) and floor exercises may be useful to maintain bone mass, muscle strength, and coordination. However, flexion exercises of the trunk should be discouraged, because they have been reported to increase the incidence of vertebral wedging in osteoporotic individuals.[151]

Goals for those with established osteoporosis should include the maintenance of bone mass, strength conditioning, increased coordination, and the reduction of back pain. Sinaki[151-154] has reviewed exercises that are safe and effective for osteoporotic subjects. Even among patients with considerable restriction, an exercise program that begins slowly and sets realistic goals can produce marked symptomatic improvement and enhance mobility. Isometric and extension exercises are probably the most useful and have been described in this setting (Figure 11–3)[152] (see also Chapter 7). The involvement of a physical therapist or exercise therapist to monitor the initiation and progress of therapy is important. For patients with gait instability, stationary cycling can be a safe aerobic activity that also can increase quadriceps strength. Exercise should be curtailed in the period immediately following a vertebral fracture, and restarted slowly as the patient's level of comfort allows, with avoidance of activities that exacerbate pain.

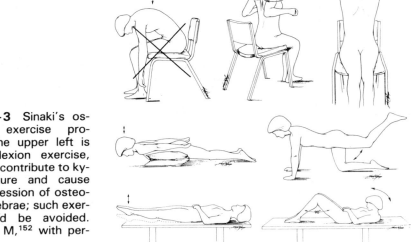

Figure 11–3 Sinaki's osteoporosis exercise program. At the upper left is a lumbar flexion exercise, which could contribute to kyphotic posture and cause more compression of osteoporotic vertebrae; such exercises should be avoided. From Sinaki M,[152] with permission.

CASE: F.J., a healthy 75-year-old woman, was seen 2 months following a compression fracture of T-10, sustained while pulling weeds in the garden. Although moderate back pain and disability were still present, she was improving. Spinal radiographs revealed anterior wedge fractures at T-7 and T-8, a compression fracture of T-10, and generalized osteopenia. She had been living alone for 10 years, and her family reported her to be alert and active but somewhat frail. In particular, she complained of episodic dizziness. The patient's family was concerned that with her established osteoporosis and a predilection for falling, exercise therapy might be contraindicated.

COMMENT: In addition to its potential for preventing bone loss, exercise may be beneficial in established osteoporosis. Specifically, exercise has been postulated to help in rehabilitation following spinal fracture, as well as providing relief in chronic back pain (see Chapter 7). Moreover, exercise may increase strength and coordination, both of potential benefit in prevention of falls and fracture.[145,146,155] Finally, several studies have suggested that regimens of modest activity may retard bone loss or increase bone mass among those with established osteoporosis.[73-84] However, these studies are not definitive and do not provide the basis for specific exercise recommendations.

Summary

Physical activity has important positive effects on skeletal health. The physiology connecting exercise and bone metabolism is an area of active study. As yet, however, findings do not allow precise training recommendations. Nutrition, hormone status, and aging all interact with physical activity to affect bone mass. The exercise prescription for bone health must be adjusted based on whether osteoporosis is being prevented or managed. For both groups, regular physical activity can be useful.

REFERENCES

1. Wolff J: The Law of Bone Remodeling (Das Gesetz der Transformation der Knochen). Springer: Berlin, 1892.
2. Biewener AA: Biomechanics of mammalian terrestrial locomotion. Science 1990; 250:1097–1103.
3. Parfitt AM: Bone remodeling and bone loss: Understanding the pathophysiology of osteoporosis. Clin Obstet Gynecol 1987; 30: 789–811.
4. Naftchi NE, et al: Mineral metabolism in spinal cord injury. Arch Phys Med Rehabil 1980; 61:139–142.
5. Stewart AF, et al.: Calcium hemostasis in immobilization: An example of resorptive hypercalciuria. N Engl J Med 1982; 306: 1136–1140.
6. Donaldson CL, et al.: Effect of prolonged bed rest on bone mineral. Metabolism 1970; 19:1071–1084.
7. Issekutz B, et al.: Effect of prolonged bed rest on urinary calcium output. J Appl Physiol 1966; 21:1013–1020.
8. Whedon GD: Disuse osteoporosis: Physiological aspects. Calcif Tissue Int 1984; 36:S146–S150.
9. Schneider VS, McDonald J: Skeletal calcium homeostasis and countermeasures to prevent disuse osteoporosis. Calcif Tissue Int 1984; 36:S151–S154.
10. Whedon GD, Mazess RB: Immobilization and bone [editorial]. Calcif Tissue Int 1983; 35:265–267.
11. Minaire P, et al.: Quantitative histological data on disuse osteoporosis. Calcif Tissue Res 1974; 17:57–73.
12. Turner RT, Bell NH: The effects of immobilization and histomorphometry in rats. J Bone Min Res 1986; 1:399–407.
13. Uhthoff H, Jaworski Z: Bone loss in response to long-term immobilization. J Bone Joint Surg 1978; 60B:420–429.
14. Uhthoff H, Sekaly G, Jaworski, Z: Effect of long-term nontraumatic immobilization on metaphyseal spongiosa in young adult and old beagle dogs. Clin Orthop 1985; 192:278–283.
15. Krolner B, Tofte B: Vertebral bone loss: An

unheeded side effect of therapeutic bed rest. *Clin Sci* 1983; 64:537–540.

16. Lanyon LE: Functional strain in bone tissue as an objective, controlling stimulus for adaptive bone remodeling. *J Biomech* 1987; 20:1083–1093.

17. Marcus R, Carte DR: The role of physical activity in bone mass regulation. *Adv Sports Med Fitness* 1988; 1:63–82.

18. Bones in space. *BMJ* 1980; 280:1288.

19. Morey ER, Baylink DJ: Inhibition of bone formation during space flight. *Science* 1978; 201:1138–1141.

20. Simmons DJ, et al.: Effect of space flight on the non-weightbearing bones of rat skeleton. *Am J Physiol* 1983; 244:R319–R326.

21. Wronski TJ, Morey ER: Effect of space flight on periosteal bone formation in rats. *Am J Physiol* 1983; 244:R305–R309.

22. Cann CE, Adachi RR: Bone resorption and mineral excretion in rats during space flight. *Am J Physiol* 1983; 244:R327–R331.

23. LeBlanc A, et al.: Bone mineral loss and recovery after 17 weeks of bed rest. *J Bone Min Res* 1990; 5:843–855.

24. Frost HM: The mechanostat: A proposed pathogenic mechanism of osteoporoses and the bone mass effects of mechanical and nonmechanical agents. *Bone Min* 1987; 2:73–85.

25. Finsen V: Osteopenia after osteotomy of the tibia. *Calcif Tissue Int* 1988; 42:1–4.

26. Frost HM: Vital biomechanics: Proposed general concepts for skeletal adaptations to mechanical usage. *Calcif Tissue Int* 1988; 42:145–156.

27. Lanyon LE: Biomechanical factors in adaptation of bone structure to function. In Uhthoff HK, ed: *Current Concepts of Bone Fragility*. Springer-Verlag: New York, 1986, pp 18–34.

28. Buckley JJ, et al.: Osteoblasts increase their rate of division and align in response to cyclic, mechanical tension in vitro. *Bone Min* 1988; 4:225–236.

29. Lips P, et al.: Lower mobility and markers of bone resorption in the elderly. *Bone Min* 1990; 9:49–57.

30. Bell NH, et al.: The effects of muscle-building exercise on vitamin D and mineral metabolism. *J Bone Min Res* 1988; 3:369–373.

31. Rodan GA: Mechanical loading deficiency and the coupling of bone formation to bone resorption. *J Bone Min Res* 1991; 6:527–529.

32. Imamura K, et al.: Continuously applied compressive pressure induces bone resorption by a mechanism involving prostaglandin E_2 synthesis. *J Cell Physiol* 1990; 144:222–228.

33. Murray DW, Rushton N: The effect of strain on bone cell prostaglandin E_2 release: A new experimental method. *Calcif Tissue Int* 1990; 47:35–39.

34. Davee AM, Rosen CJ, Adler RA: Exercise patterns and trabecular bone density in college women. *J Bone Min Res* 1990; 5:245–250.

35. Poehlman ET, Copeland KC: Influence of physical activity on insulin-like growth factor-I in healthy younger and older men. *J Clin Endocrinol Metab* 1990; 71:1468–1473.

36. Rubin CT, Lanyon LE: Regulation of bone formation by applied dynamic loads. *J Bone Joint Surg* 1984; 66:397–402.

37. Rubin CT, Lanyon LE: Bone remodeling in response to applied dynamic loads. *Trans Orthop Res Soc* 1981; 6:64.

38. Rubin CT, Lanyon LE: Regulation by bone mass by peak strain magnitude. *Trans Orthop Res Soc* 1983; 8:70.

39. Carter DR: The relationship between in vivo strains and cortical bone remodeling. In *CRC Critical Reviews in Biomedical Engineering*, Vol. 8. CRC Press: Boca Raton, FL, 1982, pp 1–28.

40. Frost HM: *Intermediary Organization of the Skeleton*, Vol. 1. CRC Press: Boca Raton, FL, 1986.

41. *Health United States*. 1984. Washington, DC: US Dept of Health and Human Services Publication PHS 85-1232.

42. Whalen RT, Carter DR, Steele CR: The relationship between physical activity and bone density. *Trans Orthop Res Soc* 1987; 12:464.

43. Carter DR: Mechanical loading histories and cortical bone remodeling. *Calcif Tissue Int* 1984; 36S:19.

44. Carter DR, Fyrie DP, Whalen RT: Trabecular bone density and loading history: Regulation of connective tissue biology and mechanical energy. *J Biomech* 1987; 20:785–794.

45. Lanyon L: Functional strain in bone tissue as an objective, and controlling stimulus for adaptive bone remodeling. *J Biomech* 1987; 20:1083–1093.

46. Viceconti M, Seireg A: A generalized procedure for predicting bone mass regulation by mechanical strain. *Calcif Tissue Int* 1990; 47:296–301.

47. Dalsky GP: The role of exercise in the prevention of osteoporosis. *Comp Ther* 1989; 15:30–37.

48. Smith EL, Gilligan C: Mechanical forces and bone. *J Bone Min Res* 1989; 6:139–173.

49. Williams JA, et al.: The effect of long-distance running upon appendicular bone mineral content. *Med Sci Sports Exerc* 1984; 16:223–247.

50. Jacobson PC, et al.: Bone density in women: College athletes and older athletic women. *J Orthop Res* 1984; 2:328–332.

51. Block JE, Genant HK, Black D: Greater vertebral bone mineral mass in exercising young men. *West J Med* 1986; 145:39–42.

52. Lane NE, Bloch DA, Jones HH: Long-distance running, bone density, and osteoarthritis. *JAMA* 1986; 255:1147–1151.

53. Jones HH, Priest JD, Hayes WC: Humeral hypertrophy in response to exercise. *J Bone Joint Surg* 1977; 59A:204–208.

54. Huddleston AL, et al.: Bone mass in life-

time tennis athletes. *JAMA* 1980; 244: 1107–1109.

55. Nilsson BE, Westlin NE: Bone density in athletes. *Clin Orthop* 1971; 77:179–182.

56. Orwoll ES, et al.: The relationship of swimming exercise to bone mass in men and women. *Arch Intern Med* 1989; 149: 2197–2200.

57. Block JE, et al.: Determinants of bone density among athletes engaged in weight-bearing and non-weightbearing activity. *J Appl Physiol* 1989; 67:1100–1105.

58. Swissa-Sivan A, et al.: Effect of swimming on bone modeling and composition in young rats. *Calcif Tissue Int* 1990; 47:173–177.

59. Swissa-Sivan A, et al.: Effect of swimming on bone growth and development in young rats. *Bone Min* 1989; 7:91–105.

60. Bevier WC, Wiswell RA, Pyka G: Relationship of body composition, muscle strength, and aerobic capacity to bone mineral density in older men and women. *J Bone Min Res* 1989; 4:421–432.

61. Pocock NA, et al.: Physical fitness is a major determinant of femoral neck and lumbar spine bone mineral density. *J Clin Invest* 1986; 78:618–621.

62. Pocock N, et al.: Muscle strength, physical fitness, and weight but not age predict femoral neck bone mass. *J Bone Min Res* 1989; 4:441–448.

63. Chow RK, et al.: Physical fitness effect on bone mass in postmenopausal women. *Arch Phys Med Rehabil* 1986; 67:231–234.

64. Oyster N, Morton M, Linnell S: Physical activity and osteoporosis in postmenopausal women. *Med Sci Sports Exerc* 1984; 16:44–50.

65. Ballard JE, McKeown BC, Graham HM: The effect of high-level physical activity (8.5 METs or greater) and estrogen replacement therapy upon bone mass in postmenopausal females, aged 50–68 years. *Int J Sports Med* 1990; 11:208–214.

66. Talmage RV, Stinnett SS, Landwehr JT: Age-related loss of bone density in nonathletic women. *Bone Min* 1986; 1:115–125.

67. Kanders B, Dempster DW, Lindsay R: Interaction of calcium nutrition and physical activity on bone mass in young women. *J Bone Min Res* 1988; 3:145–149.

68. Aloia JF, Vaswani AN, Yeh JK: Premenopausal bone mass is related to physical activity. *Arch Intern Med* 1988; 148:121–123.

69. Snow-Harter C, Bouxsein M, Lewis B: Muscle strength as a predictor of bone mineral density in young women. *J Bone Min Res* 1990; 5:589–595.

70. Sinaki M, McPhee MC, Hodgson SF: Relationship between bone mineral density of spine and strength of back extensors in healthy postmenopausal women. *Mayo Clin Proc* 1986; 61:116–122.

71. Block JE, et al.: Preventing osteoporosis with exercise: A review emphasis on methodology. *Medical Hypotheses* 1989; 30:9–19.

72. Michel BA, Bloch DA, Fries JF: Weight-bearing exercise, overexercise, and lumbar bone density over age 50. *Arch Intern Med* 1989; 149:2325–2329.

73. Smith EL, et al.: Bone involution decrease in exercising middle-aged women. *Calcif Tissue Int* 1984; 36:S129–S138.

74. Aloia JF, et al.: Prevention of involutional bone loss by exercise. *Ann Intern Med* 1978; 89:356–358.

75. Simkin A, Ayalon J, Leichter I: Increased trabecular bone density due to bone-loading exercises in postmenopausal osteoporotic women. *Calcif Tissue Int* 1987; 40: 59–63.

76. White MK, et al.: The effects of exercise on the bones of postmenopausal women. *Int Orthop* 1984; 7:209–214.

77. Sandler RB, et al.: The effects of walking on the cross-sectional dimensions of the radius in postmenopausal women. *Calcif Tissue Int* 1987; 41:65–69.

78. Krolner B, et al.: Physical exercise as prophylaxis against involutional bone loss: A controlled trial. *Clin Sci* 1983; 64:541–546.

79. Smith EL, Reddan W, Smith PE: Physical activity and calcium modalities for bone mineral increase in aged women. *Med Sci Sports Exerc* 1981; 13:60–64.

80. Margulis JY, et al.: Effect of intense physical activity on the bone mineral content in the lower limbs of young adults. *J Bone Joint Surg* 1986; 68A:1090–1093.

81. Williams JA, et al.: The effect of long-distance running upon appendicular bone mineral content. *Med Sci Sports Exerc* 1984; 16:223–227.

82. Dalsky G, Stocke KS, Ehsani AA: Weight-bearing exercise training and lumbar bone mineral content in postmenopausal women. *Ann Intern Med* 1988; 108: 824–828.

83. Chow R, Harrison JE, Notarius C: Effect of two randomized exercise programs on bone mass of healthy postmenopausal women. *BMJ* 1987; 295:1441–1444.

84. Lane NE, et al.: Running, osteoarthritis, and bone density: Initial 2-year longitudinal study. *Am J Med* 1990; 88:452–459.

85. Cavanaugh DJ, Cann CE: Brisk walking does not stop bone loss in postmenopausal women. *Bone* 1988; 9:201–204.

86. Sinaki M, et al.: Efficacy of nonloading exercises in prevention of vertebral bone loss in postmenopausal women: A controlled trial. *Mayo Clin Proc* 1989; 64:762–769.

87. Gleeson PG, et al.: Effects of weight lifting on bone mineral density in premenopausal women. *J Bone Min Res* 1990; 5:153–158.

88. Rockwell JC, et al.: Weight training decreases vertebral bone density in premenopausal women: A prospective study. *J Clin Endocrinol Metab* 1990; 71:988–993.

89. Rubin C, Bain S: Suppression of the osteo-

genic response in the aging skeleton. *J Bone Min Res* 1989; 4:S374.

90. Silbermann M, et al.: Long-term physical exercise retards trabecular bone loss in lumbar vertebrae of aging female mice. *Calcif Tissue Int* 1990; 46:80–93.

91. Steinhagen-Theissen E, Reznick A, Hilz H: Negative adaptation to physical training in senile mice. *Mech Ageing Dev* 1983; 12: 231–236.

92. Reznick A, et al.: The effect of short- and long-term exercise on aldolase activity in muscles of CW-1 and C57BL mice of various ages. *Mech Ageing Dev* 1983; 23: 253–258.

93. Severson JA, et al.: Adrenocortical function in aging exercise-trained rats. *J Appl Physiol* 1977; 43:839–846.

94. Kirk S, et al.: Effect of long-distance running on bone mass in women. *J Bone Min Res* 1989; 4:515–522.

95. Dalsky GP: Effect of exercise on bone: Permissive influence of estrogen and calcium. *Med Sci Sports Exerc* 1990; 22:281–285.

96. Bain SD, Rubin CT: Metabolic modulation of disuse osteopenia: Endocrine-dependent site specificity of bone remodeling. *J Bone Min Res* 1990; 5:1069–1075.

97. Lanyon L, Rubin C, Baust G: Modulation of bone loss during calcium insufficiency by controlled dynamic loading. *Calcif Tissue Int* 1986; 38:209–216.

98. Cummings SR, Nevitt MC: A hypothesis: The cause of hip fractures. *J Gerontol* 1989; 44:M107–M111.

99. Wickham CAC, et al.: Dietary calcium, physical activity, and risk of hip fracture: A prospective study. *BMJ* 1989; 299: 889–892.

100. Kelsey JL, Hoffman S: Risk factors for hip fracture. *N Engl J Med* 1987; 316:404–406.

101. Nevitt MC, et al.: Risk factors for recurrent nonsyncopal falls. *JAMA* 1989; 261: 2663–2668.

102. Michel BA, Bloch DA, Fires JF: Weight-bearing exercise, over-exercise, and lumbar bone density over age 50 years. *Arch Intern Med* 1989; 149:2325–2329.

103. Leichter I, et al.: Gain in mass density of bone following strenuous physical activity. *J Orthop Res* 1989; 7:86–90.

104. Margulies J, et al.: Effect of intense physical activity on the bone mineral content in the lower limbs of young adults. *J Bone Joint Surg* 1986; 68A:1090–1093.

105. Frost H: Vital biomechanics: Proposed general concepts for skeletal adaptations to mechanical usage. *Calcif Tissue Int* 1988; 42:145–156.

106. Carter D, et al.: Uniaxial fatigue of human cortical bone: The influence of tissue physical characteristics. *J Biomech* 1982; 15: 137–139.

107. Martin B, Burr D: A hypothetical mechanism for the stimulation of osteonal re-modeling by fatigue damage. *J Biomech* 1982; 15:137–139.

108. Heaney RP: Osteoporotic fracture space: An hypothesis. *Bone Min* 1989; 6:1–13.

109. Baker ER: Menstrual dysfunction and hormonal status in athletic women: A review. *Fertility Sterility* 1981; 36:691–696.

110. Abraham SF, et al.: Body weight, exercise and menstrual status among ballet dancers in training. *Br J Obstet Gynaecol* 1982; 89:507–510.

111. Frisch RE, Wyshak G, Vincent L: Delayed menarche and amenorrhea in ballet dancers. *N Engl J Med* 1980; 303:17–19.

112. Dale E, Gerlach DH, Wilhite AL: Menstrual dysfunction in distance runners. *Obstet Gynecol* 1979; 54:47–53.

113. Schwartz B, et al.: Exercise-associated amenorrhea: A distinct entity? *Am J Obstet Gynecol* 1981; 141:662–670.

114. Baker ER, et al.: Female runners and secondary amenorrhea: Correlation with age, parity, mileage, and plasma hormonal and sex-hormone-binding globulin concentrations. *Fertility Sterility* 1981; 36:183–187.

115. Loucks AB, Horvath SM: Exercise-induced stress responses of amenorrheic and eu-menorrheic runners. *J Clin Endocrinol Metab* 1984; 59:1109–1120.

116. Frisch RE, et al.: Delayed menarche and amenorrhea of college athletes in relation to age onset training. *JAMA* 1981; 246: 1559–1563.

117. Rebar RW, Cumming DC: Reproductive function in women athletes. *JAMA* 1981; 246:1590.

118. Jacobs HS: Amenorrhea in athletes. *Br J Obstet Gynaecol* 1982; 89:498–500.

119. Bullen BA, et al.: Induction of menstrual disorders by strenuous exercise in untrained women. *N Engl J Med* 1985; 312: 1349–1353.

120. Marcus R, et al.: Menstrual function and bone mass in elite women distance runners. *Ann Intern Med* 1985; 102:158–163.

121. Health H III: Athletic women, amenorrhea, and skeletal integrity [editorial]. *Ann Intern Med* 1985; 102:258–260.

122. Cann CE, et al.: Decreased spinal mineral content in amenorrheic women. *JAMA* 1984; 251:626–629.

123. Lindberg JS, et al.: Exercise-induced amenorrhea and bone density. *Ann Intern Med* 1984; 101:647–648.

124. Drinkwater BL, et al.: Bone mineral content of amenorrheic and eumenorrheic athletes. *N Engl J Med* 1984; 311:277–281.

125. Fisher EC, et al.: Bone mineral content and levels of gonadotropins and estrogens in amenorrheic running women. *J Clin Endocrinol Metab* 1986; 62:1232–1236.

126. Wolman RL, et al.: Menstrual state and exercise in determinants of spinal trabecular bone density in female athletes. *BMJ* 1990; 301:516–518.

127. Drinkwater BL, Bruemner B, Chestnut CH

III: Menstrual history as a determinant of current bone density in young athletes. *JAMA* 1990; 263:545–548.

128. Myburgh KH, et al.: Low bone density is an etiologic factor for stress fractures in athletes. *Ann Intern Med* 1990; 113: 754–759.

129. Frisch RE, Revelle R: Height and weight at menarche and a hypothesis of critical body weights and adolescent events. *Science* 1970; 169:397–399.

130. Frisch RE, McArthur JW: Menstrual cycles: Fatness as a determinant of minimum weight for height necessary for their maintenance or onset. *Science* 1974; 185: 949–951.

131. Pirke KM, et al.: The influence of dieting on the menstrual cycles of healthy young women. *J Clin Endocrinol Metab* 1985; 60:1174–1179.

132. Frusztajer NT, et al.: Nutrition and the incidence of stress fractures in ballet dancers. *Am J Clin Nutr* 1990; 51:779–783.

133. Shires R, et al.: Effects of semistarvation on skeletal homeostasis. *Endocrinology* 1980; 107:1530–1535.

134. Rigotti NA, et al.: Osteoporosis in women with anorexia nervosa. *N Engl J Med* 1984; 20:1601–1606.

135. Szmukler GI, et al.: Premature loss of bone in chronic anorexia nervosa. *BMJ* 1985; 290:26–27.

136. Treasure JL, et al.: Reversible bone in chronic anorexia nervosa. *BMJ* 1987; 474–475.

137. Warren MP, et al.: Scoliosis and fractures in young ballet dancers. *N Engl J Med* 1986; 314:1348–1353.

138. Ding J, et al.: High serum cortisol levels in exercise-associated amenorrhea. *Ann Intern Med* 1988; 108:530–534.

139. Barron JL, et al.: Hypothalamic dysfunction in overtrained athletes. *J Clin Endocrinol Metab* 1985; 60:803–812.

140. Wheeler GD, et al.: Endurance training decreases serum testosterone levels in men without change in luteinizing hormone pulsatile release. *J Clin Endocrinol Metab* 1991; 72:422–425.

141. Lindberg JS, et al.: Increased vertebral bone mineral in response to reduced exercise in amenorrheic runners. *West J Med* 1987; 146:39–42.

142. Drinkwater BL, et al.: Bone mineral density after resumption of menses in amenorrheic athletes. *JAMA* 1986; 256:380–382.

143. Riggs BL: Overview of osteoporosis. *West J Med* 1991; 154:63–77.

144. Cummings SR, Browner WS, Ettinger B: Should prescription of postmenopausal hormone therapy be based on the results of bone densitometry? *Ann Intern Med* 1990; 112:516–528.

145. Melton LJ III, Eddy DM, Johnston CC Jr: Screening for osteoporosis. *Ann Intern Med* 1990; 112:516–528.

146. Hui SL, Slemenda CW, Johnston CC Jr: Baseline measurement of bone mass predicts fracture in white women. *Ann Intern Med* 1989; 111:355–361.

147. Wasnich RD, et al.: Prediction of postmenopausal fracture risk with the use of bone mineral measurements. *Am J Obstet Gynecol* 1985; 153:745–751.

148. Cummings SR, et al.: Appendicular bone density and age predict hip fracture in women. *JAMA* 1990; 263:665–668.

149. Heaney RP, Avioli LV, Chestnut CH III: Osteoporotic bone fragility. *JAMA* 1989; 261:2986–2990.

150. Grisso JA, Baum CR, Turner BJ: What do physicians in practice do to prevent osteoporosis? *J Bone Min Res* 1990; 5:213–219.

151. Sinaki M, Mikkelsen BA: Postmenopausal spinal osteoporosis: Flexion versus extension exercises. *Arch Phys Med Rehabil* 1984; 65:593–596.

152. Sinaki M: Postmenopausal spinal osteoporosis: Physical therapy and rehabilitation principles. *Mayo Clin Proc* 1982; 57: 699–703.

153. Limburg PJ, et al.: A useful technique for measurement of back strength in osteoporotic and elderly patients. *Mayo Clin Proc* 1991; 66:39–44.

154. Sinaki M: Beneficial musculoskeletal effects of physical activity in the older woman. *Geriatr Med Today* 1989; 8:53–72.

155. Melton LJI, Chao EYS, Lane J: In Riggs BL, Melton LJI, eds: *Osteoporosis: Etiology, Diagnosis, and Management.* Raven Press: New York, 1988, pp 111–131.

PART V

Physiologic Conditions

CHAPTER 12

PREGNANCY AND EXERCISE

SIG-LINDA JACOBSON, MD, MARILYN S. PAUL, BA,
and MARK J. MORTON, MD

The cardiopulmonary system is altered uniquely during pregnancy. At rest and during exercise, the pregnant woman supplies the developing fetus, as well as herself, with oxygen and energy substrates. Also during this period, musculoskeletal and weight changes affect exercise performance and may increase the chance of injury. In this chapter, we review the physiology of exercise during pregnancy and its potential benefits, as well as conditions contraindicating higher levels of exertion. Recommendations for physical activity during pregnancy are provided to maximize the well-being of both mother and fetus.

Maternal Response to Pregnancy

WEIGHT GAIN

Weight gain during a singleton pregnancy is highly variable, averaging 12 kg.[1] Approximately 30% of this increase occurs during the first half of gestation, with a subsequent linear increase until term. The weight gain is comprised of the fetus and placenta (5 kg); increases in the uterus, breasts, and body water (4 kg); and additional body fat (3 kg). This additional weight presents an increased demand on the cardiovascular and musculoskeletal systems, and the increase in total body water may result in edema and can restrict movement of the hands and feet.

MUSCULOSKELETAL CHANGES

The expanding uterus and breasts alter a woman's center of gravity, leading to increased lumbar lordosis. This postural compensation is accentuated by joint adaptations. Beginning early in pregnancy, the connective tissue of ligaments, joints, and joint capsules is relaxed, perhaps owing to actions of estrogen and relaxin. These changes are greatest in the pelvis and contribute to the waddling gait typical of late pregnancy. Most other joints are affected as well. Low back pain is common, and the combination of a wider pelvis, increased femoral rotation, and knee joint laxity may produce knee pain.

CARDIOVASCULAR AND PULMONARY ALTERATIONS
At Rest

Cardiac output is greater during pregnancy because of increased heart rate and stroke volume.[2-7] The increase is maximal in the second trimester (an increase of 30% to 40%) and variable in the third trimester, due to postural influences on venous return.[4] Thus, supine women in late gestation have stroke volumes lower than those of postpartum supine women because pressure on the inferior vena cava lowers preload. The cause of increased resting heart rate is unknown, but the higher stroke volume appears to be related to cardiac enlargement, with a normal or slightly enhanced systolic function.[7-10] Although blood volume is greatly increased,[11] filling pressures are unchanged,[2] and arterial pressure is actually reduced in the second trimester.[12] Accordingly, vascular resistance is markedly lowered at the same time, rising toward nonpregnant levels in the third trimester.[7] The lack of increased filling pressures despite elevated blood volume may be related to increased vascular capacitance and compliance.[13] Lower vascular resistance during pregnancy reflects generalized pressor hyporesponsiveness and may be related to vasodilatory prostaglandins produced by the placenta or to endothelial derived relaxing factor produced locally in response to the pregnant state. Reduced uterine vascular resistance, associated with uterine and placental growth, plays an increasingly important role as pregnancy progresses.[14] In addition, the aorta becomes larger and more compliant during pregnancy, facilitating ventricular ejection.[15]

Pulmonary responses to pregnancy have been summarized.[16] Maternal oxygen consumption at rest increases 10% to 20% during pregnancy, but minute ventilation increases 40% to 50%, resulting in hypocarbia and a respiratory alkalosis. Maximum voluntary ventilation is unchanged. The resting hyperventilation is related to the effects of progesterone on the respiratory center. Cardiac output is increased more than the increase in oxygen consumption, resulting in a fall in arteriovenous oxygen difference during pregnancy.

During Exercise

Available data concerning work capacity during pregnancy are conflicting. Some studies suggest that maximal work may be greater, while others report that this capacity is reduced during pregnancy. Data are difficult to synthesize, because maternal fitness, type of testing, and stage of pregnancy differ among studies. Women studied during maximal upright cycle exercise toward the end of the second trimester were found to have no increase in maximal oxygen consumption and heart rate.[17] However, maximal cardiac output was greater, suggesting that arteriovenous oxygen difference at peak exercise remains lower during pregnancy than postpartum. Unfortunately, the external work performed at maximal oxygen consumption was not reported in this investigation, which limits interpretation of the findings.

Differences in exercise efficiency (oxygen uptake during fixed external work loads) have been reported during pregnancy. One report[18] found increased efficiency walking on a treadmill among women who maintained an exercise program during pregnancy. In contrast, others found consistently higher oxygen consumption at fixed work on a cycle ergometer late in the second trimester.[19] This latter finding is consistent with previous studies showing greater oxygen consumption at rest and during exercise in all trimesters of pregnancy.[20-22] Whether these discrepancies reflect differences between treadmill and cycle exercise, subject characteristics, or methodology is uncertain.

Carpenter and colleagues[23] investigated the impact of maternal weight gain during pregnancy for both sitting (cycle) and walking (treadmill) exercise, and found that oxygen consumption was greater during late pregnancy at rest and for both types of exercise, but the difference was larger for treadmill exercise. The women were reevaluated postpartum, and weight equalized to that of pregnancy. Studied in that way, 75% of the increased oxygen consumption during treadmill exercise in the third trimester of pregnancy could be accounted for by weight gain alone. Future studies will need to address subjects' fitness level, trimester of pregnancy, and type of exercise for a complete assessment of the effect of pregnancy on maximal work capacity.

During Late Gestation

In the third trimester, several factors combine to alter hemodynamics both at rest and during exercise. Uterine blood flow increases to approximately 1 L/min at end gestation.[24] This is accomplished by redistribution of blood away from nonreproductive tissues, rather than by further elevation of cardiac output. This process is associated with increased vascular resistance in nonreproductive tissues, so that the previously reduced systemic vascular resistance approaches nonpregnant values at term.[2] Arteriovenous oxygen difference widens as the extra cardiac output of early pregnancy now supplies the fetus.[2] The enlarging uterus increasingly impedes venous return from the lower extremities.[25] Coupled with the increase in venous capacitance and compliance, this may result in impaired venous return to the heart.

Only a few studies have assessed cardiac output during exercise in late gestation. These suggest that cardiac output during upright cycle exercise may be less in the third trimester than in the second trimester, primarily due to reduced stroke volume.[5] Women at 34 and 37 weeks' gestation showed greater cardiac output during exercise in late gestation than during postpartum exercise, but stroke volume either was not different or was moderately increased.[23,26] Stroke volume is labile at the initiation of cycle exercise in late gestation.[27] We interpret these data to suggest that venous return is easily compromised during late pregnancy, with resulting decreased stroke volume and limitation of cardiac output. Other factors that influence venous return during exercise, such as cutaneous vasodilation and sweating in response to increased temperature, might be expected to reduce venous return further during either prolonged exertion or exercise at higher temperatures.[28]

Response to Exercise Training

A fundamental question regarding pregnancy is whether or not the cardiovascular system can respond in the usual manner to regular exercise while already in a hyperkinetic state. This question can be approached in two ways: (1) train women during pregnancy to determine whether a typical response occurs; and (2) determine the women's response to cessation of regular exercise and observe whether conditioning effects are lost.

A training effect during pregnancy appears possible. In studies with adequate activity, regular exercise produces a typical response to training, such as a lower heart rate for a given oxygen consumption.[29,30] Conversely, a carefully performed study[31] with only two exercise sessions per week for 9 weeks, at an exercise heart rate in excess of 140 bpm, failed to alter any cardiopulmonary parameters. The latter finding suggests that it may be more difficult to improve fitness during pregnancy.

Training effects during late gestation may be difficult to demonstrate. Of 23 volunteers, 10 women were prospectively identified as fit, having performed aerobic exercise for at least 45 minutes three times a week for 2 years prior to becoming pregnant. The remainder of the volunteers were considered nonfit controls. The fit women continued to perform substantial exercise during gestation, exercising outside of structured classes 6.1 ± 3.2 hours per week before, 4.5 ± 2.2 hours per week during, and 5.2 ± 2.5 hours per week after pregnancy. The heart rate and stroke volume during upright cycle exercise were not different between fit and nonfit women at 34 to 38 weeks' gestation.[27] However, the fit women had lower resting and exercise heart rates with higher stroke volumes than the nonfit women 3 months postpartum. Thus, determination of fitness levels may be blunted by restriction of venous return during late gestation.

The effects of discontinuing regular exercise during pregnancy have not been well-examined. Clapp[18] measured the oxygen requirement of 18 recreational athletes at each work load of graded treadmill exercise. The nine women who stopped their exercise regimen while pregnant had lower cardiorespiratory efficiency than did the nine who continued regular physical activity. The respective heart rates and oxygen consumptions at fixed work loads were not reported, however. Another study found that women who stopped exercise had greater weight gain and larger babies than did women who continued endurance exercise, but these parameters were not different from those of women who had never exercised.[32]

In summary, several studies have shown that some parameters of fitness can be achieved during pregnancy. Although deconditioning likely occurs when exercise is discontinued while pregnant, supporting evidence, especially in late gestation, is incomplete.

Fetal Response to Maternal Exercise

UTERINE BLOOD FLOW

A continuous, adequate supply of oxygen and nutrients is critical for normal fetal development. It could be detrimental to the fetus if, during exercise, blood is shunted away from the uterus to working muscles. However, only one study[33] has addressed this question. Morris and colleagues injected a diffusible ion (^{24}Na) into the uterine wall and used the time for the disappearance of counts as an index of uterine blood flow. During mild, short-term cycle exercise between 32 and 40 weeks' gestation, clearance time increased 25%. The women in this investigation exercised supine, however, so that the fall in uterine blood flow may have reflected a decrease in cardiac output due to vena cava compression rather than an alteration in uterine blood flow by exercise.

Because experiments in women are limited, data from animal models have been used to make inferences about exercise's effects. Two early studies,[34,35] using ewes walking on a treadmill, concluded that exercise resulted in no change in uterine blood flow. However, only postexertional values were assessed, and neither investigator measured uterine blood flow during exercise. Subsequently, uterine blood flow has been measured in ewes just prior to discontinuing treadmill walking.[36] A 28% decrease in uterine blood flow was found during exhaustive exercise, but no change occurred at submaximal levels. Other animal studies have consistently demonstrated decreased uterine blood flow during exercise, with the change proportional to the level of exertion. Moderate-exertion walking on a treadmill produced approximately 35% decreases of uterine blood flow in ewes[37,38] and 32% decrease among Pygmy goats.[39] Another group of investigators[40] also found a 13% to 24% decrease in uterine blood flow in ewes, which correlated with the level and duration of treadmill exercise.

Blood flow to the uterus includes both myoendometrial and placental perfusion, and exercise may alter the total blood flow or differentially affect these two components. Studies in ewes and Pygmy goats at submaximal exertion have demonstrated that, while myoendometrial blood flow decreases markedly, placental perfusion, as measured by the radioactive microsphere technique, remains the same,[38] increases,[35] or decreases only slightly.[39] Thus, although uterine blood flow appears to participate in the generalized splanchnic vasoconstriction characteristic of exercise, redistribution within the uterus seems to preserve fetal blood supply. Among men, physical training results in a smaller decrease in splanchnic blood flow in response to a given work load.[41] It might be extrapolated that a smaller decrease in uterine blood flow in trained pregnant women might occur, although this has not been tested. In one study using rats,[42] uterine blood flow during exercise of trained and untrained animals did not differ.

In addition to redistribution of uterine blood flow, other mechanisms may help maintain fetal oxygenation during exertion. Nonpregnant individuals have increased hematocrits within 10 minutes of the onset of exercise.[43] Chandler and Bell[37] found a similar increase in hematocrit when pregnant ewes underwent 60 minutes of treadmill walking at a moderate level of exertion. This response increased the oxygen-carrying capacity of the blood per unit volume. Also, during moderate to maximal exercise in ewes, oxygen extraction by the uterus[37,40] and fetus[36] increases.

FETAL OXYGENATION

The critical question is whether a decrease in uterine blood flow during exercise results in a physiologically significant reduction in fetal oxygenation. Animal evidence has shown a significant decrease in fetal PO_2 during maternal exercise in ewes,[44] but other investigators observed a significant fall in fetal PO_2 only when ewes were exercised to exhaustion.[36] Similar decreases in fetal PO_2 levels were found when ewes underwent moderate, but not mild, exercise.[37] However, all of these studies have been criticized, because blood gas results were not corrected for the increases in maternal and fetal body temperatures that occur during exercise.[45] When such corrections were made, a significant decrease in fetal PO_2 was found only when ewes were run to exhaustion.[45] In these animal studies, no change in fetal base excess[36] or pH[45] was observed during exertion, further suggesting that oxygen supplies are adequate for ovine fetal metabolic demands during maternal exercise.

FETAL HEART RATE MONITORING

Continuous electronic fetal heart rate (FHR) monitoring is a widely used method to assess fetal well-being. A healthy fetus is suggested if (1) FHR is within the normal range (120 to 160 bpm), (2) the pattern is "reactive" (an increase of 15 bpm above the baseline heart rate, lasting for 15 seconds on two occasions within 20 minutes), and (3) there are no decelerations (decreases of the FHR of at least 15 bpm that return to the original baseline).[46] Abnormalities in FHR—tachycardias, bradycardias, and decelerations—can indicate fetal hypoxia.

In an attempt to detect adverse effects from maternal exercise, a number of studies have monitored FHR prior to and just after exercise.[29,47-52] These studies totaled 106 women (range, 6 to 45 per study) undertaking varying forms of exercise, which differed in intensity and duration. All investigators found statistically significant increases in FHR, but the heart rates of only a few fetuses were in the abnormal range. Although one study reported that 9 of 15 post-exercise tracings in the third trimester showed an FHR greater than 180 bpm,[47] these fetuses were monitored immediately after their mothers jogged 1.5 miles and ran up three flights of stairs. There are no data as to whether these statistically significant increases in FHR indicate hypoxia in the fetus.

Because of technical difficulties, there have been few attempts to record FHR patterns during exercise. Although fetal bradycardias have been noted with physical activity,[50,53,54] these findings can be artifacts generated by movement of the transducer while women exercise.[55,56]

Ultrasonography may provide a more reliable index of FHR during exercise. Forty-five pregnant women were studied using two-dimensional ultrasonography to record fetal cardiac activity during and after 79 maternal exercise sessions.[57] In each session, women exercised at submaximal and maximal exertion. During the submaximal exercise period, the oxygen consumption was approximately two thirds of their measured maximal aerobic power. To achieve maximal exercise, resistance was increased every 2 minutes until subjects were unable to exercise further. Only one episode of fetal bradycardia occurred during either submaximal or maximal exertion, and that single event was associated with prolonged maternal vasovagal hypotension. After discontinuance of maximal maternal exertion, 15 episodes of fetal bradycardia were noted. All fetuses had reactive non-stress tests within 30 minutes of exercise conclusion and all infants were normal at birth. Similarly, in another study, six episodes of transient fetal bradycardia occurred after 45 sessions of maximal maternal aerobic exercise.[58]

Other indices of fetal status have not shown changes during maternal exercise. When women perform treadmill walking, stationary cycling, or swimming at submaximal levels, the mean Doppler flow velocities in the fetal descending aorta,[60] systolic-to-diastolic ratio obtained with Doppler in the umbilical cord,[60] uterine artery systolic-to-diastolic ratio,[58] percentage of time spent in fetal breathing, and number of fetal movements[61] have all been similar before and after exertion.

Thus, as assessed by several different methods, no reliable indication of fetal compromise has been found during mild to moderate maternal exercise. However, as evidenced by fetal bradycardia, exhaustive or maximal exercise could result in detrimental fetal effects.[61]

HYPERTHERMIA

The developing fetus may be adversely affected by elevated maternal body temperatures. Hyperthermia has been shown to cause congenital malformations in laboratory rodents,[62,63] and retrospective human studies have associated first-trimester maternal temperatures of 38.9°C or greater with anomalies similar to those in animal studies (microcephaly, mental retardation, microphthalmia, anencephaly, hypotonia, and arthrogryposis).[64-66] It is possible, however, that the underlying disorder that caused the fever or the treatment given may have resulted in the fetal abnormality. In addition, none of the infants born to 78 women followed prospectively after a fever of at least 38.9°C in the first trimester were found to be affected.[67] Nevertheless, heat as the teratogen is suggested by case reports of similar anomalies associated with single episodes of hyperthermia from a sauna bath.[64,65] The risk to the human fetus of teratogenesis from hyperthermia is unknown, but is probably quite low.

For humans, the temperature response varies with work intensity, duration, and ambient conditions.[28,68] The amount of exercise necessary to produce an increased teratogenic effect (temperature elevation of more than 1.5°C) is approximately 43% to 86% of maximal oxygen consumption.

We have observed three women at 35 to 37 weeks' gestation as they performed 70 to 80 watts of cycle erogmetry at an environmental temperature of 20° to 22°C.[69] Their heart rates at the end of 20 minutes of pedaling averaged 78% (range, 63% to 91%) of their predicted maximal heart rate, and their rectal temperatures rose an average of 0.4°C (range, 0.2° to 0.5°) above resting levels. Fourteen weeks' postpartum, they performed the same exercise load at a similar ambient temperature. Their heart rates averaged 79% (range, 56% to

99%) of calculated maximal heart rate, and rectal temperatures increased by 0.3°C.

Our findings agree with those of Jones and colleagues,[70,71] who recorded the thermal response to treadmill exercise at 70% to 75% of both calculated maximum oxygen consumption and maximal heart rate, with controlled climate (wet bulb < 23.8°C). Four aerobically conditioned women were studied in each trimester of pregnancy and again postpartum. Core temperatures at the end of 25 minutes of exercise increased 0.6° to 1.0°C above resting levels and did not exceed 39°C. Mean core temperature responses were unchanged among trimesters and between pregnancy and postpartum. In addition, a preliminary report revealed that thermal response to exercise declined as pregnancy progressed in 15 athletic women.[72] Prior to pregnancy, the increment in rectal temperature with 20 minutes of exercise at 62% maximum preconceptional intensity was 0.6°C; at 37 weeks' gestation it was only 0.2°C greater than resting values.

Thus, consistent findings indicate that the temperature response to exercise is not greater during pregnancy, and may even be less than in the nonpregnant state. Moderate levels of exercise at usual environmental temperatures do not result in potentially dangerous increases in core body temperatures. Although there are no reports of fetal damage secondary to hyperthermia among exercising women, it seems prudent to avoid prolonged and intense exercise in warm and humid environments.[73]

FETAL GROWTH AND MISCARRIAGE

Animal studies have been used to assess the effects of maternal exercise on fetal growth. These investigations have produced conflicting results regarding the incidence of growth retardation and fetal mortality. Fetal weight was lower in pregnant guinea pigs who ran on a treadmill 60 minutes per day, but not if exercise sessions were 45 minutes or less.[74] Mice forced to run 30 minutes per day showed an increase in the number of dead and resorbed fetuses and a decrease in fetal weight,[75] and significant growth retardation was found in fetuses of rats made to swim 40 minutes per day.[76] Other investigators found no difference in fetal weights between rats run 15 minutes per day on a treadmill and nonrunning controls.[77] Growth retardation was reported to occur in Pygmy goat fetuses in multiple gestation (but not singletons) when their mothers exercised on a treadmill.[78] However, when the experiment with Pygmy goats was repeated in the same laboratory, using positive reinforcement to induce the animals to exercise, rather than aversive stimuli, there was no reduction in birth weight.[39] The authors speculated that the stress of the aversive stimuli rather than the exercise itself may have been responsible for the outcomes. Thus, the stimulus for exercise may be as important in influencing fetal growth as its intensity and duration. Extrapolating these findings to humans is difficult, because the species, exercise stimulus, and amount of exertion all may affect outcomes.

There also are several problems in assessing exercise and human pregnancy outcomes. The type and intensity of exercise vary, and thus far no study has accounted for the amount of physical activity in the woman's daily routine. Of women who exercised regularly prior to pregnancy and intended to continue, 60% stopped exercise by 28 weeks' gestation.[32] Thus, those continuing exercise to term may be a biased subset. Only one investigation has randomly assigned women to exercise and control groups.

Sustained vigorous exercise may affect fetal weight. One group of 29 women[32] exercised six or more times per week for an hour or more at an intensity greater than 50% of their maximal heart rate throughout gestation. Of babies born to these mothers, 38% had birth weights less than the 10th percentile for their gestational age, whereas only 11% of babies born to mothers who ceased exercising prior to 28 weeks' gestation had birth weights below the 10th percentile.[32] However, no significant differences were demonstrated in four other studies[29,79-81] that compared women participating in regular, mild-to-moderate exercise throughout pregnancy with nonexercising controls. In a retrospective survey,[82] no association was found between the number of miles run and birth weight of offspring among women who jogged throughout pregnancy. Likewise, no correlation was noted between birth weight and maternal physical fitness as assessed by maximum maternal heart rates achieved during submaximal exercise.[83]

Although it has long been believed that exercise can cause miscarriage, a controlled study[84] found no difference in the spontaneous abortion rate among 47 fit runners, 40 aerobic dancers, and 28 control subjects.

PRETERM LABOR AND DELIVERY

Concern has been expressed that maternal exertion may precipitate preterm labor. One investigation found a 21% incidence of preterm births (delivery at less than 37 completed weeks of pregnancy) among 29 women who exercised strenuously throughout pregnancy, compared with 9% in a group who stopped exercising prior to 28 weeks' gestation.[32] However, there was no difference in preterm births among women who participated in a moderate exercise program three times per week, compared with nonexercising controls.[29] Others found no association between the infant's gestational age at birth and the mother's weekly mileage among a group of women who ran throughout pregnancy.[82] When maternal physical fitness (as assessed by maximum heart rate achieved during submaximal cycling) was compared to gestational age of the baby at birth, no correlation was observed.[83] Finally, preterm labor may be reduced with exercise. A retrospective case-control study involving 175 women who delivered preterm and 313 women who delivered at term found an odds ratio of 0.53, or approximately half the risk (95% confidence interval, 0.36–0.78) for preterm labor in women who exercised.[85]

Attempts to define potential mechanisms of preterm labor associated with exercise have been unsuccessful. Although one group of investigators[51] noted an increase in contractions during and after mild-to-moderate treadmill exercise, others[52] found no increase in uterine activity in the ½ hour following 25 to 30 minutes of mild to moderate exertion. Likewise, no change in uterine contractions was detected in seven women after they ran 1.5 miles.[47]

In summary, unless a woman is at high risk for having a growth-retarded infant or delivering before term (see Table 12–1), there is no evidence that regular, mild-to-moderate exercise during pregnancy is harmful to her or to her baby.

Benefits of Exercise

Women have reported favorable subjective responses to regular exercise while pregnant. In a large study[79] of 845 women, the 452 exercisers reported improved self-image, relief of tension, and fewer aches and pains, especially low back pain. However, there is little objective evidence to support claims for shorter, easier labors, fewer operative deliveries, or better neonatal outcomes for exercising women. Shorter total labors were reported in multiparas who were more physically fit (as assessed by maximum heart rate achieved during a submaximal test), but not in primiparas.[83] This finding is difficult to generalize, as only 10 of 41 women were multiparas. In another study, a statistically insignificant trend for a shorter second stage of labor was found among 17 primigravidas who exercised compared with 20 who did not, and no difference was observed between 21 exercising and 27 nonexercising multiparas.[80] Three other studies[29,79,81] also found no difference in the duration of labor between women who exercised moderately and those who did not.

The reports of operative deliveries parallel those for labor. Although one investigation[79] reported a 7% incidence of cesarean section among 61 women who exercised regularly, compared to 28% in nonexercising controls, three other studies[29,32,80] found no difference in mode of delivery between exercising and nonexercising women. None of these studies commented on the number of primary versus repeat cesarean sections.

Although psychological benefits may be associated with regular exercise during pregnancy, the physical benefits for mother or infant have yet to be established. Women should be reassured that cessation of exercise is not detrimental to them or to their developing babies.

Effects of Work

The effects of recreational exercise, performed voluntarily for limited periods, may differ from the exertion associated with activities of daily living and employment. The literature on the effects of paid employment during pregnancy presents conflicting results and has been comprehensively reviewed.[86]

Employment outside the home has been associated with a decrease in birth weight. In one study, birth weights were significantly lower for children of U.S. women working outside the home after 29 weeks' gestation, and the reduction was greatest for babies born to women whose jobs required standing most of the time.[87] These results remained after controlling for gestational age, race, socioeconomic status, maternal pre-pregnancy weight, total weight gain, and blood pressure. In another investigation,[88] 731 Spanish women who worked during pregnancy were compared with 720 women who had no paid employment. After eliminating women at risk for altered fetal growth and those of low income or who performed "excessive" domestic exertion, birth weight was significantly lower for newborns of working women, particularly those who stood at work. However, birth weights were closer to control birth weights for infants born to women who quit working before the last 6 weeks of pregnancy.

Further association of low birth weight and long hours of standing has been found among obstetric residents. Women obstetricians whose first child was born during residency had significantly lighter babies than did colleagues whose first-borns were delivered before or after residency, and there was a similar trend for multiparas.[89] Similar results were found for active duty personnel when compared to the general obstetric population delivering at a U.S. Air Force hospital.[90] Of infants born to mothers on active duty, 12% weighed less than 2,500 grams, compared with 2% in the general population.

Other investigators have not found low birth weight associated with certain types of work. A prospective study[91] followed 1,507 women who presented for antenatal care to an inner city hospital in London. The authors found no correlation between birth weight at a given gestational age and the mother's physical effort or posture at work. There also was no association between birth weight and the stage of pregnancy at which the mother left work.

Although there have been reports[92,93] of an increase in the incidence of preterm births among working women, others[85,89,94,95] have found no association between employment and delivery before term. In fact, some investigators[96,97] have found better outcomes among working women. However, these women belonged to higher socioeconomic classes, attended prenatal clinics more frequently, and often had the benefit of paid maternity leave.

Because of the many variables that affect a pregnancy's outcome, studies to define the role of employment are difficult to design.[98,99] It appears that working during pregnancy does not have an adverse effect, although women who work until near term and stand all day may be more likely to have lighter babies.[100,101] The significance of this lower weight to the infant's overall well-being is unknown. Given the minimal (often nonexistent) paid maternity leave available to women in the United States and the fact that many are the sole wage earners for their families, recommendations to quit work should be made only if there is a clear risk of intrauterine growth retardation or preterm birth. The evidence to date is that there is no defined adverse outcome.

Exercise Programs During Pregnancy

If a woman is interested in participating in a program of regular exercise during pregnancy, she may ask her primary care or obstetrical provider about suitable activities. The pregnant woman needs to know (1) how to protect herself and her fetus from possible harm; (2) what programs are available, and how to choose among them; (3) how often (frequency), for how long (duration), and with what intensity to train; (4) how to monitor her response to exertion; (5) what to avoid; and (6) signs warning of impending problems. Because of the motivation to have a healthy pregnancy, her interest makes this an ideal time for an assessment of her physical activity habits and recommendation for positive change.

The main determinants of appropriate training during pregnancy are the prepregnant fitness level and considerations about the health of the mother and fetus. Women should be assessed for contraindications to exertion (Table 12–1) before advice regarding exercise is provided. If signs or symptoms develop that would contraindicate continued training, then participation in the exercise program should be halted until these are fully investigated.

Table 12-1 **CONTRAINDICATIONS TO EXERCISE IN PREGNANCY**

Absolute Contraindications	Relative Contraindications
Uterine anomaly and history of preterm fetal loss	Multiple gestation (twins)
Multiple gestation (three or more fetuses)	History of preterm labor of unknown etiology
Preterm premature rupture of membranes	First pregnancy in a woman exposed to
Incompetent cervix with or without cerclage	diethylstilbestrol
Preterm labor	Rh sensitization
Intrauterine growth retardation	Chronic hypertension
Known	Renal transplant
Suspected (until definitive studies done)	Cardiac transplant
Previous growth-retarded infant	Heart disease (New York Heart Association
Prior fetal loss and lupus anticoagulant	class I)
Pre-eclampsia	Respiratory compromise
History of early, severe pre-eclampsia	Asthma
Active systemic lupus erythematosus	Cigarette smoking
Diabetes with vascular disease	Physically strenuous, standing employment
Chronic hypertension with history of	History of back pain
superimposed pre-eclampsia	Obesity
Sickle cell anemia	Third trimester, previously sedentary
Heart disease (New York Heart Association	Unwilling or unable to exercise regularly
Class II-IV)	Acute infectious illness
Pulmonary hypertension	Fever
Marfan's syndrome	Hot, humid environment
Renal disease with hypertension or creatinine	
>0.9 mg/dL, proteinuria (>500 mg/24 hr)	
Severe kyphoscoliosis	
Vaginal bleeding of unknown etiology	
Placenta previa	
Abruptio placentae	

TRAINING INTENSITY, DURATION, AND FREQUENCY

Recommendations for the frequency, duration, and intensity of training are similar to those for nonpregnant individuals[102-104] (see Chapter 1), with a special emphasis on moderation. Heart rate is a simple indicator of exercise intensity, as there is a linear relationship between oxygen consumption and heart rate.[105-107] An exercise target heart rate of 60% to 70% of age-adjusted calculated maximum heart rate (220 bpm minus age) is the commonly used range for the pregnant woman. However, it is not clear that this is an effective calculation during pregnancy. Sixteen women were followed before, every 8 weeks during, and after a clinically normal pregnancy.[108] Heart rate was recorded by electrocardiograph during graded treadmill exercise. At the maximum exercise heart rate (140 bpm) recommended by the American College of Obstetricians and Gynecologists,[102] women exercised at an intensity that ranged from 30% to 77% of maximum oxygen consumption. Percent of maximum oxygen consumption varied both among women and between tests of the same individuals. It was concluded that heart rate alone is a poor indicator of exercise intensity during pregnancy.

The point at which the average person becomes slightly out of breath was found by Astrand and Rodahl[105] to indicate a training threshold of about 50% maximum oxygen uptake.[109] The pregnant woman can learn to estimate exercise intensity by her degree of hyperventilation, moderating exertion so that she can talk during its performance. Among men, the subjective rating of perceived exertion correlates well with percent maximum oxygen consumption, heart rate, and blood lactate concentration during exercise of constant intensity.[110] A study of 16 women showed good correlation at each trimester of pregnancy between their rating of perceived exertion and heart rate attained when performing cycle or treadmill exercise at either of two intensity levels.[111] Perceived exertion also can be used to monitor training intensity.[112] Women who are habituated to regular exercise are often accustomed to regulating the intensity of their training sessions in this way. Whether exercise intensity is regulated on the basis of heart rate, ventilation, or perceived exertion, it should remain moderate during pregnancy, to avoid potentially harmful effects of very strenuous exercise.

Appropriate Activities

Rhythmic activities utilizing large muscle groups are appropriate for cardiovascular conditioning during pregnancy (Table 12–2). Recreational activities that are intermittent or have intensities that are difficult to quantify (e.g., racquet or team sports) are best used as a supplement to physical fitness programs. Unique concerns include the importance of the warm-down phase following exercise, to prevent excessive venous pooling and hypotension. In addition, overly extended sessions may produce hypoglycemia, dehydration, and hyperthermia. Finally, pregnant women's exercise may need to diminish in duration and intensity as term approaches.

> **CASE:** M.G., a 24-year-old woman (gravida 1, para 0), was seen at 16 weeks from her last menstrual period. She was 160 cm (5'4") tall and weighed 56 kg (125 lb). Physical examination revealed no abnormalities, and her medical history was unremarkable. Uterine size was consistent with her dates, and fetal heart tones were heard. The woman had no

Table 12–2 **CONDITIONING ACTIVITIES**

Suitable in Any Program
Walking
Swimming
Bicycling
Low-impact aerobic dancing or calisthenics
Golf as adjunct to conditioning program
Racquet sports
Suitable for Women Accustomed to the Activity Before Becoming Pregnant
Jogging
Running
Cross-country skiing
For Use with Appropriate Intensity and Duration
Exercise machines that mimic movements of cycling, rowing, stair climbing, cross-country skiing

regular exercise program, but wanted to begin training so she would not get "too fat."

COMMENT: Women may be concerned about the normal weight gain of pregnancy. These patients should receive counseling regarding fetal needs for nutrition and the natural weight changes that occur during pregnancy. This woman's exercise program should begin gradually, and she will need to be followed to be sure it remains moderate and that her weight gain is appropriate.

EXERCISE PROGRAMS

If there are no contraindications to exercise (see Table 12–1), several options are available, including maternal exercise classes, instructions from books or videotapes, an individualized regimen, or some combination of these (Table 12–3). The advantages and disadvantages of different types of training programs are outlined in Table 12–4.

An exercise class designed specifically for pregnant women has advantages. The camaraderie that develops among participants encourages regular attendance. Class structure sets the duration of the conditioning component, while facilitating monitoring of intensity to keep each woman's exercise within the mild-to-moderate range. Women can be instructed in maneuvers to assist overall flexibility and muscle strength, and in how to avoid potentially harmful

Table 12–3 **EXERCISE PROGRAMS FOR PREGNANT WOMEN**

Exercise Classes
Exercise classes for pregnant women
Aquatic exercise classes
Low- or mid-impact aerobics classes (with modification)
Introductory fitness classes (with modification)
Stretching or yoga classes (as adjunct to conditioning program)
The YMCA has a national program of prenatal exercise called "You & Me, Baby." Other community resources include the YMCA, YWCA, and Jewish Community Center; fitness or exercise clubs; city or county community education or parks and recreation departments; hospital obstetric departments; and religious organizations. Check with them for current availability of programs.
Guided Individual Programs
Books
Susan L. Regnier: *Exercises for Baby and Me*. Meadowbrook Press: Deephaven, MN, 1989. Available at YMCA facilities offering the "You & Me, Baby" classes or from Meadowbrook Press (800) 338-2232.
Femmy DeLyser: *Jane Fonda's New Pregnancy Workout and Total Birthing Program*. Simon & Schuster: New York, 1989. Available in bookstores.
Recordings
ACOG: *Pregnancy Exercise Program* [audiocassette]. Feeling Fine Programs: Los Angeles, 1985. Available from Feeling Fine Programs (800) 423-0102.
ACOG: *Pregnancy Exercise Program* [video]. Feeling Fine Programs: Los Angeles, 1985. Available from Feeling Fine Programs (800) 423-0102.
Fox Hills Video: *Kathy Smith's Pregnancy Workout* [video]. Heron Communications: Los Angeles, 1989. Available in bookstores and video stores.
Warner Home Video: *Jane Fonda's Workout: Pregnancy, Birth and Recovery* [video]. Warner Communications: Burbank, CA, 1983. Available in bookstores and video stores.

Table 12–4 **ADVANTAGES AND DISADVANTAGES OF DIFFERENT PREGNANCY EXERCISE PROGRAMS**

Exercise Class
+ Provides supervision
+ May promote regular exercise
− Peer pressure may encourage overexertion

Books and Recordings
+ Can be used anytime
− Modification for individual needs may be difficult
− May include inappropriate exercises (such as those performed supine or twists)
+ Some conform with ACOG guidelines

Individual Program
+ Best for women accustomed to regular exercise
− Requires the most self-discipline and self-monitoring
+ May be used as adjunct to class, books, or tapes

Key: + = advantage; − = disadvantage.

movements. In addition, instructors can assist participants in modifying routines to meet specific individual requirements.

For some women, a program of individual home exercise may be preferred or, depending on facilities, may be the only alternative. Books, audiotapes, and videotapes of exercise routines for pregnant women are available (see Table 12–3), and their worth should be judged in the same way as classes: Is the information sound, understandable, and current? Are any harmful movements or practices taught? Is moderation stressed, with no pressure to keep up with a demonstrator's cadence or a musical beat? Are role models realistic and appropriate in garb and demeanor? Are the routines easily modified to suit an individual's changing needs?

Whatever program is followed, certain exercises should be avoided (Table 12–5). Because of potential joint damage, jumping, bouncing, and twisting movements (e.g., standing diagonal toe touches) should be avoided unless performed in a slow and controlled manner. Exercises to strengthen abdominal

Table 12–5 **EXERCISE ACTIVITIES TO AVOID DURING PREGNANCY**

Avoid Throughout Pregnancy
Jumping, bouncing, twisting
Competitive events
High-altitude sports
Contact sports
Heavy weight-lifting
Scuba diving
Board and platform diving
Exercise in hot, humid conditions
May Become Unsafe as Pregnancy Progresses
Volleyball
Gymnastics
Horseback riding
Water skiing
Alpine skiing
Ice skating
Exercise performed supine

muscles are typically performed supine, and in that position, the uterus and contents can interfere with maternal venous return; this activity should be eliminated as pregnancy progresses. The pelvic tilt offers an improvement on the sit-up, and can be performed at any convenient time while standing or sitting.[102] To avoid fetal risk, we advise women to avoid activities that risk trauma or that involve extremes of temperature or marked alterations in barometric pressure.

CASE: S.Y., a 30-year-old woman (gravida 2, para 1), whose first infant weighed 4,280 grams (9 lb, 10 oz), was recently diagnosed as having gestational diabetes. She had not previously performed regular exercise, was employed at home, and at the time of the examination was at 22 weeks' gestation. Her weight was 91 kg (203 lb), and her height 155 cm (5'2"). She was placed on a diabetic diet and required 12 units of intermediate-acting insulin every morning and 8 units at bedtime to keep fasting and preprandial blood glucose values less than 100 mg/dL.

COMMENT: Because of concerns about adverse fetal effects, exercise for pregnant diabetic women usually has been discouraged, but as discussed in Chapter 8, exercise can improve insulin sensitivity. Physical activity has been recognized as adjunctive therapy for gestational diabetes.[113] Prior to recommending exercise, however, the clinician should evaluate the woman for any contraindication, and the activity should be appropriate for her prepregnancy fitness level. An exercise class for pregnant women can be especially helpful, allowing close supervision of exercise as well as a chance for socializing with other pregnant women. If classes are unavailable, walking (provided she were interested in it) would be an appropriate, easily regulated training mode. The patient and her pregnancy should be followed closely by her obstetrician and primary care provider.

Exercise also has been studied for pregnant women with type I (insulin-dependent) diabetes. A prospective, randomized trial of moderate exercise for diabetic women was conducted.[114] Thirteen women who walked 20 minutes after each meal were compared with 21 control women randomized to no exercise. There was a trend for better glucose control and lower infant birth weights in the exercise group, but differences were not statistically significant. Importantly, there were no adverse outcomes in the exercise group.

GUIDELINES FOR WOMEN WHO EXERCISE REGULARLY

Although most women can continue moderate exercise during pregnancy, extremely active women may present additional concerns. Conservative recommendations[102,103] may prove frustrating to the athlete or more highly trained woman. During pregnancy, the intensity and duration of training should be reduced to avoid potential deleterious effects on uterine blood flow. The maintenance of prepregnancy fitness, rather than a significant increase in performance, is an appropriate goal. Highly trained nonpregnant individuals were able to maintain training-induced gains in maximal oxygen consumption with a duration and frequency of exercise reduced by as much as two thirds,[115,116] and intensity by almost one third,[117] but this has not been tested in pregnant women.

CASE: G.J. is a 30-year-old woman who exercised by swimming 1 mile 2 to 3 times a week. She had a positive serum pregnancy test 4½ weeks after her last menstrual period. This is her first pregnancy, and she has no medical problems.

COMMENT: G.J. can be encouraged to continue regular exercise and should be advised that she may feel the need to diminish the intensity or duration of the workouts as pregnancy progresses. She should be reassured that there is no harm in continuing her exercise, nor would she cause problems by stopping exercise for the remainder of the pregnancy.

CASE: D.L., a 28-year-old competitive distance runner (gravida 1, para 0), developed spotting at 12 weeks' gestation. A viable fetus was demonstrated by ultrasonography.

COMMENT: This woman should discontinue exercise. Although there is no well-documented evidence that exercise increases the rate of spontaneous pregnancy loss, it is a common belief. Whatever the outcome, cessation of exercise will allow her to feel that she is doing what is best for her fetus. If it is determined by her physician that she may resume physical activity (for example, no further bleeding and a normal fetus after 4 to 6 weeks), she should do so gradually and perhaps aim for a reduced intensity. Replacing some of her running with low-impact training (e.g., walking or swimming) would be appropriate.

CASE: J.B., a 30-year-old woman (gravida 4, para 3) with three children at home, worked in a power plant, moving 50-pound drums and climbing scaffolding. Her past medical history was unremarkable, and her prior pregnancies were uncomplicated. Uterine examination was consistent with dates.

COMMENT: Rather than adding recreational exercise, it is appropriate to reduce her risk of work injury. Important questions include: (1) Are alternative duties available to her without loss of job security? (2) Does she expect to receive maternity leave? (3) Can she return postpartum to the same job level? and (4) Does she wish to do so? If the answers to these questions are no, she might want to consider leaving that particular job late in the second trimester or early in the third.

Summary

An exercise prescription for the pregnant woman will be one that is individualized and specific to her situation. The formulation of a physical activity regimen considers the woman's risk status, evaluates her previous and recent exercise habits, and includes monitoring of her exertion and the pregnancy's status. Heart rate, the usual marker of exercise intensity, may be unreliable, and perceived exertion should be used instead. In addition, women should be encouraged to participate in their care by assessing their responses to training. The resulting dialogues during regular prenatal visits will offer an opportunity for health care providers to influence habits and attitudes relating to health and fitness at a time in a woman's life when she may be most receptive to such advice.

REFERENCES

1. Hytten FE: Weight gain in pregnancy. In Hytten FE, Chamberlain G, eds: *Clinical Physiology in Obstetrics.* Blackwell Scientific Publications: Oxford, England, 1980, pp 208–209.
2. Bader RA, et al.: Hemodynamics at rest and during exercise in normal pregnancy as studied by cardiac catheterization. *J Clin Invest* 1955; 34:1524–1536.
3. Roy SB, et al.: Circulatory effects of pregnancy. *Am J Obstet Gynecol* 1966; 96:221–225.
4. Walters WAW, MacGregor WG, Hills M: Cardiac output at rest during pregnancy and the puerperium. *Clin Sci* 1966; 30:1–11.
5. Ueland K, et al.: Maternal cardiovascular dynamics, IV: The influence of gestational age on the maternal cardiovascular response to posture and exercise. *Am J Obstet Gynecol* 1969; 104:856–864.
6. Atkins AFJ, et al: A longitudinal study of cardiovascular dynamic changes throughout pregnancy. *Eur J Obstet Gynecol Reprod Biol* 1981; 12:215–224.
7. Robson SC, et al.: Serial study of factors influencing changes in cardiac output during human pregnancy. *Am J Physiol* 1989; 256:H1060–H1065.
8. Katz R, Karliner JS, Resnick R: Effects of a natural volume overload state (pregnancy) on left ventricular performance in normal human subjects. *Circulation* 1978; 58:434–441.
9. Laird-Meeter K, et al.: Cardiocirculatory adjustments during pregnancy: An echocardiographic study. *Clin Cardiol* 1979; 2:328–332.
10. Rubler S, Damani PM, Pinto ER: Cardiac size and performance during pregnancy estimated with echocardiography. *Am J Cardiol* 1977; 40:534–540.
11. Hytten FE, Paintin GB: Increase in plasma volume during normal pregnancy. *J Obstet Gynaecol Br Commonw* 1963; 70:402–407.
12. MacGillivray I, Rose GA, Rowe B: Blood pressure survey in pregnancy. *Clin Sci* 1969; 37:395–407.
13. Davis LE, et al.: Vascular pressure–volume relationships in pregnant and estrogen-treated guinea pigs. *Am J Physiol* 1989; 257:R1205–R1211.
14. Hytten FE, Leitch I: *The Physiology of Human Pregnancy,* ed 2. Blackwell Scientific Publications: Oxford, England, 1971; pp 92–100.
15. Hart MV, Morton MJ, Hosenpud KD: Aortic function during normal human pregnancy. *Am J Obstet Gynecol* 1986; 154:887–891.
16. Artal R, et al.: Pulmonary responses to exercise in pregnancy. In Artal R, Wiswell RA, eds: *Exercise in Pregnancy.* Williams & Wilkins: Baltimore, 1986, pp 147–154.
17. Sady SP, et al.: Cardiovascular response to cycle exercise during and after pregnancy. *J Appl Physiol* 1989; 66:336–341.
18. Clapp JF III: Oxygen consumption during treadmill exercise before, during, and after pregnancy. *Am J Obstet Gynecol* 1989; 161:1458–1564.
19. Sady MA, et al.: Cardiovascular response to maximal cycle exercise during pregnancy and at two and seven months postpartum. *Am J Obstet Gynecol* 1990; 162:1181–1185.
20. Knuttgen HG, Emerson K: Physiological response to pregnancy at rest and during exercise. *J Appl Physiol* 1974; 36:549–553.
21. Pernoll ML, et al.: Oxygen consumption at rest and during exercise in pregnancy. *Respir Physiol* 1975; 25:285–293.
22. Hutchinson PL, Cureton KJ, Sparling PB: Metabolic and circulatory responses to running during pregnancy. *Phys Sportsmed* 1981; 9:55–61.
23. Carpenter MW, et al.: Effect of maternal weight gain during pregnancy on exercise performance. *J Appl Physiol* 1990; 68:1173–1176.
24. Lunell NE, et al.: Uteroplacental blood flow in pre-eclampsia measurements with indium-113m and a computer-linked gamma camera. *Clin Exp Hypertens* 1982; 1(B):105–117.
25. Kerr MG, Scott DB, Samuel E: Studies of the inferior vena cava in late pregnancy. *BMJ* 1964; 1:532–533.
26. Pivarnick JM, et al.: Cardiac output responses of primigravid women during exercise determined by the direct Fick technique. *Obstet Gynecol* 1990; 75:954–959.
27. Morton MJ, et al.: Exercise dynamics in late gestation: Effects of physical training. *Am J Obstet Gynecol* 1985; 152:91–97.
28. Rowell LB: Human cardiovascular adjustments to exercise and thermal stress. *Physiol Rev* 1974; 54:75–159.
29. Collings CA, Curet LB, Mullin JP: Maternal and fetal responses to a maternal aerobic exercise program. *Am J Obstet Gynecol* 1983; 145:702–707.
30. Erkkola R: The influence of physical training during pregnancy on physical work capacity and circulatory parameters. *Scand J Clin Lab Invest* 1976; 35:747–754.
31. Ihrman K: A clinical and physiological study of pregnancy in a material from northern Sweden, VIII: The effect of physical training during pregnancy on the circulatory adjustment. *Acta Soc Med Upsal* 1960; 65:335–347.
32. Clapp JF III, Dickstein S: Endurance exercise and pregnancy outcome. *Med Sci Sports Exer* 1984; 16:556–562.
33. Morris N, et al.: Effective uterine blood flow during exercise in normal and pre-eclamptic pregnancies. *Lancet* 1956; 2:481–484.
34. Orr J, et al.: Effect of exercise stress on carotid, uterine, and iliac blood flow in pregnant and nonpregnant ewes. *Am J Obstet Gynecol* 1972; 114:213–217.

35. Curet LB, et al.: Effect of exercise on cardiac output and distribution of uterine blood flow in pregnant ewes. *J Appl Physiol* 1976; 40:725–728.
36. Clapp JF III: Acute exercise stress in the pregnant ewe. *Am J Obstet Gynecol* 1980; 136:489–499.
37. Chandler KD, Bell AW: Effects of maternal exercise on fetal and maternal respiration and nutrient metabolism in the pregnant ewe. *J Develop Physiol* 1981; 3:161–178.
38. Bell AW, et al.: Effects of exercise and heat stress on regional blood flow in pregnant sheep. *J Appl Physiol* 1986; 60:1759–1764.
39. Hohimer AR, et al.: Effect of exercise on uterine blood flow in the pregnant pygmy goat. *Am J Physiol* 1984; 246:H207–H212.
40. Lotgering FK, Gilbert RD, Longo LD: Exercise responses in pregnant sheep: Oxygen consumption, uterine blood flow, and blood volume. *J Appl Physiol* 1983; 55: 834–841.
41. Clausen JP, Trap-Jensen J: Effects of training on the distribution of cardiac output in patients with coronary artery disease. *Circulation* 1970; 42:611–624.
42. Jones MT, et al.: Effects of training on reproductive tissue blood flow in exercising pregnant rats. *J Appl Physiol* 1990; 69: 2097–2103.
43. Greenleaf JE, et al.: Plasma [Na⁺], [Ca²⁺], and volume shifts and thermoregulation during exercise in man. *J Appl Physiol* 1977; 43:1026–1032.
44. Emmanouilides GC, et al.: Fetal responses to maternal exercise in the sheep. *Am J Obstet Gynecol* 1972; 112:130–137.
45. Lotgering FK, Gilbert RD, Longo LD: Exercise responses in pregnant sheep: Blood gases, temperatures, and fetal cardiovascular system. *J Appl Physiol* 1983; 55: 842–850.
46. Freeman RK, Gorite TJ: Antepartum fetal monitoring. In *Fetal Heart Rate Monitoring.* Williams & Wilkins: Baltimore, 1981, pp 113–129.
47. Hauth JC, Gilstrap LC, Widmer K: Fetal heart rate reactivity before and after maternal jogging during the third trimester. *Am J Obstet Gynecol* 1982; 142: 545–547.
48. Collings C, Curet LB. Fetal heart rate response to maternal exercise. *Am J Obstet Gynecol* 1985; 151:498–501.
49. Clapp JF III: Fetal heart rate response to running in midpregnancy and late pregnancy. *Am J Obstet Gynecol* 1985; 153: 251–252.
50. Artal R, et al.: Fetal heart rate responses to maternal exercise. *Am J Obstet Gynecol* 1986; 155:729–733.
51. Cooper KA, et al.: Fetal heart rate and maternal cardiovascular and catecholamine responses to dynamic exercise. *Aust NZ J Obstet Gynaecol* 1987; 27:220–223.
52. Veille J-C, et al.: The effect of exercise on uterine activity in the last eight weeks of

pregnancy. *Am J Obstet Gynecol* 1985; 151:727–730.
53. Artal R, et al.: Fetal bradycardia induced by maternal exercise. *Lancet* 1984; 2: 258–260.
54. Jovanovic L, Kessler A, Peterson CM: Human maternal and fetal responses to graded exercise. *J Appl Physiol* 1985; 58:1719–1722.
55. Paolone AM, et al.: Fetal heart rate measurement during maternal exercise: Avoidance of artifact. *Med Sci Sports Exerc* 1987; 19:605–609.
56. O'Neill ME, et al.: "Pseudo" fetal bradycardia during maternal exercise (letter). *J Appl Physiol* 1987; 62:849–850.
57. Carpenter MS, et al.: Fetal heart rate response to maternal exertion. *JAMA* 1988; 259:3006–3009.
58. Watson WJ, et al.: Fetal responses to maximal swimming and cycling exercise during pregnancy. *Obstet Gynecol* 1991; 77: 382–386.
59. Pijpers L, Wladimiroff JW, McGhie J: Effect of short-term maternal exercise on maternal and fetal cardiovascular dynamics. *Br J Obstet Gynaecol* 1984; 91:1081–1086.
60. Hume RF, et al.: Fetal umbilical artery Doppler flow response to graded maternal aerobic exercise. Presented at the Ninth Annual Meeting of the Society of Perinatal Obstetricians, 1989.
61. Platt LD, et al.: Exercise in pregnancy, II: Fetal responses. *Am J Obstet Gynecol* 1983; 147:487–491.
62. Kilham L, Ferm VH: Exencephaly in fetal hamsters following exposure to hyperthermia. *Teratology* 1978; 14:323–326.
63. Edwards MJ: Congenital defects in guinea pigs: Fetal resorptions, abortions, and malformations following induced hyperthermia during early gestation. *Teratology* 1969; 2:313–328.
64. Smith DW, Clarren SK, Harvey MAS: Hyperthermia as a possible teratogenic agent. *J Pediatr* 1978; 92:878–883.
65. Miller P, Smith DW, Shepard T: Maternal hyperthermia as a possible cause of anencephaly. *Lancet* 1978; 1:519–520.
66. Fraser FC, Skelton J: Possible teratogenicity of maternal fever (letter). *Lancet* 1978; 2:634.
67. Clarren SK, et al.: Hyperthermia: A prospective evaluation of a possible teratogenic agent in man. *J Pediatr* 1979; 95: 81–83.
68. Rowell LB, Blackmon JR, Bruce RA: Indocyanine green clearance and estimated hepatic blood flow during mild to maximal exercise in upright man. *J Clin Invest* 1964; 43:1677–1690.
69. Morton MJ, Paul MS, unpublished data.
70. Jones RL, Botti JJ, Anderson WM: Thermoregulation in moderately exercising, aerobically conditioned women. Presented at the Fourth Annual Meeting of the Society of Perinatal Obstetricians, 1984.

71. Jones RL, et al.: Thermoregulation during aerobic exercise in pregnancy. *Obstet Gynecol* 1985; 65:340–345.
72. Clapp JF, Kelm L, Philbin C: Thermal responses to rest and endurance exercise during pregnancy. Presented at the 37th Annual Meeting of the Society for Gynecological Investigation, 1990.
73. McMurray RG, Katz VL: Thermoregulation in pregnancy: Implications for exercise. *Sports Med* 1990; 10:146–158.
74. Nelson PS, Gilbert RD, Longo LD: Fetal growth and placental diffusing capacity in guinea pigs following long-term maternal exercise. *J Devel Physiol* 1983; 5:1–10.
75. Terada M: Effect of physical activity before pregnancy on fetuses of mice exercised forcibly during pregnancy. *Teratology* 1974; 10:141–144.
76. Levitsky LL, et al.: Metabolic response to fasting in experimental intrauterine growth retardation induced by surgical and nonsurgical maternal stress. *Biol Neonate* 1977; 31:311–315.
77. Blake CA, Hazelwood RL: Effect of pregnancy and exercise on actomyosin, nucleic acid and gycogen content of the rat heart. *Proc Soc Exper Biol Med* 1971; 136:632–636.
78. Dhindsa DS, Metcalfe J, Hummels DH: Responses to exercise in the pregnant Pygmy goat. *Respir Physiol* 1978; 32:299–311.
79. Hall DC, Kaufmann DA: Effects of aerobic and strength conditioning on pregnancy outcomes. *Am J Obstet Gynecol* 1987; 157:1199–1203.
80. Kulpa PJ, White BM, Visscher R: Aerobic exercise in pregnancy. *Am J Obstet Gynecol* 1987; 156:1395–1403.
81. Fort PL, Fort IL: The relationship of maternal exercise on labor, delivery and health of the newborn. *J Sports Med Phys Fitness* 1991; 31:95–99.
82. Jarrett JC, Spellacy WN: Jogging during pregnancy: An improved outcome? *Obstet Gynecol* 1983; 61:705–709.
83. Pomerance JJ, Gluck L, Lynch VA: Physical fitness in pregnancy: Its effect on pregnancy outcome. *Am J Obstet Gynecol* 1974; 119:867–876.
84. Clapp JF III: The effects of maternal exercise on early pregnancy outcome. *Am J Obstet Gynecol* 1989; 161:1453–1457.
85. Berkowitz G, et al.: Physical activity and the risk of spontaneous preterm delivery. *J Reprod Med* 1983; 28:581–588.
86. Saurel-Cubizolles MJ, Kaminski M: Work in pregnancy: Its evolving relationship with perinatal outcomes. *Soc Sci Med* 1988; 22:431–442.
87. Naeye RL, Peters EC: Working during pregnancy: Effects on the fetus. *Pediatrics* 1982; 69:724–727.
88. Alegre A, et al.: Influence of work during pregnancy on fetal weight. *J Reprod Med* 1984; 29:334–336.
89. Grunebaum A, Minkoff A, Blake D: Pregnancy among obstetricians: A comparison of births before, after, and during residency. *Am J Obstet Gynecol* 1987; 157:79–83.
90. Fox ME, Harris RE, Brekken AL: The active-duty military pregnancy: A new high-risk category. *Am J Obstet Gynecol* 1977; 129:705–707.
91. Rabkin CS, et al.: Maternal activity and birth weight: A prospective, population-based study. *Am J Epidemiol* 1990; 131:522–531.
92. Saurel-Cubizolles MJ, et al.: Pregnancy and its outcome among hospital personnel according to occupation and working conditions. *J Epidemiol Community Health* 1985; 39:129–134.
93. Mamelle N, Laumon B, Lazar P: Prematurity and occupational activity during pregnancy. *Am J Epidemiol* 1984; 119:309–320.
94. Meyer BA, Daling J: Activity level of mother's usual occupation and low infant birth weight. *J Occup Med* 1985; 27:841–847.
95. Klebanoff MA, Shiono PH, Carey JC: The effect of physical activity during pregnancy on preterm delivery and birth weight. *Am J Obstet Gynecol* 1990; 163:1450–1456.
96. Murphy JF, et al.: Employment in pregnancy: Prevalence, maternal characteristics, perinatal outcome. *Lancet* 1984; 1:1163.
97. Saurel MJ, Kaminski M: Pregnant women at work (letter). *Lancet* 1983; 1:475.
98. Selevan SG: Design considerations in pregnancy outcome studies of occupational populations. *Scand J Work Environ Health* 1981; 7(Suppl 4):76–82.
99. Joffe M: Biases in research on reproduction and women's work. *Int J Epidemiol* 1985; 14:118–123.
100. Peoples-Sheps MD, et al.: Characteristics of maternal employment during pregnancy: Effects on low birthweight. *Am J Public Health* 1991; 81:1007–1012.
101. Launer LJ, et al.: The effect of maternal work on fetal growth and duration of pregnancy: A prospective study. *Br J Obstet Gynaecol* 1990; 97:62–70.
102. ACOG Home Exercise Programs: *Exercise During Pregnancy and the Postpartum Period*. American College of Obstetricians and Gynecologists: Washington, DC, 1985.
103. ACOG Home Exercise Programs: *Safety Guidelines for Women Who Exercise*. American College of Obstetricians and Gynecologists: Washington, DC, 1986.
104. American College of Sports Medicine: *Guidelines for Exercise Testing and Prescription*, ed 3. Lea & Febiger: Philadelphia, 1986.
105. Åstrand P-O, Rodahl K: *Textbook of Work Physiology: Physiological Basis of Exercise*, ed 2. McGraw-Hill: New York, 1977.
106. Hellerstein HK, Ader R: Relationship be-

tween per cent maximal oxygen uptake (% max $\dot{V}O_2$) and per cent maximal heart rate (% MHR) in normals and cardiacs (ASHD). *Circulation* 1971; 43(suppl II):71–76.

107. Wilmore JH, Haskell WL: Use of the heart rate–energy expenditure relationship in the individualized prescription of exercise. *Am J Clin Nutr* 1971; 24:1186–1192.

108. Clapp JF, Betz L, Philbin C: Cardiovascular adaptations to treadmill exercise before, during and after pregnancy. Presented at the 35th Annual Meeting of the Society for Gynecological Investigation, 1989.

109. American College of Sports Medicine: *Resource Manual for Guidelines for Exercise Testing and Prescription.* Lea & Febiger: Philadelphia, 1988.

110. Ekblom B, Goldbarg AN: The influence of physical training and other factors on the subjective rating of perceived exertion. *Acta Physiol Scand* 1971; 83:399–406.

111. Pivarnik JM, Lee W, Miller JF: Physiological and perceptual responses to cycle and treadmill exercise during pregnancy. *Med Sci Sports Exerc* 1991; 23:470–475.

112. Borg GA: Psychophysical bases of perceived exertion. *Med Sci Sports Exerc* 1982; 14:377–381.

113. Summary and recommendations of the Second International Workshop-Conference on Gestational Diabetes Mellitus. *Diabetes* 1985; 34(suppl 2):123–126.

114. Hollingsworth DR, Moore TR: Postprandial walking exercise in pregnant-dependent (type I) diabetic women: Reduction of plasma lipid levels but absence of a significant effect on glycemic control. *Am J Obstet Gynecol* 1987; 157:1359–1363.

115. Hickson RC, Rosenkoetter MA: Reduced training frequencies and maintenance of increased aerobic power. *Med Sci Sports Exerc* 1981; 13:13–16.

116. Hickson RC, et al.: Reduced training duration effects on aerobic power, endurance, and cardiac growth. *J Appl Physiol* 1982; 53:225–229.

117. Hickson RC, et al.: Reduced training intensities and loss of aerobic power, endurance, and cardiac growth. *J Appl Physiol* 1985; 58:492–499.

PART VI

Chronic Medical Illnesses

CHAPTER 13

EXERCISE AND PULMONARY DISEASE

ALAN F. BARKER, MD

Prior to the mid-1960s, rest was considered an important strategy for pulmonary patients, to allow "diseased" lungs to heal. During the past 25 years, however, supervised and self-administered exercise programs have become integral therapy for most patients with chronic obstructive pulmonary disease (COPD).[1,2] Today, only those with hypercapnia are prescribed rest as management for their advanced pulmonary disease.

In this chapter, I review the cardiorespiratory response to physical exertion and exercise testing to evaluate individuals with exertional dyspnea. I present the components of exercise training for patients with COPD, the proper use of oxygen supplementation, and the management of exercise-induced asthma.

Cardiorespiratory Response to Exercise

Exercise requires coordination of the cardiovascular, respiratory, and musculoskeletal systems. During physical activity, the cardiovascular and pulmonary systems must respond to support the increased gas exchange requirements that result from muscle metabolism (also see Chapter 5). Muscle blood flow is augmented to deliver more oxygen and remove carbon dioxide (CO_2)

produced by muscular activity. The sequence of events during exercise includes the following:

1. Cardiac output increases, through both higher stroke volume and heart rate. When stroke volume becomes maximal, subsequent cardiac output elevation is due to further heart rate increases.

2. In the pulmonary circulation, unperfused arterial segments open, allowing improved ventilation (V) and perfusion (Q) matching (V/Q) and more efficient oxygen intake (Vo_2) and CO_2 elimination.

3. As CO_2 is added to venous blood from exercising muscles, the initial response is a linear increase in ventilation to remove this product of cellular respiration. The coupling is so efficient that arterial CO_2 and pH change little during mild and moderate exercise. During aerobic metabolism, muscle CO_2 production is directly related to oxygen consumption via substrate utilization. With higher-intensity exercise, lactic acid accumulation triggers additional CO_2 formation due to buffering of hydrogen ion (lactate) by bicarbonate. This leads to an accelerated response in minute ventilation (VE) in relation to oxygen uptake. The steep inflection in the linear relation between minute ventilation and oxygen uptake is termed the ventilatory threshold. Only with extreme exercise and high lactic acid production does metabolic acidemia ensue.[3]

At rest, the major factor for VE stimulation is arterial CO_2 ($Paco_2$), which depends on ventilatory control from brain stem respiratory centers, as well as on the amount of functioning lung parenchyma. An inefficient lung bellows and ventilation-perfusion (V/Q) mismatching, as with emphysema, will contribute to reduced ventilation and an elevation of $Paco_2$, especially during exercise.[3]

The oxygen supply to skeletal muscles is dependent on arterial perfusion and O_2 content. Anemia will directly lower oxygen-carrying capacity, whereas the reduced oxygen affinity for hemoglobin, as occurs with acidemia, allows more oxygen release for muscular work. Perfusion can be affected by untoward physiologic conditions or drugs that reduce cardiac output, increase vascular resistance, or result in blood flow distribution abnormalities.[4]

Evaluation of Dyspnea

Lung disease is a generic term that can indicate many disorders. The majority of individuals with chronic pulmonary dyspnea will have one of three disorders: COPD, asthma, or interstitial lung disease. A brief review of these disorders facilitates interpretation of exercise testing and management.

PULMONARY DISEASE AND EXERCISE LIMITATIONS

Chronic Obstructive Pulmonary Disease

Most patients with COPD have a combination of emphysema and chronic bronchitis. With asthma or reactive airway disease, abnormalities include increased airway resistance and hyperinflation.[5] These abnormalities usually are intermittent and reversible if acute attacks are promptly controlled. Asthma is included among the obstructive lung diseases, and many patients with emphysema and bronchitis have a component of reversible broncho-spasm. However, it is useful to maintain the term COPD for the chronic, more irreversible diseases caused by years of cigarette smoking.

The physiologic hallmark of COPD is expiratory airflow obstruction. With chronic bronchitis, this obstruction mainly is due to narrow airways caused by inflammation, edema, and excessive secretions. Emphysema results from de-struction of alveoli and loss of elastic tethering, leading to airway collapse and increased airflow resistance.

Exercise tests of individuals with pulmonary and cardiac disease are pre-sented later. Although the patient with COPD often has a normal or near-nor-mal PaO_2 at rest, exercise can lead to hypoxemia by stressing the reduced air space reserve and magnifying the $\dot{V}/Q$ imbalance. This will limit exercise capacity and result in early fatigue. For those with this problem, supplemental oxygen administration during exercise (discussed in detail later) can correct hypoxemia, delay anaerobic metabolism, and allow greater exercise.

The ability to exercise with COPD is limited by various abnormalities, listed in Table 13–1. Although the major defect in COPD is fixed airway obstruction, reversible components are often present, including pulmonary secretions and airway smooth-muscle reactivity. Maximal ventilation is re-duced during exercise, potentially reducing exercise capacity.

The normal resting minute ventilation ($\dot{V}E$) is usually 5 to 7 L/min. How-ever, due to $\dot{V}/Q$ mismatching, patients with COPD can have a resting $\dot{V}E$ of 11 to 13 L/min. An excessive increase in ventilation for oxygen consumption at various work loads is a hallmark of COPD. Among normal individuals, the O_2 cost of breathing at rest is 2.5 mL/min or 1% to 2% of the total body consump-tion; this may increase to 10% of O_2 consumption with COPD.[6,7] In severe COPD, the increased demand for respiratory muscle perfusion potentially steals oxygen from peripheral muscles or even the heart.[6,8] Since those with more severe COPD have greater $\dot{V}/Q$ abnormalities, they can exhibit oxygen desaturation during physical activity. Lowered oxygen saturation can contrib-ute to stimulation of ventilation (hypoxic drive), resulting in a greater feeling of breathlessness. As $\dot{V}/Q$ mismatching increases, CO_2 may be retained, leading to respiratory acidosis.

Both chronic bronchitis and emphysema result in lung hyperinflation and air trapping.[9,10] The diaphragm is stretched and flattened, reducing its ability to expand the thorax further and creating a mechanical disadvantage for the ventilatory muscles. Maximal contractile force and negative inspiratory pres-sures are reduced. The thoracic-wall elastic recoil, which assists inspiratory rib

Table 13–1 **FACTORS RESULTING IN EXERCISE LIMITATION AMONG PATIENTS WITH COPD**

Airway obstruction
Ventilation/perfusion imbalance (leading to hypox-
    emia and hypercapnia)
Hypoxemia
Altered chest mechanics
Increased work of breathing
Deconditioned state

cage expansion, also is impaired.[6,11] Increased rib cage dimensions direct forces downward, working against outward expansion.[5,11] As more time is spent during muscle contraction, blood supply to the diaphragm may be impeded.[12] The resultant elevated work of breathing causes higher intrathoracic pressures and even greater reductions in capillary blood flow.[13,14]

Because of impaired lung response, patients may not continue previous physical activity levels, owing to sensations of breathlessness. As lung function worsens, exercise may be curtailed altogether, leading to a more sedentary lifestyle. The reduced activity results in lowered aerobic fitness and greater levels of dyspnea at similar work loads.

Pulmonary Fibrosis

Other types of pulmonary disease affect the ability to exercise. Interstitial pulmonary fibrosis includes a group of disorders (e.g., pneumoconiosis, rheumatic disease) initially characterized by polymorphonuclear inflammation in terminal airways and interstitial lymphocytic infiltration. Latter stages include fibroblastic infiltration, collagen deposition, and scarring.[15] Dyspnea is a universal symptom, crackles are present on chest auscultation, and radiographs show diffuse reticulonodular infiltrates. Unlike individuals with COPD and asthma, those with interstitial pulmonary fibrosis have small, restricted, stiff lungs. This results in an elevated diaphragmatic dome, with its movement impeded by parenchymal scarring and adhesions. Because of noncompliant lungs, hypoxemia, and limited ability to increase $\dot{V}E$ during physical activity, aerobic capacity is reduced.

PULMONARY FUNCTION TESTING

Pulmonary function testing can confirm a suspected disorder and assist in quantitating the respiratory impairment. The forced vital capacity (FVC) is normal or only slightly reduced in ventilatory obstruction. Timed expiratory volumes and flow rates, including forced expiratory volume in 1 second (FEV_1); forced expiratory flow, mid-expiration phase ($FEF_{25\%-75\%}$); and FEV_1/FVC, will be reduced below 80% of predicted in obstructive lung diseases. The FEV_1 is the most reproducible test for airway obstruction.

Unlike obstructive diseases, restrictive disorders, such as interstitial pulmonary fibrosis, will show a significant decrease in FVC. FEV_1 is reduced in proportion to FVC, so that FEV_1/FVC and expiratory flow rates are relatively unchanged.

Because physical exertion involves interaction among pulmonary, cardiac, and muscle function, resting spirometry provides an imprecise estimate of exercise capacity. In general, the patient with mild reductions in FEV_1 ($FEV_1 > 65\%$ predicted) often has no pulmonary limitations, and the patient with severe impairment ($FEV_1 < 50\%$ predicted) has limited ventilatory reserve and reduced exercise capability.[16] Patients with $FEV_1 < 30\%$ of predicted are short of breath at rest.

RESPIRATORY MUSCLE ASSESSMENT

Respiratory muscle static or isometric strength is quantitated by the inspiratory pressure (measured by a manometer) generated at functional residual capacity (the end of a normal exhalation). Patients with COPD usually have a 15% to 30% reduction in producing this pressure.[17,18] Distinguishing the difference between respiratory muscle weakness and fatigue is difficult but important, as the former may improve with training while the latter requires rest. Respiratory muscle weakness usually is manifest as reduced inspiratory pressures and compensated hypercapnia (increased $PaCO_2$ with normal or compensated pH on arterial blood gas). Fatigue is distinguished by worsening hypoxemia and uncompensated hypercapnia or respiratory acidosis (increased $PaCO_2$ and decreased or uncompensated pH).

Dynamic respiratory muscle function is quantitated by the maximal voluntary ventilation (MVV). The dyspnea index, used in exercise testing, is the relationship between demand, or measured minute ventilation, and capacity, or MVV: dyspnea index (DI) = $\dot{V}E/MVV$. Maximum voluntary ventilation often is estimated by multiplying the FEV_1 by 35, or by other formulas using pulmonary function measurements.[19,20] In general, individuals do not experience dyspnea until the DI is greater than 0.55. A very high DI during exercise suggests respiratory limitations as a cause for breathlessness. Pulmonary dyspnea is indicated by a DI value near 1, without attaining the ventilatory threshold while the maximal heart rate response is lower than predicted.

EXERCISE TESTING FOR DYSPNEA EVALUATION

Some individuals with normal spirometry will have dyspnea only with exercise. Exercise testing may help identify an abnormality or a specific diagnosis. Dynamic exercise testing can take several forms, but usually is performed by either cycle ergometry or treadmill walking.[21-23] Treadmill testing is used extensively in cardiac evaluation, and walking is a familiar activity. However, because the patient's upper body is relatively stationary during cycling, it is easier to monitor blood pressure, collect expired gases, and perform arterial blood gas analysis using that technique. In general, the tests are comparable, although cycle exercise often results in a slightly lower $\dot{V}O_2$ because less muscle mass is used during the activity. Cycling also may underestimate the exercise desaturation that occurs with self-paced walking.[22]

Parameters of gas exchange can be measured during and after exercise. These values help to define pulmonary and cardiac impairment. Oxygen desaturation during exercise, as monitored by digital oximetry or arterial blood gas analysis, documents the limited lung reserve in COPD and pulmonary fibrosis.

This effect in COPD is partly due to $\dot{V}/Q$ imbalance and reduced diffusion, in addition to the limited ventilatory reserve and rise in PcO_2.[24] When expired air is assessed during exercise, an increase in dead space or wasted ventilation (increased CO_2 in collected gases) indicates pulmonary vasculature loss, a consequence of destructive respiratory disorders.

If the syndrome of exercise-induced asthma (discussed in detail later) is suspected, patients can be exercised breathing air cooled by a heat-exchanging coil. When increased obstructive impairment is noted after exercise ($\geq 15\%$ reduction in FEV_1 from baseline), exercise-induced asthma is likely.[25]

> **CASE:** L.C., a 69-year-old woman with a history of hypertension and smoking, noted dyspnea on exertion when walking with her husband during his cardiac rehabilitation classes. She had no symptoms of cough or sputum production. Resting spirometry revealed mild ventilatory

obstruction (FEV$_1$ = 1.61, or 65% of predicted), with a normal FVC. During exercise testing, her electrocardiogram (ECG) did not demonstrate evidence of ischemia. However, at the end of exercise, her DI was high (0.99), and she was unable to reach an anaerobic or ventilatory threshold (the VE-to-Vo$_2$ relationship remained linear).

COMMENT: Although somewhat unexpected because her FEV$_1$ value was not greatly reduced, this patient clearly had a pulmonary limitation to exercise. Comparisons between patients with cardiac and pulmonary disease offer insights into the etiology of exercise limitations.[19,20]. Table 13–2 includes some of the expected differences at rest and during exercise between cardiac and respiratory impairment.

Pulmonary Rehabilitation

In addition to physical activity, a comprehensive pulmonary rehabilitation program includes nutritional support and cigarette-smoking cessation.[1,2] For some individuals, components can include respiratory muscle training, bronchodilator therapy, and oxygen supplementation. The type of resources available for exercise rehabilitation vary considerably. Some individuals, by themselves or with family or friends, have the motivation to plan and carry out all or parts of an exercise program. Other patients need professional rehabilitation programs, which may include physicians, nurses, and respiratory therapists. Often these programs are limited to larger communities and can be expensive. Modifications of the comprehensive rehabilitation may be available through a hospital, workplace, or local affiliate of the American Lung Association.

EXERCISE TRAINING

The long-term benefits of exercise training for individuals with COPD have not been established. Most controlled studies of patients with respiratory dysfunction have been less than 3 months in duration.[26] In the short term, documented exercise benefits have included increased endurance and improved maximal performance, along with reduced hospitalizations[27] and enhanced ability to walk and maintain household activities.[28,29,30] Table 13–3 summarizes uncontrolled and controlled rehabilitation studies. To maintain improvements, continued training is critical, as benefits disappear in 1 to 2 months if regular exercise is stopped.[31] In addition to functional indices, almost all studies have observed that exercise allows patients with COPD to feel better about themselves, their families, and their overall outlook on life.[32,33]

Ideal modes of aerobic exercise for a respiratory patient include walking and swimming. During swimming, most arm and leg muscles are used, and there are few orthopedic limitations to this activity. Swimming also should be encouraged for those with reactive airway component to COPD. Exercise-induced bronchospasm is less likely, since swimming is normally performed indoors where the temperatures and humidity are high. However, the elderly may be unfamiliar with swimming or may not have access to the warm, shallow pools necessary for exercise. Specific upper-extremity training may be helpful for individuals who have limitations to walking or leg exercise.[40]

Table 13-2 **PHYSIOLOGIC PARAMETERS AT REST AND WITH MAXIMAL EXERCISE (Lung Disease vs. Cardiac Disease)**

	PO_2 or O_2 saturation		$\dot{V}E$		VD/VT		O_2-pulse*		ECG	
	Rest	Exerc	Rest	Exerc	Rest	Exerc	Rest	Exerc	Rest	Exerc
COPD	N or ↓	↓	N or ↑	↑↑	N	↑↑	N	↑	N	↓ HR (MAX)
Interstitial fibrosis	N or ↓	↓	N or ↑	↑	N	↑↑	N	↑	N	↓ HR (MAX)
Coronary artery disease	N	N	N	↓ (MAX)	N	N	N	↑–↓	N or ST–T change	ST–T change; arrhythmia

Key: $\dot{V}E$ = minute ventilation; VD/VT = ratio of dead space to tidal volume; ECG = electrocardiogram; COPD = chronic obstructive pulmonary disease; N = normal; ↑ = decrease; ↑ = increase; HR = heart rate; MAX = at maximum exertion or exercise.

*O_2-pulse = ratio of oxygen consumption to heart rate (HR) at any level of exercise. It is a reflection of stroke volume.

Table 13-3   **RESULTS OF EXERCISE REHABILITATION PROGRAMS FOR PATIENTS WITH CHRONIC OBSTRUCTIVE PULMONARY DISEASE**

Author	Number of Patients	Duration of Exercise Program	Endurance*	Increased Maximum Oxygen Uptake
		Without Control Group		
Niederman, et al.[29]	33	9 weeks	Increased	No
Holle, et al.[30]	54	6 weeks	Increased	Yes
ZuWallack, et al.[34]	50	6 weeks	Increased	NA
Chester, et al.[35]	21	4 weeks	NA	No
Swerts et al.[35a]	27	8 weeks	Increased	NA
Mungall and Hainsworth[36]	10	12 weeks	Increased	NA
Carter et al.[36a]	59	12 weeks	Increased	Yes
		With Control Group		
Cockcroft, Saunders, and Berry[37]	18 E 16 C	6 months	Increased	No
McGavin et al.[38]	12 E 12 C	12–27 weeks	Increased	Yes
Sinclair and Ingram[39]	17 E 16 C	10 months	Increased	NA

*Endurance = distance on a timed walk or over a measured distance.
Key: E = exercise group, C = control group, NA = not available.

The advantages of walking include its familiarity, ability to be performed alone, and lack of expense. For some, a treadmill,[21] bicycle,[22] or 12-minute walk[41,42] can be the form of training. The 12-minute walk test is simple and reproducible.[42] An individual is asked to walk at a rapid pace on a level course for 12 minutes. The distance walked is measured. The results have been used as a motivator and objective gauge for rehabilitation programs.[43,44]

Among those with severe COPD, additional techniques for rehabilitation should include "energy conservation." This requires a well-planned daily routine and an efficient home situation, such as avoidance of stair climbing, minimizing heavy lifting, and alternating lengthy tasks (e.g., vacuuming) with periods of rest. Consultation with an occupational or physical therapist may be necessary to develop appropriate exercise programs.

Adverse consequences may occur during or after exercise in patients with COPD. No matter what mode of exercise, those with COPD should begin at low intensity and duration, slowly increasing to a duration of 20 to 40 minutes. Initially, patients may only be able to exercise for a few minutes; a schedule of training, rest, and resumed training should be established to enhance the conditioning effect. The duration of continuous activity is increased at weekly intervals until the patient can complete 20 minutes of exercise. Conditioning should commence with sessions at least three times a week, but patients should be encouraged to train each day. Finally, the intensity of exercise can be increased after a training regimen has been established (in 4 to 6 weeks), to improve fitness levels and functional capacity.

The diaphragm can fatigue due to failure of contractile processes or neuromuscular transmission.[45] Fatigue may be manifest as metabolic (lactic) acidosis, complicating a previously compensated respiratory acidosis. Arterial hypoxemia,[46-48] hypercapnia,[49] and hypotension[50] may occur. For these reasons, supervision with monitoring of heart rate, blood pressure, and arterial saturation are integral in the early days or weeks of programs designed to improve strength and endurance. Patients exercising alone or without medical supervision should be educated about heart rate monitoring, indications of fatigue, and who to contact if adverse events occur.

Those with COPD may have decompensation due to respiratory infection or other illness. During these periods rest is necessary. Resumption of exercise should be encouraged as soon as possible to prevent loss of previous strength or endurance gains.

NUTRITIONAL SUPPLEMENTATION

Malnutrition, as manifest by weight loss and reduced muscle mass, has been recognized in 20% of individuals with severe COPD.[51-53] Muscle mass loss alters both peripheral and diaphragmatic muscles and can contribute to exercise limitations. Inadequate nutrition often is due to appetite suppression, increased fuel requirement for respiratory muscle work,[54] and adverse side effects of medications. In addition, chronic systemic steroid therapy, frequently used in asthma and COPD, can heighten muscle protein catabolism, increase adiposity, and decrease strength and endurance.[55-57] When energy expenditure is increased further by physical activity, occasional nutritional supplementation should be encouraged to maintain adequate diet.

Nutritional supplementation of COPD patients has yielded conflicting results. Several studies have shown no improvement in weight, respiratory muscle strength, or pulmonary function.[52,53,58,59] Certain supplements caused patients to reduce their usual dietary intake because of attendant bloating and dyspepsia. However, when patients were placed in the controlled setting of a research unit and given an intake in excess of caloric needs, weight gain and improved respiratory muscle strength occurred.[60]

There is a concern about carbohydrate supplementation for COPD patients with elevated arterial P_{CO_2}. Since glucose metabolism produces more CO_2 per mole than fat does, hypercapnia and acidosis may ensue during high-carbohydrate feeding among those with limited ventilatory reserve. This phenomenon has been a problem during parenteral feedings of patients on mechanical ventilators,[61] as well as for ambulatory COPD patients.[62] Because of this concern, a higher percentage of calories should be derived from fat. For these patients, nutritional supplements should contain approximately 45% fat (preferably unsaturated), 35% carbohydrate, and 20% protein.[62,63]

ELIMINATION OF CIGARETTE SMOKING

Cessation of cigarette smoking is a crucial ancillary step, allowing stabilization, if not improvement, in pulmonary function. If smoking is stopped by those with few pack-years, impaired pulmonary function may normalize.[64,65] The benefits and success of smoking cessation strategies have been reviewed.[66]

Approximately 80% of those who stop smoking gain a relatively small amount of weight.[67] However, the increased weight can adversely affect exercise performance and breathing.[66] Regular exercise may reduce the level of weight gain. Although several studies have suggested that physical training does not help an individual stop cigarette smoking,[68-70] a recent investigation[71] of 20 women treated with smoking cessation techniques and regular exercise found that physical conditioning helped maintain smoking cessation.

RESPIRATORY MUSCLE TRAINING

For normal individuals and those with mild ventilatory impairment, respiratory function does not limit exercise. However, respiratory muscle weakness can be a limiting factor in patients with COPD. Respiratory muscle training has the potential to improve pulmonary function and exercise capacity.[72-74] A training program to improve muscle strength usually consists of two components: mechanical resistive loading and pharmacologic muscle stimulation.

A popular exhalation exercise is pursed-lip breathing.[75] This technique is used to reduce the sensation of dyspnea and relieve anxiety. Subjects are instructed to purse their lips during exhalation, applying back or expiratory positive pressure. This method can reduce airway collapse, increase tidal volume, and decrease respiratory rate. Short-term studies have shown improved oxygenation and reduced CO_2 levels, but breathing patterns have not been standardized or the work of breathing measured.[72] The technique is not natural for many patients, and long-term benefits are unclear.

Most respiratory muscle training strategies emphasize inspiratory muscles, as they provide the power to inflate the lungs. A variety of inspiratory resistive devices have been introduced. These are designed so that the patient inspires through tubes or mouthpieces of varying sizes. Some have fixed orifices, while others employ variable orifice sizes that the patient can adjust (Figure 13–1A).

Another inspiratory training strategy is threshold loading, in which the force behind an inspiratory valve is increased (see Figure 13–1B). Although these devices are relatively simple to use, inexpensive, and give positive reinforcement, efficacy has been difficult to document. Outcomes usually are measured as an increase in the ability to tolerate a smaller orifice or length of time in inspiration. A beneficial outcome is the ability to take longer and deeper breaths, which adds to patient comfort.[72]

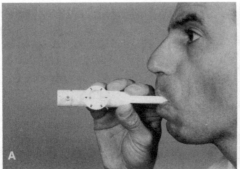
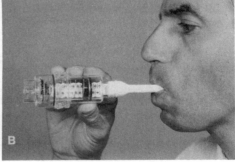

Figure 13–1 Two types of inspiratory muscle trainers. (*A*) The resistance can be increased by the gauge on the side; supplemental oxygen can be added through the end-piece (Pflex). (*B*) An adjustable spring-loaded valve blocks air flow to a desired threshold (Threshold).

Resistive and threshold loading do not alter resting pulmonary function,[72] but most studies in patients with COPD show an increase in respiratory muscle performance as measured by decreased dyspnea and increased inspiratory pressures.[76-80] In a subgroup of a set of investigations assessed by meta-analysis, five studies that ensured appropriate inspiratory training revealed significant improvement in functional status.[80a]

Voluntary isocapnic hyperventilatory training has been shown to improve endurance in patients with COPD. This technique, which can be performed at home, stimulates higher ventilation by breathing from a special elastic bag containing room air with additional carbon dioxide. In one study,[81] as part of a comprehensive home rehabilitation program, patients performed either goal-oriented walking or isocapnic hyperventilation. Walking improved endurance without changing respiratory strength. However, isocapnic hyperventilation enhanced both exercise performance and respiratory muscle strength.

All studies of respiratory muscle training have been short-term (weeks to a few months). It is unknown whether long-term use will induce fatigue or continue to improve clinical performance. Specific respiratory muscle training has a role in exercise programs as long as the emphasis is on inspiratory loading and using techniques to increase the volume of each breath.[72] This form of training may be most helpful in COPD patients whose ambulation is limited.

PHARMACOLOGIC THERAPY

The major limiting symptom during exercise in patients with COPD is shortness of breath. Opiates and alcohol have been used by patients to relieve the sensation of breathlessness.[82] However, because of their potential for causing respiratory depression and addiction, their use is not recommended.

Use of bronchodilators will benefit individuals with asthma or chronic bronchitis with a reactive component, and their use should be attempted in almost all patients with COPD. Although theophylline's role in the management of COPD has become less prominent,[83] it has been a mainstay of therapy. Theophylline is a bronchodilator (relaxes airway smooth muscles), promotes right ventricular contraction, stimulates respiratory drive, induces a mild diuresis, reduces dyspnea, and stimulates mucociliary transport.[84,85]

Early studies of respiratory muscle performance showed that theophylline augmented diaphragmatic contractility of paralyzed patients.[86] The same effect can be demonstrated among normal individuals during prolonged, intense exercise.[87] More recently, aminophylline decreased diaphragmatic fatigue and increased transdiaphragmatic pressure (a measure of diaphragm strength) for patients with severe COPD manifest by hypoxemia and hypercapnia.[88] In another study,[89] patients with severe COPD treated with theophylline had less dyspnea and decreased arterial CO_2, along with increased Po_2, as compared to a placebo group. Because only small changes in pulmonary function occurred, this effect was not felt to be due to reversal of bronchoconstriction. In summary, orally administered theophylline improves measures of respiratory muscle performance, affects airway tone, and reduces the level of dyspnea.[89,90]

Inhaled beta agonists improve airway tone and pulmonary function in many patients with COPD. This effect alone will augment gas exchange, allowing greater ability to exercise. Specific effects on either diaphragmatic or peripheral muscle performance are not known. Other medications, such as aerosolized or systemic steroids, play a role in reducing airway inflammation and improving pulmonary function. Use of steroids by the aerosol route has become a major component of asthma and COPD therapy. Use of systemic steroids has been minimized because of weight gain and myopathy, among other side effects.

OXYGEN SUPPLEMENTATION

When chronic, resting hypoxemia ($PaO_2 < 60$ mm Hg or oxygen saturation $< 88\%$) is present, patients will benefit when supplemental oxygen is administered 17 to 24 hours per day. Those benefits include improved exercise tolerance and neuropsychological function, as well as a reduction in pulmonary hypertension, reactive erythrocytosis, and mortality.[91,92]

Individuals with resting oxygen saturations above 90% may desaturate during exercise. If spirometry shows an $FEV_1/FVC \geq 0.50$, oxygen saturation typically does not fall with exercise. Most patients with an $FEV_1/FVC \leq 0.50$ will desaturate with exercise, however, and should be studied with oximetry.[93,94] Greater hypoxemia leads to increased pulmonary hypertension, reduced oxygen delivery, and respiratory muscle fatigue.[95] Oxygen via nasal cannula will relieve dyspnea and increase endurance in some patients.[96,97]

> **CASE:** M.R., a 67-year-old retired salesman, was seen because of increased breathlessness. Over the past 6 months, he gave up fishing, could no longer push a grocery cart, and stopped walking in the evening. His wife also noted that he began taking long afternoon and evening naps. He had smoked two packs of cigarettes a day for 45 years, stopping 1 year ago.
>
> On physical examination, he was 173 cm (5'9") tall and weighed 68 kg (150 lb). His heart rate was 106 bpm, and his blood pressure was 110/70 mm Hg. Auscultation of the chest revealed decreased breath sounds at the lung bases. His jugular venous pressure was increased. There was 2+ ankle edema and mild acrocyanosis. Laboratory studies showed a hematocrit level of 50%, with a normal white blood cell count. His chemistry battery was normal except for a slightly increased aspartate aminotransferase level. Chest radiograph showed flattened diaphragms and decreased markings in the upper chest. Spirometry showed FVC = 90%, $FEV_1 = 35\%$, with $FEV_1/FVC = 0.30$. These were interpreted as severe obstructive impairment. Room air arterial blood gas results were pH = 7.38, $PCO_2 = 45$ mm Hg, and $PO_2 = 50$ mm Hg. (Calculated O_2 saturation was 85%.) Walking down the hallway increased his heart rate to 130 bpm, while his oxygen saturation fell to 78%. The ECG showed p-pulmonale and right axis deviation.
>
> A diagnosis of COPD and cor pulmonale with right heart failure was made. He was treated with diuretics and supplemental continuous oxygen at 1.5 L/min. Over the next 3 weeks, his ankle edema disappeared, and he experienced a return of his previous energy level. He stopped napping, returned to fishing, and started thrice-weekly walks. In addition, he could work in the yard, play with the grandchildren, and help with vacuuming. Results of spirometry were unchanged.
>
> **COMMENT:** A decrease in exercise capabilities accompanied by end-organ insufficiency (fatigue, napping, or loss of interests) may be evidence

of cor pulmonale with right heart failure and hypoxemia. Continuous supplemental oxygen will improve quality of life and longevity in such patients.[91] Oxygen supplementation is available in canister systems, which allows easy ambulation, many kinds of physical activities, and travel.

Exercise-induced Asthma

The syndrome of exercise-induced asthma may be an isolated phenomenon in otherwise asymptomatic individuals, or a major limitation among those with asthma. It is characterized by transient airflow obstruction several minutes into or following exercise.[97a] This is usually between 5–10 minutes after the activity. The current popularity of jogging, running, and brisk walking in outdoor weather has uncovered exercise-induced asthma in many individuals. During exercise, higher $\dot{V}E$ is accompanied by airway water loss and a resultant increase in mucus osmolarity.[98] Exercise in cold and dry climatic conditions (e.g., jogging on a winter day) can provoke bronchospasm, whereas exercise in warmer temperatures with high humidity (such as swimming) is less likely to stimulate asthma.[99]

The temporal relationship of symptoms to exercise is important. Symptoms of exercise-induced asthma do not arise at the start of exercise or during the accelerative phase but begin during deceleration or after exercise has stopped. Classic examples include the onset of cough or shortness of breath in an individual during the time-out of a soccer or basketball game. The symptoms may last 20 minutes, occasionally preventing the return to physical activity. Symptom timing will help distinguish the syndrome from cardiac or other chronic respiratory disease. The dyspnea of exercise-induced asthma also can include coughing that begins as exercise accelerates and ameliorates with reduced intensity or cessation of exercise.

The symptoms of exercise-induced asthma can be reproduced in the laboratory with hyperventilation and cold air challenge. A reduction in FEV_1 or peak expiratory flow rate of 10% or a 25% reduction of $FEF_{25\%-75\%}$, suggests exercise-induced asthma. In some subjects, the genesis of the condition is more complex, as exposure to other triggering factors such as automobile exhaust, industrial pollutants, and aeroallergens contributes to airway hyperresponsiveness.

Regular exercise remains an integral part of health care for individuals with exercise-induced asthma.[100] Avoiding strenuous exercise in cold, dry air often is a necessity, although it may be a difficult choice for the dedicated jogger, skier, or bicyclist. Use of a paper mask, nose breathing, and prolonged deceleration during a lengthy run are sometimes useful aids, in addition to medication, to prevent exercise-induced asthma.[101] Chronic use of inhaled beta-2 agonists is effective in preventing or ameliorating the symptoms, but beta-2 agonists also can be administered effectively 15–30 minutes before an outdoor race or game. Cromolyn MDI is either the first or second choice and, if given 30 minutes before vigorous activity, will reduce bronchospasm without producing the tremor or chronotropic side effects found with inhaled beta agonists. Systemic medications, including oral beta-2 agonists and theophylline components, are preventive, but muscle tremor, elevated heart rate, and nausea may occur and interfere with athletic performance.[102] Calcium channel blockers also can be used. Some individuals have to alter their exercise style or location to indoor sports. Swimming may be an acceptable alternative for asthmatic exercise enthusiasts.

> **CASE:** G.K., a 30-year-old nurse, was self-referred due to exertional dyspnea. She related a history of hay fever and springtime wheezing most of her life. She was a frequent backpacker, jogger, and bicyclist. The previous fall, she developed "bronchitis" with coughing and wheezing that persisted for 3 weeks. Four weeks later, she returned to jogging but after 200 yards stopped secondary to cough, chest congestion, and dyspnea. The same symptoms recurred each time she tried jogging or bicycling. On physical examination several days later, the only pertinent finding was auscultatory chest wheezing with forced exhalation. Spirometry showed FEV_1 of 71% predicted and FEV_1/FVC of 64%. The chest radiograph was normal, and skin-prick tests to a battery of antigens were negative.
>
> For the next 3 months, she could perform only limited outdoor strenuous exercise, and her fitness was regained by swimming. Then in the spring, two puffs of albuterol metered-dose inhaler and cromolyn were initiated before each exercise session. Gradually the duration of each run was increased without symptoms.

> **COMMENT:** Asthma is a common disorder affecting 3% to 5% of the adult population, while wheezing after exercise occurs in 15% of adults.[103] Viral respiratory illnesses are the most frequent cause of asthma exacerbations, and symptoms and signs can persist for up to 6 months after the infection. Exercise-induced asthma can be prevented by the prior administration of beta agonists and cromolyn. Although cromolyn is not a bronchodilator, it has stabilizing effects on airway function when given before exercise. Many athletes with exercise-induced asthma prefer cromolyn, because they avoid the occasional tremor and feelings of anxiety that are side effects of beta agonists.

Summary

The airways, lung parenchyma, diaphragm, and peripheral muscles can be affected by respiratory disease. These abnormalities will often lead to exertional dyspnea. Resting spirometry and exercise testing can define the defects, gauge the level of impairment, and assess the need for therapeutic interventions. An exercise test also can be used as a motivating device for reconditioning programs. Effective rehabilitation of the individual with COPD is performed with a comprehensive approach. This includes smoking cessation, bronchodilator administration to improve pulmonary function, inspiratory exercises to enhance respiratory muscle strength, and graded ambulation (with oxygen supplementation as needed) to increase endurance and functional abilities.

REFERENCES

1. Sahn SA, Nett LM, Petty TL: Ten-year follow-up of comprehensive program for severe COPD. *Chest* 1980; 77:311–314.
2. Moser KM, et al.: Results of a comprehensive rehabilitation program: Physiologic and functional effects on patients with chronic obstructive pulmonary disease. *Arch Intern Med* 1980; 140:1596–1601.
3. Wasserman K, et al.: *Principles of Exercise Testing and Interpretation.* Lea & Febiger: Philadelphia, 1987, pp 3–26.
4. Brown SE, Caschari RJ, Light RW: Arte-

rial oxygenation desaturation during meals in patients with severe chronic obstructive pulmonary disease. *South Med J* 1983; 76:194–198.

5. Martin J, et al.: The role of respiratory muscles in the hyperinflation of bronchial asthma. *Am Rev Respir Dis* 1980; 121:441–447.

6. Donahoe M. et al.: Oxygen consumption of the respiratory muscles in normal and in malnourished patients with chronic obstructive pulmonary disease. *Am Rev Respir Dis* 1989; 140:385–391.

7. McGregor M, Becklake MR: The relationship of oxygen cost of breathing for respiratory mechanical work and respiratory force. *J Clin Invest* 1961; 40:971–989.

8. Levison H, Cherniack RM: Ventilatory cost of exercise in chronic obstructive pulmonary disease. *J Appl Physiol* 1968; 25:21–27.

9. Thurlbeck WM: *Chronic Airflow Obstruction in Lung Disease.* WB Saunders: Philadelphia, 1976.

10. Dodd DS, Brancatisano T, Engel LA: Chest wall mechanics during exercise in patients with severe chronic airflow obstruction. *Am Rev Respir Dis* 1984; 129:33–38.

11. Sharp JT: The respiratory muscles in chronic obstructive pulmonary disease. *Am Rev Respir Dis* 1986; 136:1089–1091.

12. Roussos C, et al.: Fatigue of inspiratory muscles and their synergic behavior. *J Appl Physiol* 1979; 46:897–904.

13. Buchler B, et al.: Effects of pleural pressure and abdominal pressure on diaphragmatic blood flow. *J Appl Physiol* 1985; 58:691–697.

14. Juan G, et al.: Effect of carbon dioxide on diaphragmatic function in human beings. *N Engl J Med* 1984; 310:874–879.

15. Schwarz MI, King TE Jr: *Interstitial Lung Disease.* BC Decker: Toronto, 1988, pp 1–13.

16. American Thoracic Society: Evaluation of impairment/disability secondary to respiratory disorders. *Am Rev Respir Dis* 1986; 133:1205–1209.

17. Black LF, Hyatt RE: Maximal static respiratory pressures in generalized neuromuscular disease. *Am Rev Respir Dis* 1985; 132:42–47.

18. Rochester DF, Braun, NM: Determinants of maximal inspiratory pressure in chronic obstructive pulmonary disease. *Am Rev Respir Dis* 1985; 132:42–47.

19. Clark RSH, Freedman S, Campbell, EJH: The ventilatory capacity of patients with chronic airway obstruction. *Clin Sci* 1969; 36:307–316.

20. Dillard TA, Piantadosi S, Rajagopal KR: Prediction of ventilation at maximal exercise in chronic airflow obstruction. *Am Rev Respir Dis* 1985; 132:230–235.

21. Pineda H, Haas F, Axen K: Treadmill exercise training in chronic obstructive pulmonary disease. *Arch Phys Med Rehabil* 1986; 67:155–158.

22. Cockcroft A, et al.: Arterial oxygen desaturation during treadmill and bicycle exercise in patients with chronic obstructive airway disease. *Clin Sci* 1985; 68:327–332.

23. Gallagher CG: Exercise and chronic obstructive pulmonary disease. *Med Clin North Am* 1990; 74:619–641.

24. Dantzker DR, G'Alonzo GE: The effect of exercise on pulmonary gas exchange in patients with severe chronic obstructive pulmonary disease. *Am Rev Respir Dis* 1986; 69:1135–1139.

25. Cropp GJA: The exercise bronchoprovocation test: Standardization of procedures and evaluation of response. *J Allergy Clin Immunol* 1979; 64:627–633.

26. Hughes RL, Davison R: Limitations of exercise reconditioning in COLD. *Chest* 1983; 83:241–249.

27. Hudson LD, Tyler ML, Petty TL: Hospitalization needs during an outpatient rehabilitation program for severe chronic airway obstruction. *Chest* 1976; 70:606–610.

28. Carter R, et al.: Exercise conditioning in the rehabilitation of patients with chronic obstructive pulmonary disease. *Arch Phys Med Rehabil* 1988; 69:118–122.

29. Niederman MS, et al.: Benefits of a multidisciplinary pulmonary rehabilitation program. *Chest* 1991; 99:798–804.

30. Holle RHO, et al.: Increased muscle efficiency and sustained benefits in an outpatient community hospital-based pulmonary rehabilitation program. *Chest* 1988; 94:1161–1168.

31. Coyle EF, et al.: Time course of loss of adaptations after stopping prolonged intense endurance training. *J Appl Physiol* 1984; 57:1857–1864.

32. Dudley DL, et al.: Psychosocial concomitants to rehabilitation in chronic obstructive pulmonary disease (3 parts). *Chest* 1980; 77:413–420, 544–551, 677–684.

33. Cockroft AE, et al.: Psychological changes during a controlled trial of rehabilitation in chronic respiratory disability. *Thorax* 1982; 37:413–416.

34. ZuWallack RL, et al.: Predictors of improvement in the 12-minute walking distance following a six-week outpatient pulmonary rehabilitation program. *Chest* 1991; 99:805–808.

35. Chester EH, et al.: Multidisciplinary treatment of chronic pulmonary insufficiency. *Chest* 1977; 72:695–702.

35a. Swerts PM, et al.: Exercise reconditioning in the rehabilitation of patients with chronic obstructive pulmonary disease: A short- and long-term analysis. *Arch Phys Med Rehabil* 1990; 71(8):570–573.

36. Mungall IPF, Hainsworth R: An objective assessment of the value of exercise training to patients with chronic obstructive airways disease. *Q J Med* 1980; 49:77–85.

36a. Carter R, et al.: Exercise conditioning in the rehabilitation of patients with chronic obstructive pulmonary disease. *Arch Phys Med Rehabil* 1988; 69(2):118–122.

37. Cockcroft AE, Saunders MJ, Berry G: Randomized controlled trial of rehabilitation in chronic respiratory disability. *Thorax* 1981; 36:200–203.

38. McGavin CR, et al.: Physical rehabilitation for the chronic bronchitic: Results of a controlled trial of exercise in the home. *Thorax* 1977; 32:307–311.

39. Sinclair DJM, Ingram CG: Controlled trial of supervised exercise training in chronic bronchitis. *BMJ* 1980; 280:519–521.

40. Lake FR, et al.: Upper-limb and lower-limb exercise training in patients with chronic airflow obstruction. *Chest* 1990; 97:1077–1083.

41. Guyatt GH, et al.: Effect of encouragement on walking test performance. *Thorax* 1984; 39:818–822.

42. McGavin CR, Gupta SP, McHardy GJR: Twelve-minute walking test for assessing disability in chronic bronchitis. *BMJ* 1976; 1:822–823.

43. Faryniarz K, Mahler DA: Writing an exercise prescription for patients with COPD. *J Respir Dis* 1990; 11:638–644.

44. Reis AL, Archibald CJ: Endurance exercise training at maximal targets in patients with COPD. *J Cardiopul Rehab* 1987; 7:594–601.

45. Grassino A, et al.: Inspiratory muscle fatigue as a factor limiting exercise. *Bull Eur Physiopathol Respir* 1979; 15: 105–111.

46. Minh VD, et al.: Hypoxemia during exercise in patients with chronic obstructive pulmonary disease. *Am Rev Respir Dis* 1979; 120:787–794.

47. Refferstin B, et al.: Circulatory transport of oxygen in patients with chronic airflow obstruction exercising maximally. *Am Rev Respir Dis* 1982; 125:426–431.

48. Young IH, Woolcock AJ: Arterial blood gas tension changes at the start of exercise in chronic obstructive pulmonary disease. *Am Rev Respir Dis* 1979; 119: 213–221.

49. Ingram RH Jr, Miller RB, Tate LA: Ventilatory response to carbon dioxide and to exercise in relation to the pathophysiologic type of chronic obstructive pulmonary disease. *Am Rev Respir Dis* 1972; 105:541–551.

50. Schrijen F, et al.: Pulmonary and systemic hemodynamic evaluation in chronic bronchitis. *Am Rev Respir Dis* 1978; 117:25–31.

51. Braun SR, et al.: The prevalence and determinants of nutritional changes in chronic obstructive pulmonary disease. *Chest* 1984; 85:358–363.

52. Braun SR, et al.: Predictive clinical value of nutritional assessment factors in COPD. *Chest* 1984; 85:353–357.

53. Schols AMWJ, et al.: Nutritional state and exercise performance in patients with chronic obstructive lung disease. *Thorax* 1989; 44:937–944.

54. Goldstein S, et al.: Energy expenditure in patients with chronic obstructive pulmonary disease. *Chest* 1987; 91:222–224.

55. Askari A, Vignos PJ Jr, Moskowitz RW: Steroid myopathy in connective tissue disease. *Am J Med* 1976; 61:485–492.

56. Melzer E, Souhrada JF: Decrease in respiratory muscle strength and static lung volumes in obese asthmatics. *Am Rev Respir Dis* 1980; 121:17–22.

57. Swinburn CR, et al.: Adverse effect of additional weight on exercise against gravity in patients with chronic obstructive airways disease. *Thorax* 1989; 44:716–720.

58. Lewis MI, Belman MJ, Darr-Uyemua L: Nutritional supplementation in ambulatory patients with chronic obstructive pulmonary diseases. *Am Rev Respir Dis* 1987; 135:1062–1068.

59. Openbrier DR, et al.: Factors affecting nutritional status and the impact of nutritional support in patients with emphysema. *Chest* 1984; 85(suppl):67S–68S.

60. Wilson DO, et al.: Nutritional intervention in malnourished patients with emphysema. *Am Rev Respir Dis* 1986; 134: 672–677.

61. Covelli HD, et al.: Respiratory failure precipitated by high carbohydrate loads. *Ann Intern Med* 1981; 95:579–585.

62. Brown SE, et al.: Exercise performance following a carbohydrate load in chronic airflow obstruction. *J Appl Physiol* 1985; 58:1340–1346.

63. Angelillo VA, et al. Effects of low- and high-carbohydrate feedings in ambulatory patients with chronic obstructive pulmonary disease and chronic hypercapnia. *Ann Intern Med* 1985; 103: 883–885.

64. Tashkin DP, et al.: The UCLA population studies of chronic obstructive respiratory disease. *Am Rev Respir Dis* 1984; 130: 707–715.

65. US Surgeon General Report. *The Health Consequences of Smoking: Chronic Obstructive Lung Disease.* Rockville, MD: US Dept of Health and Human Services, Office on Smoking and Health; 1984. DHHS publication PHS 84–50205.

66. Fisher EB Jr, et al.: Smoking and smoking cessation. *Am Rev Respir Dis* 1990; 142: 702–720.

67. Williamson DF, et al.: Smoking cessation and severity of weight gain in a national cohort. *N Engl J Med* 1991; 324:739–745.

68. Hill JS: Effect of a program of aerobic exercise on the smoking behavior of a group of adult volunteers. *Can J Public Health* 1985; 76:183–186.

69. Taylor CB, et al.: Smoking cessation after acute myocardial infarction: The effects

of exercise training. *Addict Behav* 1988; 13:331–335.

70. Russell PO, et al.: The effects of physical activity as maintenance for smoking cessation. *Addict Behav* 1988; 13:215–218.

71. Marcus BH, et al.: Usefulness of physical exercise for maintaining smoking cessation in women. *Am J Cardiol* 1991; 68:406–407.

72. Pardy RL, Reid WD, Belman MJ: Respiratory muscle training. *Clin Chest Med* 1988; 9:287–296.

73. Aldrich TK: The application of muscle endurance training techniques to the respiratory muscles in COPD. *Lung* 1985; 163:15–22.

74. Levine S, Weiser P, Gillen J: Evaluation of a ventilatory muscle endurance training program in the rehabilitation of patients with COPD. *Am Rev Respir Dis* 1988; 133:400–406.

75. Tiep BL, et al.: Pursed-lips breathing training using ear oximetry. *Chest* 1986; 90:218–221.

76. Larson JL, et al.: Inspiratory muscle training with a pressure threshold breathing device in patients with chronic obstructive pulmonary disease. *Am Rev Respir Dis* 1988; 138:689–696.

77. Flynn MG, et al.: Threshold pressure training, breathing pattern, and exercise performance in chronic airflow obstruction. *Chest* 1989; 95:535–540.

78. Belman MJ, Shadmehr R: Targeted resistive ventilatory muscle training in chronic obstructive pulmonary disease. *J Appl Physiol* 1988; 65:2726–2735.

79. Harver A, Mahler DA, Daubenspech JA: Targeted inspiratory muscle training improves respiratory muscle function and reduces dyspnea in patients with chronic obstructive pulmonary disease. *Ann Intern Med* 1989; 111:117–124.

80. Chen HI, Dukes R, Martin BJ: Inspiratory muscle training in patients with chronic obstructive pulmonary disease. *Am Rev Respir Dis* 1985; 131:251–255.

80a. Smith K, et al.: Respiratory muscle training in chronic airflow limitation: A meta-analysis. *Am Rev Respir Dis* 1992; 145: 533–559.

81. Ries AL, Moser KN: Comparison of isocapnic hyperventilation and walking exercise training at home in pulmonary rehabilitation. *Chest* 1986; 90: 285–289.

82. Woodcock AA, et al.: Effects of dihydrocodeine, alcohol, and caffeine on breathlessness and exercise tolerance in patients with chronic obstructive lung disease and normal blood gases. *N Engl J Med* 1981; 305:1611–1616.

83. Lam A, Newhouse MT: Management of asthma and chronic airflow limitation: Are methylxanthines obsolete? *Chest* 1990; 98:44–52.

84. Hendeles L, Weinberger M: Theophylline: A "state of the art" review. *Pharmacother* 1983; 3:1–44.

85. Bukowsky M, Nakatsu K, Hunt PW: Theophylline reassessed. *Ann Intern Med* 1984; 101:63–73.

86. Nochromovitz ML, et al.: Conditioning of the diaphragm with phrenic stimulation after prolonged disease. *Am Rev Respir Dis* 1988; 130:685–688.

87. Murciano D, et al.: Effects of theophylline and enprofylline on diaphragmatic contractility. *J Appl Physiol* 1987; 63:51–57.

88. Murciano D, et al.: Effects of theophylline on diaphragmatic strength and fatigue in patients with chronic obstructive pulmonary disease. *N Engl J Med* 1984; 311: 349–353.

89. Murciano D, et al.: A randomized, controlled trial of theophylline in patients with severe chronic obstructive pulmonary disease. *N Engl J Med* 1989; 320: 1521–1525.

90. Mahler DA, et al.: Sustained-release theophylline reduces dyspnea in nonreversible obstructive airway disease. *Am Rev Respir Dis* 1985; 131:22–25.

91. Nocturnal Oxygen Therapy Trial Group: Continuous or nocturnal oxygen therapy in hypoxemic chronic obstructive lung disease. *Ann Intern Med* 1980; 93: 391–398.

92. Grant I, et al.: Neuropsychologic findings in hypoxemic chronic pulmonary disease. *Arch Intern Med* 1982; 142:1470–1476.

93. Ries AL, Farrow JT, Clausen JL: Pulmonary function tests cannot predict exercise-induced hypoxemia in chronic obstructive pulmonary disease. *Chest* 1988; 93:454–459.

94. Carlin BW, Clausen JL, Ries AL: The use of cutaneous oximetry in the prescription of long-term oxygen therapy. *Chest* 1988; 94:239–241.

95. Pardy RL, Bye PTP: Diaphragmatic fatigue in normoxia and hyperoxia. *J Appl Physiol* 1985; 58:738–742.

96. Bye PTP, et al.: Ventilatory muscle function during exercise in air and oxygen in patients with chronic airflow limitation. *Am Rev Respir Dis* 1985; 132:236–240.

97. Bradley BL, et al.: Oxygen-assisted exercise in chronic obstructive lung disease. *Am Rev Respir Dis* 1978; 118:239–243.

97a. Virant FS: Exercise-induced bronchospasm: Epidemiology, pathophysiology, and therapy. *Med Sci Sports Exerc* 1992; 24(8):851–855.

98. McFadden ER Jr: Respiratory heat and water exchange: Physiologic and clinical implications. *J Appl Physiol* 1983; 54: 331–336.

99. Fitch KD, Morton AR: Specificity of exercise in exercise-induced asthma. *BMJ* 1971; 4:555–581.

100. Haas F, et al.: Effect of aerobic training on forced expiratory airflow in exercising

asthmatic human. *J Appl Physiol* 1987; 63:1230–1235.

101. Shurman-Ellstein R, et al.: The beneficial effect of nasal breathing on exercise-induced bronchoconstriction. *Am Rev Respir Dis* 1978; 118:65–73.

102. Anderson SD, et al.: An evaluation of pharmacotherapy for exercise-induced asthma. *J Allergy Clin Immunol* 1982; 64:612–624.

103. Dodge RR, Burrows B: The prevalence and incidence of asthma and asthma symptoms in a general population. *Am Rev Respir Dis* 1980; 122:567–575.

CHAPTER 14

EXERCISE FOR INDIVIDUALS WITH END-STAGE RENAL DISEASE

PATRICIA PAINTER, PhD

Patients with end-stage renal disease (ESRD) treated with dialysis have extremely low exercise tolerance compared to healthy individuals of the same age.[1-5] In general, little effort has been made to improve these patients' functional capacity, above providing dialysis or renal transplantation. The American College of Cardiology's rehabilitation goals for patients with cardiovascular disease include optimizing functional capacity and improving emotional adjustment to illness.[6] These goals also are applicable to patients with renal impairment. Although several studies indicate that functional capacity can be increased in dialysis patients, no general guidelines have been established. The goals of this chapter are to review the literature on exercise and renal disease, suggest appropriate and practical exercise programs for this patient group, and identify barriers that may exist in programming exercise for these patients.

Exercise Tolerance

Exercise capacity is reduced in ESRD, as estimated from work loads achieved and by directly measuring maximal oxygen consumption (VO_{2max}).[1-4] The VO_{2max} values reported for dialysis patients are consistently lower than

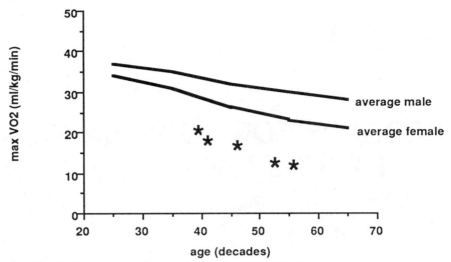

Figure 14−1 Maximal oxygen uptake value of ESRD patients compared to normal. Connected points are the average values for each decade of age in the normal population. Asterisks represent values reported in various studies of dialysis patients.[1−4,11]

established normal values for sedentary individuals (Figure 14−1).[7] In studies that have measured VO_{2max} as a part of exercise training programs, the levels ranged from 15.4 to 23.6 mL/kg per min (4.4 to 6.7 metabolic equivalents [METs]).[1−4] Patients in these studies typically had no associated medical problems, such as diabetes or heart disease, and may have had higher values than average dialysis populations. We found in a large cross-section of dialysis patients that maximal values averaged only 3.5 METs.[8] Thus, even among uncomplicated patients, exercise capacity is severely limited, with maximal achievable energy expenditure comparable to levels required for the usual activities of daily living.

Uremia appears to affect exercise ability directly, as aerobic capacity improves with successful transplantation. Patients who have received a renal transplant have maximal oxygen uptakes similar to those of normal sedentary individuals.[6,9] Several factors may limit the ability of uremic patients to transport and utilize oxygen. Figure 14−2 shows the normal transport of oxygen to the working muscles and the primary control of these functions. The right side of the figure indicates the steps in this sequence that may be affected by uremia. It is apparent that both central (cardiac output, arterial oxygen content) and peripheral (muscle oxygen extraction) abnormalities may reduce expected levels of peak oxygen consumption.

Recent evidence[10,11] suggests that central factors may be a major limitation for oxygen uptake. Patients undergoing dialysis have blunted heart-rate responses to exercise; they do not achieve the expected age-predicted maximal values. Most can achieve only 70% of predicted maximal levels. Kettner and colleagues[12] have reported that heart rates among these patients at any relative level of exercise are 20% lower than in normal individuals. Assessment of dialysis patients' cardiac outputs reveals that maximal stroke volumes are within expected values,[10,11] making the low maximal heart rate the major

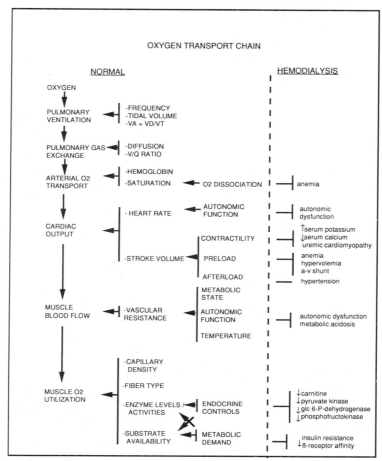

Figure 14–2 Physiologic systems and controls involved in the transport of oxygen from the atmosphere to the working muscles in healthy subjects (*left*), and factors that may affect oxygen transport (and thus $V_{O_{2max}}$) in patients with chronic renal failure (*right*).

limitation for maximal cardiac output. After renal transplantation, a normal maximal heart rate returns.[6,10]

Lower total arterial oxygen content is another contributor to the reduction in $V_{O_{2max}}$. Moore and others[11] have shown that muscle oxygen extraction is actually quite high among uremic patients, resulting in lower venous oxygen contents at maximal exercise than in normal individuals.[11] However, since the anemia associated with chronic renal failure limits oxygen delivery to muscles, a patient's total oxygen consumption is reduced. Patients who received human recombinant epoietin alfa have increased their maximal oxygen uptake when the hemoglobin was normalized,[13] although $V_{O_{2max}}$ still remained below normal. In addition, the $V_{O_{2max}}$ does not always parallel increased hemoglobin,[13] suggesting that other factors contribute to the lowered exercise capacity.

Fatigue is a common symptom of ESRD patients, and symptoms are improved by the use of epoietin alfa. Although erythropoietin increases exercise capacity, it will not produce the skeletal muscle changes that occur with exercise training. Thus, the optimal treatment would be to increase the hemoglobin with erythropoietin, which will facilitate exercise training (i.e., patients will be able to train at higher levels without fatiguing). Exercise training may have the potential to greatly enhance and even normalize functional capacity in these patients.

Several abnormalities that accompany uremia may affect muscle metabolism and contribute to peripheral limitations in oxygen consumption. These include altered calcium metabolism (reduced conversion to active vitamin D and excessive parathyroid hormone)[14] and cellular membrane integrity,[15] abnormal substrate availability (abnormal lipid and carbohydrate metabolism),[16,17] and insufficient intracellular buffering with consequent acidosis.[18] Even following dialysis and correction of acidosis, energy metabolism parameters (ATP, phosphocreatine, and total adenine nucleotide) measured in skeletal muscle biopsies remain significantly lower than normal.[18]

Exercise Training

HEMODIALYSIS PATIENTS

Several investigators have reported results of physical training among dialysis patients. A consistent finding has been improvement in exercise capacity, with the average increase in VO_{2max} ranging from 21% to 42%.[1,2,4] These studies have typically included uncomplicated patients who participated in supervised exercise programs of stationary cycling, walking, or walk-jogging. Two investigations had patients exercise using a stationary cycle during the hemodialysis treatment (Figure 14–3),[19,20] and similar increases in functional capacity were reported. Effects seem to plateau after a few months, as programs that varied from 10 weeks to 12 months[1,2,4,15,16] showed comparable VO_{2max} increases (21% to 30%). These findings suggest that the disease may limit the amount of improvement.

Maximal aerobic capacity may not be the only index of increased functional ability. In the only large-scale program that included patients with other

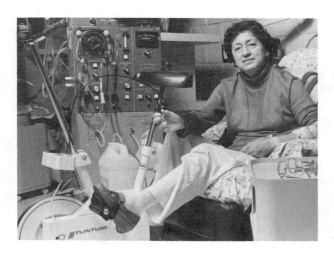

Figure 14–3 Bicycle setup for exercising during the hemodialysis treatment.

complicating medical problems, such as diabetes and cardiovascular disease, only small absolute changes in peak exercise capacity (20%, or an increase of 0.7 MET) were observed after training.[21] Prior to conditioning, most patients were able to cycle continuously for only 5 to 10 minutes. However, at the end of the training period, all patients were cycling continuously for 30 minutes or more. Thus, although cardiorespiratory changes, as reflected by maximal oxygen uptake, may be limited, peripheral adaptations may occur that allow improved performance during submaximal exercise and enable significant improvements in endurance.

> **CASE:** C.D., a 40-year-old, fully employed man, had been on dialysis for 5 years. He was a little-league football referee. Before training, he was able to officiate only one game per weekend as a result of fatigue. After 3 months of regular exercise training, he increased his officiating to three games each weekend.

> **COMMENT:** Submaximal improvements can translate into significant gains in ability to perform activities of daily living. Unpublished data from participants in our study revealed that 98% experienced less joint stiffness, 95% reported more muscle strength, and 86% reported improved endurance. Most believed that their leg strength increased within 6 to 8 weeks of initiating the cycling program.[21]

In addition to benefits in functional capacity, some studies have observed improved lipid levels and blood pressure control with training. Goldberg and colleagues[22] reported improvements in lipid profiles (lower triglycerides, increased high-density lipoprotein fraction), blood pressure control, and glucose tolerance among hemodialysis patients who participated in 12 months of exercise training. However, kidney function is not changed, and there is no evidence that anemia is improved.

> **CASE:** E.S., a 28-year-old man, had been treated with hemodialysis for 8 years. He was employed part-time as a grounds keeper (i.e., raking leaves, shoveling snow). He was treated with hydralazine and propranolol for hypertension. Before a conditioning program, he underwent exercise testing. During his initial test, he achieved a maximal level of 6 METs with peak systolic blood pressure of 260 mm Hg. He then began a regimen of regular exercise, which enabled him to discontinue all antihypertensive medication after just 3 months. Follow-up exercise testing performed after 3 and 6 months of training revealed significantly lower systolic pressures during submaximal work loads and at maximal exercise (Figure 14–4).

> **COMMENT:** As discussed in Chapter 2, regular exercise training can reduce blood pressure. Hagberg and colleagues[23] reported significantly improved blood pressure control, with decreased medication requirements, in six patients undergoing hemodialysis over a 12-month conditioning period. In another study,[19] exercise training during dialysis treatment resulted in significant improvement in blood pressure control in five of eight hypertensive patients, allowing for reduced medication requirements.

Not all studies have shown improvements in coronary risk factors with exercise training, suggesting that other factors associated with renal disease may override the beneficial effects of physical activity. For example, in one large clinical program,[16] no changes were observed in lipid profiles over 6 months of conditioning. The lack of response to this particular program may

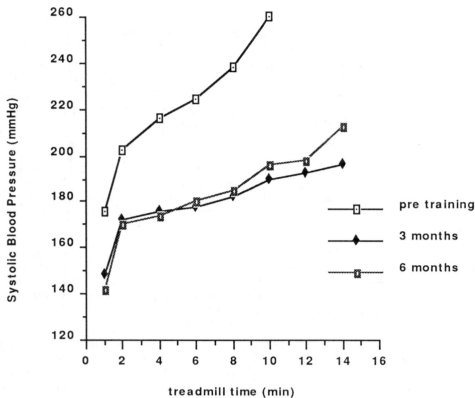

Figure 14–4 Systolic blood pressure responses to graded exercise tests of the same protocol before training and after 3 months and 6 months of exercise training. Antihypertensive medications before exercise were propranolol 80 mg qd and hydralazine 50 mg qd; no medications were needed after 3 and 6 months. (From Painter et al,[19] p. 89, with permission, copyright S. Karger AG, Basel.)

have been due to the low training intensity (2 to 2.5 METs), which may have been an insufficient stimulus to elicit risk-factor improvement. The absence of beneficial effects also may indicate that the effect of the underlying azotemia on lipid metabolism prevents the usual metabolic consequences of training. Thus, the results of any exercise program can vary depending on the training regimen and comorbidity among the patients involved.

RENAL TRANSPLANT RECIPIENTS

The exercise capacity of renal transplant recipients also can be improved with regular exercise. Researchers have reported significant increases in both estimated and measured VO_{2max} in renal transplant recipients following training.[24,25] Miller and coworkers[24] incorporated 10 renal transplant recipients into a cardiac rehabilitation program soon after transplantation (average, 17 days after surgery). These volunteers were supervised during treadmill exercise and stationary cycling for an average of 15 sessions over 6 weeks. Peak METs increased from 5.1 to 9.7. After 2 years of home exercise, the estimated intensity increased further to 10.9 METs.

In another study,[25] 16 patients began training several years after transplantation. These individuals were involved in stretching, walking, jogging, and calisthenics at an intensity of 60% to 85% of maximal heart rate, 3 days per week for 6 months. The measured VO_{2max} increased 25% over the 6-month period. This program also incorporated strength measurements of the hamstring and quadriceps muscles. Peak torque (a measure of strength) generated by the quadriceps and hamstring muscle groups improved 16% and 32%, respectively. Thus, in addition to endurance capacity, strength can be enhanced by many of those who have received renal transplantation after appropriate training.

Because immunosuppressive therapy with corticosteroids may weaken muscles, strength training may have particular benefits following transplantation. Isokinetic training has resulted in strength increases for these patients. In one study,[26] 12 renal transplant patients trained with isokinetic resistance three times per week for 50 days. Before conditioning, patients had a 36% higher fat-to-muscle ratio than normal individuals, as determined by computed tomography. Also, peak torque and total work output were 20% lower than normal before conditioning. Following training, significant increases in mid-thigh muscle area were observed, accompanied by a normalization of peak torque and total work output in both the quadriceps and hamstring muscle groups.

No studies have assessed the effect of exercise training on cardiovascular risk factors among renal transplant patients. Other potential benefits awaiting investigation among this group include the effects of exercise therapy on weight control, immunosuppression, return-to-work status, and quality of life.

> **CASE:** J.B., a 42-year-old woman who received a kidney transplant 2 years ago, complained of "lack of energy." She was a mother of five, three of whom were still at home. J.B. was unable to keep up with her mother, an active 72-year-old. Following transplantation, J.B. gained 16 kg (35 lb), which concerned her. She had always been thin, and friends and family consistently commented on her increased body weight.
>
> She began a program of walking (3 days each week) at the local YMCA and was given intensive dietary counseling. J.B. modified her eating habits to maintain a low-fat (20% of calories from fat) and low-calorie (800 kcal) diet. Over 3 months, she lost 9 kg (20 lb). As her energy level increased, she began walking each day. In addition, she was able to keep up with her mother, and her children said that she was always "on the go," something they had not seen since her kidneys failed 5 years before. At a symposium on transplantation, J.B. stated that she "thought her new life would begin when she got her transplant, but it didn't start until she began her exercise program."
>
> **COMMENT:** The benefits of regular exercise can complement the metabolic improvements associated with renal transplantation.

Exercise Testing and Renal Disease

The diagnostic value of electrocardiographic (ECG) exercise testing among dialysis patients has been questioned.[27,28] These individuals have low exercise tolerance, which may reduce their ability to achieve a level of myocardial stress adequate to detect ischemia. Maximal heart rates usually are below 85% of the age-predicted value,[28] and the latter level is needed to ensure adequate myocardial stress for diagnostic reliability. In addition, patients undergoing hemodialysis typically have abnormal resting ECGs, which may affect the interpretation of changes during exercise. Alterations with exertion can relate to left ventricular hypertrophy, volume overload, or anemia, and may not be indicative of ischemia.

No studies have compared the exercise ECG with angiographic data in nondiabetic uremic patients. Among those with diabetes and uremia, the sensitivity of the exercise ECG appears to be reduced. Although 11 of 20 patients studied by Orie and colleagues[29] had significant coronary narrowing, only two had positive exercise ECGs, resulting in a sensitivity of 18%. Thallium imaging after infusion of dipyridamole (or a similar challenge) may be preferred to detect coronary ischemia, because this method does not rely on achieving a myocardial stress through physical exertion.[22]

The current standard recommendation by the American College of Sports Medicine[30] and the American Heart Association[31] is that exercise testing is required before starting exercise training for patients at high risk, and those undergoing dialysis. However, since their peak exercise tolerance is similar to that of activities of daily living, their energy expenditure during training will be similar to the activities required at home. Therefore, exercise training places these patients at no greater risk than customary daily exertion. This presents a dilemma for professionals developing exercise programs for dialysis patients. Dipyridamole thallium imaging may be the most appropriate screening technique if program policy requires diagnostic information about myocardial ischemia. Otherwise, it may be more practical to monitor the patient's blood pressure and ECG at the prescribed perceived exertion level for the initial training sessions. This will in some way assess both ischemic and hemodynamic responses to the prescribed exercise intensity.

Renal transplant recipients are typically the most clinically stable patients with ESRD. Depending on the center, most, especially those at high risk for coronary disease, undergo a thorough cardiovascular evaluation prior to transplantation. Thus, it may not be necessary to repeat a cardiac evaluation soon after surgery unless symptoms of coronary insufficiency are present. However, as exercise capacity and heart rate response to exercise are normalized after transplantation, symptoms may develop when higher levels of myocardial stress are undertaken. Because of these changes and increased exercise capacity, ECG stress-test sensitivity is increased. If training is not initiated within several months following transplantation, a symptom-limited maximal exercise test should be performed prior to training.

Recommendations for Exercise

Although the optimal exercise prescription for patients with ESRD has not been defined, a program should consider instruction on the mode, frequency, duration, intensity, and progression of training. Exercise recommendations also must contain information on timing in relation to dialysis treatments. The following guidelines and suggestions have been developed from reported studies and from experience reported by patients and by staff involved in training patients with ESRD.

TYPE OF EXERCISE

Types of exercise used for individuals with ESRD include walking, walk-jogging, and stationary cycling. These activities utilize large muscle groups in a rhythmic manner. Non-weightbearing activities, such as stationary cycling, may be more appropriate for patients with extreme muscle weakness, bone disease, peripheral neuropathy, or severe visual impairment (who are at risk of falling). Following kidney transplantation, immunosuppressive treatment with corticosteroids increases the risk of joint deterioration and muscle weakness. Thus, non-weightbearing activity also may be prescribed to avoid the excessive joint stresses associated with jogging or other jarring activities. Progression to weightbearing activities can be considered as muscle strength increases. Although swimming and water exercises are not contraindicated, patients treated with peritoneal dialysis will require vigilant care of the catheter site after each session.

TIMING OF EXERCISE

The decision about when to train must take into account the physiologic changes associated with dialysis treatments. Patients undergoing hemodialysis typically feel better on nondialysis days. Several studies have incorporated exercise during this time.[1,2] Unfortunately, poor exercise compliance on non-dialysis days has been noted, with less than half of patients attending more than 50% of sessions.[3] It is not realistic to expect patients to undergo dialysis for 3 to 4 hours, 3 days per week, and attend a supervised exercise program on other days. Thus, since exercise training must be performed on a regular basis to be effective, it is reasonable to have patients participate in exercise on their dialysis days. Training during hemodialysis treatments using a stationary cycle (see Figure 14–3) may allow for supervision without further disrupting the individual's routine and therefore should enhance participation.

Chronic ambulatory peritoneal dialysis (CAPD) is a form of treatment in which dialysis fluid is introduced into the peritoneal cavity through a permanently placed catheter in the abdominal wall. Dialysis takes place through the peritoneal membranes. Fluid is exchanged by the patient every 4 to 6 hours. Usually fluid is present in the abdomen at all times. CAPD patients may choose to exercise in the "empty" condition, however, which relieves intra-abdominal pressure on the catheter and may prevent catheter-site irritation. In this state, movement during exercise can be enhanced, enabling the patient to achieve a higher training intensity. Many report feeling more comfortable during exercise if they have "drained out," although some note abdominal discomfort when completely "drained" and therefore only drain partially for exercise. Exercise in the empty condition can be accomplished by draining the abdomen of the dialysis fluid and either attaching a sterile empty bag to the catheter or capping it off and removing the bag. The newer catheters make this easier than did earlier systems. Nevertheless, this procedure should be carefully discussed and performed only with guidance from the CAPD team.

FREQUENCY AND DURATION OF EXERCISE

Training frequency typically is three times per week, on nonconsecutive days. However, since exercise intensity among dialysis patients is low, they may improve more and minimize joint stiffness by daily activity. Inconsistencies in training frequency, with long breaks, should be avoided if possible. The deconditioning effect associated with exercise cessation may be exacerbated by uremia or dialysis treatments, or by prednisone therapy for transplant patients.

Those who are only able to exercise for short periods may train two or more times daily to achieve the recommended 30 to 45 minutes of activity each day. Initially most patients will be able to exercise continuously for 5 to 15 minutes. Increasing the duration by 1 to 2 minutes each session (or each week, depending on individual tolerance) is recommended. At first, patients may require an interval approach to their training, with 2-minute work intervals and 1 minute of rest. They then can progress gradually by increasing the work interval and decreasing the length of the rest periods (each session or each week, according to individual tolerance) until they are able to exercise continuously for 30 minutes.

INTENSITY OF EXERCISE

The exercise intensity is frequently the most difficult aspect to prescribe. Among healthy individuals, a heart-rate prescription is developed from the predicted or measured maximal heart rate (see Chapter 1). However, this approach is not applicable for dialysis patients. As discussed, heart rates may not consistently reflect exercise intensity, because of fluid status, timing of antihypertensive medications, and the effects of uremia on maximal heart rate.[8] Also, if exercise is incorporated during the hemodialysis treatment, the heart rate may fluctuate depending on the rate and amount of fluid removal. Therefore, exercise intensity is most effectively prescribed using ratings of perceived exertion, which will accommodate the variability in physiologic status of the patient (see Chapter 1). Patients should be able to carry on a conversation during exercise and avoid over-exertion. Adequate cool-down is also essential, especially if the training takes place during hemodialysis.

For psychological and motivational purposes, it may be helpful to have patients exercise at a low intensity until they are able to increase their duration of exercise to between 20 to 30 minutes. This progression gives the patient positive feedback as the minutes of exercise increase. Also, if training takes place during dialysis, others can become aware of the program, providing additional reinforcement for exercising patients.

Transplant recipients typically achieve normal maximal exercise heart rates. Therefore heart-rate prescriptions for exercise intensity can be used, starting at the lower level (60% of maximal predicted or measured heart rate) and gradually progressing to 80% or 85% of the maximal value. Ratings of perceived exertion should be used in addition to the heart-rate prescription, especially if patients are prescribed beta-adrenergic blocking agents, which will reduce submaximal heart rates at fixed external work loads.

Barriers to Exercise Training

Individuals with ESRD have limited functional abilities, and there are several barriers to regular physical conditioning, despite its potential benefits. Exercise training for dialysis or transplant patients is not reimbursed by Medicare, unless the patient has a diagnostic classification that would qualify him or her for cardiac rehabilitation. In addition, many dialysis patients experience frequent medical problems that result in hospitalization, making it difficult to sustain a regular exercise program. Despite the studies presented in this chapter, no randomized clinical trial has been conducted to appropriately assess the cost and clinical benefits of exercise training among dialysis patients.

Dialysis is a passive therapy, typically administered by health care providers. The attitudes of ancillary health care personnel can reinforce patients' views of themselves as chronically ill. This also is reflected in the Social Security Administration's classification of dialysis patients as disabled. Rehabilitation professionals may have to work diligently to reverse the perceptions of the patients, families, and staff of their status, and reinforce the patients' ability to participate in regular physical activity. In light of these realities, it is important to develop reasonable expectations as to what exercise training may or may not accomplish. A program of exercise has the potential to influence attitudes of health care workers and patients in a positive manner by showing what results can be achieved through training.

SUMMARY

Patients with ESRD have a marked reduction in exercise capacity. A program of regular physical activity can enhance functional capacity and improve the ability to perform daily living tasks. Training requires a specific individualized prescription, along with reinforcement and close follow-up. Although prior illness and chronic use of immunosuppressive drugs can result in limitations in endurance and strength after transplantation, exercise can improve these parameters as well.

Providers of ESRD therapy should be encouraged to facilitate patients' responsibility in improving their own functional capacity by providing convenient and appropriate programs for regular exercise. This aspect of patient care offers an exciting challenge for the future.

REFERENCES

1. Goldberg AP, et al.: Therapeutic benefits of exercise training for hemodialysis patients. *Kidney Int* 1983; 516:S303–S309.
2. Zabetakis PM, et al.: Long-duration submaximal exercise conditioning in hemodialysis patients. *Clin Nephrol* 1982; 18:17–22.
3. Shalom R, et al.: Feasibility and benefits of exercise training in patients on maintenance dialysis. *Kidney Int* 1984; 25:958–963.
4. Painter PL, et al.: Exercise capacity in hemodialysis, CAPD, and renal transplant patients. *Nephron* 1986; 42:47–51.
5. Evans RW, et al.: The quality of life of patients with end-stage renal disease. *N Engl J Med* 1985; 312:553–559.
6. Parmley WW: Recommendations of the American College of Cardiology on cardiovascular rehabilitation. *Cardiology* 1986; 7:4–5.
7. American Heart Association Committee on Exercise: *Exercise Testing and Training of Individuals with Heart Disease or at High Risk for Its Development: A Handbook for Physicians.* American Heart Association: Dallas, 1977.
8. Painter PL: Exercise during hemodialysis: Participation rates. *Dialysis Transplant* 1986; 17:21–26.
9. Painter PL, et al.: Exercise tolerance changes following renal transplantation: *Am J Kidney Dis* 1987; 10:452–456.
10. Painter PL, et al.: Improvement in maximal oxygen uptake and cardiac output soon after renal transplantation. (Unpublished data)
11. Moore GE, et al.: Determinants of maximal oxygen uptake in patients with end-stage renal disease: On and off dialysis. *Med Sci Sports Exerc* 25(1):18–23, 1993.
12. Kettner A, et al.: Cardiovascular and meta-

bolic responses to submaximal exercise in hemodialysis patients. *Kidney Int* 1984; 26: 66–71.

13. Mayer G, et al.: Working capacity is increased following recombinant human erythropoietin treatment. *Kidney Int* 1988; 43:525–528.
14. Bratbar N: Skeletal myopathy in uremia: Abnormal energy metabolism. *Kidney Int* 1982; 24(suppl 16):S81–S86.
15. Cunningham JN, et al.: Resting transmembrane potential difference in normal subjects and severely ill patients. *J Clin Invest* 1971; 50:49–53.
16. Metcoff J, et al.: Cell metabolism in uremia. *Am J Clin Nutr* 1978; 30:1627–1634.
17. Nakao T, et al.: Impaired lactate production by skeletal muscle with anaerobic exercise in patients with chronic renal failure. *Nephron* 1982; 31:111–115.
18. Del Canale S, et al.: Muscle energy metabolism in uremia. *Metabolism* 1986; 35: 981–983.
19. Painter PL, et al.: Effects of exercise training during hemodialysis. *Nephron* 1986; 43: 87–92.
20. Moore GE, et al.: Exercise training for hemodialysis patients: Selection of appropriate participants. (Submitted for Publication)
21. Painter PL, et al.: Clinical experience with exercise training during dialysis. (Unpublished data)
22. Goldberg AP, et al.: Exercise training reduces coronary risk and effectively rehabilitates hemodialysis patients. *Nephron* 1986; 42:311–316.
23. Hagberg JM, et al.: Exercise training im-
proves hypertension in hemodialysis patients. *Am J Nephrol* 1983; 3:209–212.
24. Miller TD, et al.: Graded exercise testing and training after renal transplantation: A preliminary study. *Mayo Clin Proc* 1987; 62:773–777.
25. Kempeneers GLG, et al.: The effects of an exercise training program in renal transplant recipients (abstract). Presented at South African Transplant Society; August 1987.
26. Horber FF, et al.: Evidence that prednisone-induced myopathy is reversed by physical training. *J Clin Endocrinol Metab* 1985; 61: 83–88.
27. Rostrand SG, Rutsky EA: Cardiac disease in dialysis patients. In Nissenson A, ed: *Dialysis Therapy.* CV Mosby: St. Louis. In press.
28. Painter PL, et al.: Exercise testing in patients with chronic renal disease. (Unpublished data)
29. Orie JE, et al.: Thallium 201 myocardial perfusion imaging and coronary arteriography in asymptomatic patients with end-stage renal disease secondary to juvenile onset diabetes mellitus. *Transplant Proc* 1986; 27:1709–1710.
30. American College of Sports Medicine: *Guidelines for Exercise Testing and Exercise Prescription,* ed 3. Lea & Febiger: Philadelphia, 1985.
31. Joint American College of Cardiology/American Heart Association Task Force on Assessment of Cardiovascular Procedures (Subcommittee on Exercise Testing): Guidelines for exercise testing. *Circulation* 1986; 74:653A–667A.

CHAPTER 15

EXERCISE AND CANCER

MARYL L. WINNINGHAM, PhD

Over 1 million Americans are diagnosed with cancer each year.[1] Approximately half of these patients will survive 5 years or more, and many will experience functional limitations as a result of disease, treatment, or both.[2] Although exercise is advocated as having both preventive and therapeutic benefits, only recently has physical activity been suggested for cancer prevention and rehabilitation of patients with malignant neoplasms.

Exercise as Cancer Prevention

A sedentary lifestyle may increase the risk of developing certain cancers. In a 14-year study from Sweden,[3] 16,477 subjects were observed for physical activity levels and colon cancer. The greatest risk of colon cancer was among those assessed as having low physical activity levels during occupational and recreational periods. There were no gender differences, and the relationship between a sedentary lifestyle and risk was still present after controlling for age. Similarly, an inverse relationship between colon cancer and physical activity was found among men in the Framingham study.[4]

Other prospective studies[5-7] have examined physical activity levels and cancer. Over 12,500 men and women between ages 25 and 74 were examined during 1971–1975, with activity levels determined by questionnaire.[5] Subjects were reassessed during 1982–1984. After controlling for confounders, such as body mass index and cigarette smoking, those who were highly active in nonrecreational periods had lower rates of colorectal and lung cancer (men) and lower rates of cervical and breast cancer (women). In addition, men who engaged in regular recreational exercise had lower rates of prostate cancer.

Although a beneficial relationship between exercise and lower cancer rates has been demonstrated, it is not yet clear what volume (intensity × duration × frequency) of physical activity is necessary to reduce the risk of cancer. In an attempt to determine the amount of physical activity that will reduce cancer incidence, an investigation[6] by questionnaire of Harvard alumni suggests that more than 4,0000 kcal of weekly energy expenditure are necessary to decrease development of prostate cancer. This level of exercise would be comparable to walking or jogging more than 5.5 miles each day. A threshold of activity was necessary, as lower amounts of exercise were of no benefit. However, quantifying amounts of exercise by questionnaire is subjective and often results in overestimation by younger subjects and lower activity levels among the elderly.[7] Blair and colleagues[8] directly determined fitness levels by treadmill testing. Subjects were separated into five levels of fitness. Those in the lowest quintile of fitness had higher mortality rates due to cardiovascular disease and cancer than individuals who were more fit, after an average 8-year follow-up. However, benefits were present for those in the next-lowest fitness level and, unlike the college alumni study,[6] a graded reduction in cancer death rates was found among those with greater fitness. It was estimated that benefits could accrue from just 30 to 60 minutes of brisk walking each day.[8]

Thus, an emerging body of evidence suggests a strong inverse association between higher levels of fitness or greater amounts of physical activity and cancer occurrence or mortality. However, more evidence is necessary to determine the quantity of exercise necessary to provide this benefit.

POTENTIAL PROTECTIVE MECHANISMS

The mechanism for the observed lower cancer rates and mortality due to exercise is unknown. One proposed general mechanism attempts to link reduced cancer and coronary disease. This theory suggests that the potential benefit is due to lower serum iron levels among exercisers.[9] Since iron may act as a catalyst for oxygen-free-radical–induced tissue damage, lower iron levels could induce less tissue injury, resulting in less coronary disease and lower cancer rates. A possible mechanism for exercise-induced protection from colorectal carcinoma may be that greater physical activity reduces stool transit time, decreasing local contact between colonic mucosa and fecal carcinogens.[3] With regard to prostate cancer, high testosterone levels can help initiate or promote its growth. Since exercise reduces testosterone levels, regular physical activity may delay or assist in preventing prostate cancer.[6] Primary prevention of breast cancer by exercise could occur through reducing ovulatory cycles and altering women's hormonal milieu.[10]

Exercise Implications of Malignant Neoplasms

Unlike many other chronic illnesses, which have a single etiology or identifiable pathology, the generic term *cancer* includes diverse diseases that can arise in any organ or body tissue. Knowledge about cancer, its complications, course, and treatments is important for the development of safe and effective exercise programs. Although research is limited, studies indicate that individuals with cancer who enter a supervised exercise program may have improved emotional status and fewer somatic symptoms, as well as decreased fatigue and greater functional capacity. The following discussion will address issues involved in applying exercise training to the management of individuals with cancer.

EXTENT OF DISEASE

The classification of malignant tumors is complex and depends on their site, histogenic origin, and extent and distribution of metastases. Increasingly, the TNM staging system is used to define a malignant tumor. "T"—tumor— represents the primary tumor, and is followed by the numbers 1 through 4, indicating the size or extent of spread beyond local anatomic boundaries. "N" stands for regional lymph node involvement, and "M" represents extent of metastasis.[11]

An individual's cancer staging will have implications for possible exercise–disease complications. For example, a tumor occurring in bone may increase the chance of fracture. Patients with multiple myeloma, the most common primary bone tumor among adults, are particularly susceptible to fractures from mechanical stress. Pulmonary tumors can result in impaired gas exchange. Hepatic tumors may be responsible for metabolic and coagulation disturbances.

Although tumors can produce damage by invasion or mechanical compression of normal tissues, they also can cause paraneoplastic syndromes, such as inappropriate antidiuretic hormone production or a variety of neurologic syndromes.[12] In addition, patients with cancer are at risk for several emergent conditions. Cancer-related emergencies include spinal cord compression, superior vena cava syndrome, bowel obstruction, increased intracranial pressure, pericardial or pleural effusion, and venous thrombosis.[12-14] Thus, complaints of neck or back pain, which otherwise might not require evaluation, must be assessed carefully in these individuals.

Nutritional issues are important among patients with cancer. Various nutrient deficiencies can occur secondary to the decreased caloric intake produced by the mechanics of certain tumors, tumor–host competition, and the effects of chemotherapy.[15] Awareness of a patient's nutritional status will allow appropriate supplementation to maintain caloric balance when exercise is prescribed.

Surgery for tumor excision or debulking, as well as the implantation of therapeutic devices such as radiation implants or Hickman catheters, is common in this population. Since cancer and related therapies can retard healing, it is important that vigorous activity be avoided until the incision site is well healed. It is wise to request written consent from the surgeon for patient participation in exercise programs.

EFFECTS OF DRUG THERAPY

In many chronic illnesses, the drug treatment promotes or supports normal physiologic functioning. Cancer treatments, however, may inhibit or be toxic to normal function. Cancer chemotherapies potentially interfere with exercise capacity and can create conditions that may affect patient safety in a training program. Knowing an individual's drug treatment, its mode of action, and its common side effects is essential in developing an exercise prescription. Table 15–1 lists the names, classes of action, indications, and side effects of common antineoplastic agents.

Both the tumor and its management can affect immunologic function and risk for infection. Often, factors released by tumor cells suppress the general immune response of the host. It is not unusual for the infectious complications of cancer or its therapy to be the ultimate cause of patient death.[16] For that reason, it is important that the cancer patient's environment be evaluated for sources of infection. In particular, respiratory tubing, mouthpieces, and facemasks* used for the collection of respiratory gases in graded exercise testing are a potential source of infection and must be sterile. Symptoms of an infection or fever require evaluation prior to exercise.

Common side effects of antineoplastic therapy may have an impact on the ability to exercise. Bone marrow suppression, resulting in anemia, can lead to tachycardia, decrease oxygen-carrying capacity, and exacerbate cardiac ischemia. This may necessitate a reduction in exercise intensity or even its cessation. Drugs exhibiting cardiotoxic effects (cardiomyopathy, arrhythmias, and transient electrocardiographic changes) include dactinomycin, daunorubicin, cyclophosphamide, doxorubicin, and mitoxantrone.[17-19] Monitoring of cumulative dosage and noninvasive cardiac assessment may be appropriate. Because use of many antineoplastic agents results in arrhythmias,[20] it is also prudent to discourage moderate or vigorous activity for 36 hours after intravenous chemotherapy.

Bleomycin, carmustine, busulfan, and other related drugs can lead to pulmonary toxicity. Serial pulmonary function tests are useful in identifying subclinical and progressive deterioration[21-22] that can have an impact on gas exchange and exercise capacity. The neurotoxic effects of certain agents can result in sensorimotor deficits,[23] which can also influence the ability to exercise.

Finally, medications that produce severe nausea and vomiting may result in dehydration and electrolyte abnormalities.

> **CASE:** J.Z., a 22-year-old man, was diagnosed as having non-Hodgkin's lymphoma. He was placed on the ProMACE/CytaBOM protocol (low doses of cyclophosphamide, doxorubicin [Adriamycin], etoposide, prednisone, cytarabine, bleomycin, vincristine [Oncovin], and methotrexate) at intervals of 21 days. He continued to exercise vigorously, often bicycling more than 20 miles per day, swimming 1 mile, and lifting weights 3 days per week.
>
> After his third course of treatment, he began complaining of numbness in his hands and feet, noting that the numbness in his hands seemed to be worse immediately after weight lifting. He met with an oncology exercise physiologist once a week to monitor his progress. Coaching included teaching how he could assess his own hydration status, warning him about a tendency toward bleeding and infection during certain periods in the chemotherapy cycle, cautioning him against weight

---

*Facemasks are preferred as a comfort measure whenever possible because cancer patients often suffer from stomatitis and xerostomia.

Table 15–1 **COMMON ANTINEOPLASTIC AGENTS AND THEIR SIDE EFFECTS**

Drug Name	Class of Action	Indications	Common Side Effects*
5-Fluorouracil	Pyrimidine antimetabolite	Breast, bladder, colon, liver, ovarian, pancreatic, gastric, prostate, and basal cell skin CA	N&V, bone marrow suppression, possible cardiac ischemia, GI bleeding, cerebellar dysfunction
Bleomycin	Generates free radicals	Squamous cell CA of the head and neck, lymphomas, testicular CA, melanoma, lung CA	Pulmonary pneumonitis and fibrosis, oral ulcerations, acute anorexia, N&V, kidney damage, bone marrow suppression
Cisplatin	Cross-links DNA	Hodgkin's and non-Hodgkin's lymphomas; multiple myeloma; prostate, ovarian, and testicular CA; melanoma	Severe N&V; mild bone marrow suppression; hemolytic anemia; hearing loss; peripheral neuropathy; hypertension; azotemia; renal magnesium, calcium, potassium, and phosphorus wasting
Cyclophosphamide	Alkylator	Breast, lung, endometrial, and testicular CA; Hodgkin's and non-Hodgkin's lymphomas; leukemia; multiple myeloma	Hyponatremia, pulmonary fibrosis, moderate bone marrow suppression, N&V, hemorrhagic cystitis, interstitial pneumonitis, somnolence, confusion; augments doxorubicin-associated cardiotoxic effects; potent immunosuppressant
Doxorubicin	DNA intercalator, generates free radicals	Breast, bladder, thyroid, lung, and ovarian CA; acute leukemia; Hodgkin's and non-Hodgkin's lymphomas	Stomatitis, esophagitis, severe bone marrow suppression, cardiomyopathy (esp. with radiotherapy to mediastinum), cardiac arrhythmias, potentiation of other anticancer therapy side effects

Continued

Table 15–1 **COMMON ANTINEOPLASTIC AGENTS AND THEIR SIDE EFFECTS**—*Continued*

Drug Name	Class of Action	Indications	Common Side Effects*
Dactinomycin	DNA intercalator	Choriocarcinoma, melanoma, testicular tumors, Wilms' tumor, rhabdomyo-sarcoma, Ewing's sarcoma	Severe bone marrow suppression, fever, myalgias, fatigue, GI ulcerations, anorexia, N&V, decreased calcium level
Methotrexate	Inhibits dihydrofolate reductase	Acute leukemia; sarcomas; breast, colon, lung, and testicular CA; lymphomas	Azotemia, hematuria, interstitial pneumonitis, photosensitivity, nausea, severe bone marrow suppression, neurotoxicity (including paresis and leuko-encephalopathy), GI ulceration, hepatotoxicity
Vinblastine	Inhibits tubulin function	Hodgkin's and non-Hodgkin's lymphomas; testicular, breast, renal, and head and neck CA	Photophobia, leukopenia, neurotoxicity (including paresthesias and peripheral neuropathy), increased radiation injury to GI tract
Vincristine	Mitotic arrest, inhibits tubulin function	Acute leukemia; Hodgkin's and non-Hodgkin's lymphomas; brain, testicular, breast, and cervical CA; Wilms' tumor	Photophobia, neuropathy, paresthesias, muscle wasting, leukopenia, local injection phlebitis, uric acid nephropathy
Hydrocortisone†	Hormonal therapy, lymphocyte glucocorticoid receptor binding	Acute lymphoblastic leukemia, Hodgkin's lymphoma, breast CA, multiple myeloma	Osteoporosis, myopathy, impaired wound healing, glucose intolerance, electrolyte disturbances, fluid retention

*Assume fatigue to be a major side effect with all treatments.
†Although not an antineoplastic agent, is frequently used in treatment.
Key: CA = cancer, N&V = nausea and vomiting, GI = gastrointestinal.

lifting in the 24 hours before laboratory tests, and suggesting that he use the open palm of his hands to push up the handgrips on the resistance machines.

Following this advice, he had no problems with his exercise regimen during his treatment, except for feelings of exceptional fatigue for 2 to 3 days after his chemotherapy. The general loss of feeling in his hands and feet improved while he continued to receive chemotherapy. He is now disease-free 3 years post-treatment and continues his exercise program.

COMMENT: Dosage of chemotherapy is often governed by the results of laboratory tests, which can indicate the degree of toxicity resulting from treatment. Because vigorous activity can result in temporary leukocytosis and abnormalities in serum enzymes,[24] exercise should not be undertaken the day blood is drawn for laboratory tests. Similarly, heavy activity such as weight lifting or distance running should not be performed for 24 to 36 hours before assessment of serum enzyme levels.

Although no studies have addressed the value of strength training or maintenance exercise for cancer patients, it seems logical that low-intensity resistance exercise, such as that recommended by the American College of Sports Medicine,[25] would help maintain the strength necessary for activities of daily living and perhaps minimize the loss of lean body mass that is prevalent among cancer patients even when cachexia is not present. Because of the neurotoxic effects of specific drugs, patients may experience an impairment in tactile sense, as well as in gripping ability. For this reason, weight machines that are fixed in place may be safer than free weights, especially in the conditioning of large muscle groups.

EFFECTS OF RADIATION THERAPY

Clinical symptoms encountered by patients receiving radiation therapy include anorexia, nausea or vomiting, diarrhea, urinary dysfunction, skin toxicity, xerostomia, and stomatitis.[26,27] Thoracic radiation may result in pericarditis and pneumonitis, which can progress to pulmonary fibrosis. These may develop weeks or even months after therapy has been terminated. Furthermore, radiation treatments prior to, concomitant with, or following chemotherapy may potentiate the toxic effects of either therapy.[27]

CASE: E.M., a 29-year-old man, had been diagnosed at age 23 with Hodgkin's disease. He had an exploratory laparotomy that included splenectomy and lymph node dissection. Afterward, he received several weeks of radiation therapy to the thorax and was placed on the MOPP protocol (mechlorethamine, vincristine [Oncovin], procarbazine, and prednisone). He achieved a complete remission. While mowing the lawn at age 25, he had chest pain, which proved to be an anterior myocardial infarction (MI). Soon after his MI, he underwent two-vessel coronary bypass surgery for vessels with 95% obstruction.

After recovery from his surgery, he was referred to a cardiac rehabilitation program. Following discharge from this program, he continued to run 3 miles 4 days per week and has remained disease-free for the past 5 years, with no further evidence of coronary artery disease.

COMMENT: Late effects of cardiac radiation include accelerated atherosclerosis leading to coronary ischemia and MI. An enlarged heart and increased cardiothoracic ratio also have been reported in patients after radiation treatment for Hodgkin's disease.[28-30]

Exercise as Management

Cancer patients may benefit both physically and psychologically from regular exercise. The improved oxygen-utilizing capacity that accompanies aerobic conditioning can result in increased work capacity and efficiency. Results from the limited number of empirical studies applying principles of aerobic exercise to cancer patients have been encouraging.

CLINICAL EVIDENCE OF EFFICACY

In a study of individuals who had been diagnosed with cancer in the previous 5 years, Buettner[31] reported that those who exercised three times per week for 8 weeks (n = 7) showed significant improvement in fitness levels (VO_2 at a heart rate [HR] of 150 bpm) over control subjects (n = 10). Further, the fitness program produced significant positive personality changes as measured by the Cyclothymia, Surgency and Self-sufficiency scales on the Cattell Sixteen Personality Factor Questionnaire. Only 2 of the 17 subjects were receiving treatment for cancer during their participation in the study.[31]

A retrospective study[32] compared women with breast cancer who exercised to women with breast cancer who did not participate in regular physical activity. Groups were of similar age, education, and employment, and did not differ in stage of disease, type of treatment, time since diagnosis, or pre-existing health conditions that could limit exercise. Exercisers reported a higher quality of life than nonexercisers.

Since chronic disease patients often suffer from fatigue and debilitation, Winningham[33] designed a moderate-intensity, cycle ergometry exercise protocol, Winningham aerobic interval training (WAIT), which enables patients to benefit from a full 20 minutes of aerobic conditioning from their first session without inducing fatigue, stiffness, or soreness. The subject is entered in the WAIT protocol at an upper work load that induces an HR response of 60% to 85% of the HR reserve, calculated from the highest HR achieved on a preliminary, graded cycle ergometer exercise test. Each exercise level of the protocol consists of a set of higher–lower (12.5-watt increment) work loads for a set number of minutes. With improved leg strength, the time spent at lower intensity is reduced and time at the higher intensity is increased. Improved endurance, reflected in a lower HR response to the exercise prescription, is an indication to increase the resistance levels. This protocol has been used on a variety of deconditioned clinical groups, including cancer patients.

In a study of women undergoing adjuvant chemotherapy for breast cancer, MacVicar and Winningham[34] found that exercising patients (n = 6) and exercising healthy subjects (n = 6) made comparable gains in functional capacity in response to 10 weeks of the WAIT protocol, three times per week, compared with a control group of nonexercising patients (n = 4), who exhibited a slight loss. Both the patients and healthy women showed improvement in total mood disturbance scores on the Profile of Mood States, while the cancer-patient controls demonstrated a worsening score.[34]

More recently, 16 breast-cancer patients received adjuvant chemotherapy and engaged in the same type of exercise program, 12 received chemotherapy but did not exercise, and 14 exercised but did not have chemotherapy. Those engaged in exercise training demonstrated a significant decrease in reports of nausea on Derogatis' Symptom Checklist-90, revised.[35] Another study of 45 patients with stage II breast cancer who were receiving adjuvant chemotherapy showed a 40% increase in functional capacity (Vo_{2max}) in the exercising group (n = 18) participating in the WAIT protocol, compared with the placebo (n = 11) and control (n = 16) groups.[36]

> **CASE:** D.D., a 38-year-old rehabilitation nurse, discovered a mass in her left breast during a self-examination. She underwent a mastectomy and lymph node dissection (T2, N2, M0) for breast carcinoma. After this, she was placed on the CMF protocol (cyclophosphamide, methotrexate, and 5-fluorouracil), receiving intravenous chemotherapy once a week for a year.
>
> After 3 months of therapy, she was referred to an oncology exercise program. Following 10 weeks' participation on an aerobic, cycle ergometry protocol (60% to 85% of HR_{max}), she showed a 28% improvement in oxygen uptake. She purchased a cycle ergometer and continued to exercise three times per week on her own for the duration of that year.
>
> Within weeks of completing the CMF protocol, she found another rapidly growing tumor in her chest wall. She was placed on high-dose doxorubicin. Two months later, a computed tomography (CT) scan revealed evidence of metastasis in her ribs, and she received radiation therapy. At this time, she came to the exercise physiologist for coaching on continuing her exercise program. It was suggested that she monitor her pulse for rate and rhythm on awakening, to check for possible doxorubicin toxicity. A reduced training heart rate (approximately 60% of HR_{max}) was recommended.
>
> Because the rib metastases resulted in referred back pain, she found she could sleep better in a recliner. She placed her cycle ergometer next to her recliner so she could intermittently cycle and rest. During this time, she continued to work full-time. Despite continued treatment with radiation and doxorubicin, subsequent CT scans showed metastatic spread to her thoracic vertebrae and lungs. Medical personnel were amazed that she was still working. She told them that she thought the exercise was responsible for giving her the energy to continue working. Since the disease process continued to worsen and she was having increased pain, she made the decision to discontinue treatments. She continued to use her cycle ergometer for brief periods (5 minutes at a time) several times a day even after she had to quit working. She continued to live independently and care for herself until shortly before her death.
>
> **COMMENT:** This patient demonstrates that, with appropriate modification, exercise may be used to maintain functional capacity in individuals suffering from late-stage cancer. Hospice nurses often report an improved quality of life in patients who stay active as long as possible versus those who resort to bed rest earlier in the course of their disease.

Exercise Prescription

The development of rehabilitation strategies that could benefit patients with cancer has been hindered by the view that these individuals are doomed and incurable. As a result, many patients who could benefit from judicious programs of physical activity are still being advised to "take it easy" and "get plenty of rest" by well-meaning families and health professionals. Appropriate exercise can stimulate or maintain the body's functional capacity, whereas unnecessary rest in chair or bed inevitably results in progressive fatigue and weakness.

The principles of the exercise prescription and guidelines for training programs have been presented in detail in Chapter 1. To be safe and effective for cancer patients, the exercise prescription should consider the individual's medical and functional status, as well as the type of cancer and its management. For those individuals undergoing treatment, it is necessary to monitor therapeutic response and disease progression throughout their participation in an exercise program.

EXERCISE HISTORY

Information regarding the following variables should be obtained:
- performance status
- whether the person has other illnesses independent of the cancer (e.g., cardiovascular disease, pulmonary disease, or diabetes)
- status of the cancer (type, extent, and location of the malignant neoplasm, and the location and extent of metastasis)
- complications resulting from the tumor and metastatic site(s)
- type of therapy
- actual or potential complications resulting from the therapy.

Establishing the patient's performance status provides a useful index of his or her ability to participate in an exercise program. Clinical ratings of performance status are based on degree of functional independence and are often classified according to the Zubrod or Karnofsky scales[37] (Table 15–2).

INTENSITY AND DURATION OF TRAINING

Standard aerobic conditioning is only recommended for individuals of Zubrod 0 or 1 (Karnofsky 70% to 100%) status. Patients who are fully functional and had an active lifestyle prior to their diagnosis should be encouraged to continue what they enjoy doing, with the exercise therapist assuming the role of coach.

> **CASE:** R.R., a 36-year-old marathoner, underwent a left mastectomy with axillary lymph node dissection. Because the biopsy revealed several

Table 15–2 **PERFORMANCE STATUS CLASSIFICATION: ZUBROD AND KARNOFSKY SCALES**

Activity and Symptoms	Zubrod Scale	Karnofsky Scale (%)
Normal activity, no restrictions	0	90–100
Symptomatic but ambulatory, able to engage in self-care	1	70–80
Ambulatory >50% of time, needs occasional assistance	2	50–60
Ambulatory <50% of time, requires nursing care	3	30–40
Bedridden, may require hospitalization	4	10–20

positive lymph nodes, she received radiation therapy prior to starting chemotherapy with the CMFP protocol (cyclophosphamide [Cytoxan], methotrexate, 5-fluorouracil, prednisone). Immediately following her final radiation treatment, she developed symptomatic radiation pneumonitis requiring hospitalization. Although the pneumonitis resolved, residual pulmonary fibrosis remained. When chemotherapy was initiated, she expressed frustration from being "out of shape and getting fatter." After referral to an oncology exercise program, she participated in an aerobic, interval-training program (the WAIT protocol) three times per week, with her heart rate between 60% and 85% of HR_{max} attained on the pre-test. Other than occasional lowering of her white blood cell count below 3,500/mm^3, she tolerated therapy without problems. After 10 weeks her VO_{2max} increased 27%, with a decrease in percent body fat from 32% to 28%.

Following her chemotherapy, she continued to do well on a program of jogging 3 miles three times a week, swimming a fourth of a mile twice a week, and occasionally participating in "fun runs." Of the exercise program, she said, "After my mastectomy and especially after the pneumonitis, I was afraid of 'overdoing it.' I felt my body had betrayed me. This program helped me to gain confidence in my body again and encouraged me to continue to exercise."

COMMENT: The tendency toward weight gain in women undergoing chemotherapy for breast cancer has been reported as one of the most distressing side effects. Moderate-intensity, aerobic interval-training exercise at 60% to 85% of heart rate reserve three times per week can have a moderating effect on the problem of weight gain, stabilizing subcutaneous body fat stores and increasing lean body weight in women on chemotherapy for breast cancer.[38]

Those individuals with some functional impairment (Zubrod 2 or Karnofsky 50% to 60%) may benefit from a program that begins with brief-duration exertion. A regimen of 5- to 10-minute walk-rest intervals two or three times per day builds stamina. Exercise sessions are increased in duration, with a goal of 30 minutes of nonstop walking without dyspnea. This limited exercise program is especially important in preventing the effects of bed rest, which can contribute to a decline in performance status.

Zubrod 2 individuals may participate in a more intense program (with training heart rate at 60% to 75% of HR_{max}) if supervision and monitoring are available. If these patients participate in standard cardiopulmonary rehabilitation programs, it is important to supplement the training with information specific to the malignant process, special precautions, and treatment effects.

EXERCISE MODE

In deciding which type of exercise to prescribe, the issue of safety must come first, followed by patient preference and convenience. Exercise restrictions may be, in part, based on routine laboratory values (Table 15–3). In patients with low platelet counts or possible bone metastases, rope jumping, jogging, or running may lead to hemarthrosis or stress fractures, and should be avoided. Although exercise injuries such as stress fractures or shin splints may present as a positive radionuclide bone scan,[39] it also is true that metastatic bone tumors can masquerade as injury.[40] Active patients at risk for bone

Table 15−3 **EXERCISE RESTRICTION BASED ON COMPLETE BLOOD COUNT**

White blood cell count <3,000 cells/mm³
Check absolute granulocyte count.

Absolute granulocyte count <2,500 cells/mm³
Take infection precautions.
Patient should avoid crowded areas.
Patient should not use shower rooms, pools, saunas, or hot tubs due to associated risk of infection.

Platelet count <50,000 cells/mm³
Restrict activity due to risk of bleeding.

Hemoglobin <10 g/dL
No vigorous activity.

metastases or stress fractures (as with multiple myeloma) should be counseled into activities such as bicycling or swimming, to reduce the possibility of fracture. However, it is important to consider that use of public spas and recreation centers presents a potential for infection. Swimming, in particular, can present select health risks,[41,42] particularly for an immunologically compromised individual.

Unless contraindicated, walking is a key component of activities of daily living and is the recommended activity for those with no prior exercise experience. The cycle ergometer also is a preferred training method. The equipment requires little space, is relatively inexpensive and mobile, and permits precise regulation of exercise intensity.

The intensity of exertion is guided by heart rate (HR). However, the calculated exercise HR prescription from a measured or predicted maximal heart rate[25] may be affected by two characteristics common to cancer patients: (1) the resting HR tends to be high, and (2) aerobic capacities are reduced. It is not unusual for ambulatory cancer patients to have maximal METs ranging from 3 to 5. Thus, the HR reserve used in standard exercise prescription HR calculations represents a relatively narrow range, and using a percentage maximal heart rate may be useful as a guide to training intensity.

For patients with no metabolic abnormalities or cardiopulmonary disease, an exercise HR intensity between 60% and 85% of HR_{max} can lead to improvement, if the work is interval (discontinuous, intermittent, or ratio). The higher−lower ratio exercise may be preferable for individuals with functional limitations and easy fatigability. The WAIT protocol, mentioned earlier, is effective for patients with a wide range of capabilities; most patients with Zubrod 1 to 2 functional status are able to perform a full 20-minute aerobic conditioning workout during their first exercise session without post-exercise feelings of fatigue, stiffness, or soreness. Additional contraindications to exercise are listed in Table 15−4.

For patients who are deconditioned following surgery or prolonged, debilitating treatments (Zubrod 2 to 3), a bicycling or walking program can improve aerobic abilities. Among these individuals, it is sufficient to have the HR range approximately 60% of HR_{max}, keeping the walking to shorter periods and resting between sessions. When training intensity is lower and the duration

Table 15–4 **CONTRAINDICATIONS TO EXERCISE**

Any bony or back pain of recent onset
Dyspnea of sudden onset
Intravenous chemotherapy within previous 24
  hours
Muscular weakness of recent onset
Nausea onset during exercise
Severe nausea or vomiting within previous
  24–36 hours
Unusual fatigability
Febrile illness
Cachexia

shorter, exercise should be prescribed more frequently. Zubrod 2 to 3 patients will profit from several short walks of 5 to 10 minutes per day. As endurance improves, the duration can be increased to 30 to 60 minutes.

Many debilitated individuals find that exertional fatigue and weakness overwhelms them without warning. To determine the starting point for Zubrod 2 to 3 patients, ask individuals how far they can walk before feeling fatigued. Whatever distance they can walk, place a chair halfway. Have them walk to the chair, rest until they feel recovered, then walk back. They should rest for awhile, then repeat the exercise. The goal is to gently exert without reaching exhaustion. By repeating this several times daily, it is possible to prevent or mitigate numerous complications resulting from bed rest. If the disease process is stable, it may be possible to increase the walking time every 2 to 3 days by 1 minute each direction, every session. If the disease process is progressive, the goal is to maintain the patient's endurance for as long as possible.

Sometimes treatment regimens render a patient unable to stand for several days, but recovery is often rapid on cessation of each cycle of therapy. Such patients may progress from Zubrod 3 to Zubrod 1 to 2 within a week. The goal is to prevent as much deconditioning as possible, with more aggressive rehabilitation efforts between chemotherapy administration.

Zubrod 0 to 2 patients on a walking program can continue to increase speed until their exercise HR reaches 80% of HR_{max}. Younger individuals without contraindications may wish to progress to a walk-jog program at this point. On an interval-ratio cycle ergometry program, such as the WAIT protocol, the work load can be gradually increased in increments of ¼ kilopond-meter or 12.5 watts; in addition, time spent at a higher ratio can be increased as leg fatigue lessens (i.e., longer time at the higher versus the lower work load). In the exercise studies mentioned previously, Zubrod 0 to 1 subjects progressed to a higher ratio each week or to a higher work load when their exercise HR no longer reached the 75% to 85% range. Ratio and work load progression should not both be made at once.

After a difficult treatment or infectious illness, patients often ask when they can start back on their exercise program. The first day they feel better can be misleading, since patients may feel full of energy when they wake up but feel exhausted by midday. To avoid over-exertion while still recovering, an empiric rule is to advise "Wait until you feel better one day, then wait one more day," before returning to the regular exercise program. When resuming participation in the program, drop the exertional level back to that of 1 week prior to the interruption and monitor heart rate closely. If the heart rate is higher than 75% of HR_{max}, reduce the exertional level further. If the heart rate is within 60% to 75% of HR_{max}, the patient should stay at that level for at least two sessions before progressing.

Summary

Regular physical activity may reduce the rate of developing certain cancers. In addition, aerobic exercise has been found to promote functional capacity or fitness, as well as to produce positive emotional changes in people with cancer. Before applying the standard principles of exercise prescription to cancer patients, the following information should be obtained: (1) performance level, (2) the existence of other chronic conditions such as cardiopulmonary disease or diabetes, (3) status of the cancer, (4) complications resulting from the tumor and metastatic site, (5) type of therapy, and (6) actual or potential complications resulting from the therapy. Use of moderate-intensity, interval-ratio aerobic exercise can prevent many of the consequences of bed rest and promote feelings of energy without inducing fatigue. For patients with treatment-resistant cancer, appropriate exercise may be a means of retaining functional capacity, independence, and quality of life for as long as possible. For patients who go into remission or who are "cured," exercise can be a rehabilitative tool to restore them to optimal functioning after treatment.

REFERENCES

1. Boring CC, Squires TS, Tong T: Cancer statistics, 1992. CA 1992; 42(1):19–38.
2. Kurtzman SH, Garner B, Kelner WS: Rehabilitation of the cancer patient. Am J Surg 1988; 155:791–803.
3. Gerhardsson M, Floderus B, Norell SE: Physical activity and colon cancer risk. Int J Epidemiol 1988; 17(4):743–746.
4. Ballard-Barbash R, et al.: Physical activity and risk of large bowel cancer in The Framingham Study. Cancer Res 1990; 50(12): 3610–3613.
5. Albanes D, Blair A, Taylor PR: Physical activity and risk of cancer in the NHANES 1 population. Am J Public Health 1989; 79(6): 744–750.
6. Lee IM, Paffenbarger RS, Hsieh CC: Physical activity and risk of prostatic cancer among college alumni. Am J Epidemiol 1992; 135(2):169–179.
7. Drury TF, ed.: Assessing Physical Fitness and Physical Activity in Population-Based surveys. Washington, DC: US Government Printing Office; 1989. US Dept Health and Human Services, Public Health Service, publication DHS 89-1253.
8. Blair SN, et al.: Physical fitness and all-cause mortality: A prospective study of healthy men and women. JAMA 1989; 262(17):2395–2401.
9. Lauffer RB: Exercise as prevention: Do the health benefits derive in part from lower iron levels? Med Hypothesis 1991; 35: 103–107.
10. Bernstein L, et al.: The effects of moderate physical activity on menstrual cycle patterns in adolescence: Implications for breast cancer prevention. Br J Cancer 1987; 55(6): 681–685.
11. Henson DE: Staging for cancer: New developments and importance to pathology. Arch Pathol Lab Med 1985; 109:13–16.
12. Goodman TL: Oncologic emergencies. In Rosenthal S, Carignan JR, Smith BD, eds: Medical Care of the Cancer Patient. WB Saunders: Philadelphia, 1987, pp 345–357.
13. Johnson BL, Gross J: Handbook of Oncology Nursing. John Wiley & Sons: New York, 1985, pp 399–534.
14. Glover DJ, Glick JH: Metabolic oncologic emergencies. CA 1987; 37(5):302–320.
15. Munro HN: Tumor–host competition for nutrients in the cancer patient. J Am Diet Assoc 1977; 71(10):380–384.
16. Pitot HC: Fundamentals of Oncology, ed 3. Marcel Dekker: New York, 1986, p. 440.
17. Ali MK, Ewer MS: Cancer and the Cardiopulmonary System. Raven Press: New York, 1984, pp 40–100.
18. Kaszyk LK: Cardiac toxicity associated with cancer therapy. Oncol Nurs Forum 1986; 13(4):81–88.

19. Tokaz LK, VonHoff DD: The cardiotoxicity of anticancer agents. In Perry MC, Yarbro JW: *Toxicity of Chemotherapy*. Grune & Stratton: Orlando, Fla., 1984, pp 199–226.
20. Unverferth DV, Balcerzak SP, Neidnart JA: Ventricular arrhythmias following intravenous cancer chemotherapy (abstract). *Clin Res* 1983; 31(4):742A.
21. Ginsberg SJ, Comis RL: The pulmonary toxicity of antineoplastic agents. In Perry MC, Yarbro JW: *Toxicity of Chemotherapy*. Grune & Stratton: Orlando, Fla., pp 227–268.
22. Wickham R: Pulmonary toxicity secondary to cancer treatment. *Oncol Nurs Forum* 1984; 13(2):68–77.
23. Kaplan RS: Neurotoxicity of antitumor agents. In Perry MC, Yarbro JW: *Toxicity of Chemotherapy*. Grune & Stratton: Orlando, Fla., 1984, pp 365–431.
24. Robertson AJ, et al.: The effect of strenuous physical exercise on circulating blood lymphocytes and serum cortisol levels. *J Clin Lab Immunol* 1981; 5:53–57.
25. American College of Sports Medicine: *Guidelines for Exercise Testing and Prescription*, ed 4. Lea & Febiger: Philadelphia, 1991, p 179.
26. Hilderley L: Radiotherapy. In Groenwald SL: *Cancer Nursing: Principles and Practice*. Jones & Bartlett: Boston, 1987, pp 320–347.
27. Lewis CL: Principles of radiation oncology. In Rosenthal S, Carignan JR, Smith BD: *Medical Care of the Cancer Patient*. WB Saunders: Philadelphia, 1987, pp 63–78.
28. Perrault DJ, Levy M, Herman JD: Echocardiographic abnormalities following cardiac radiation. *J Clin Oncol* 1985; 3(4):546–551.
29. Pohjola-Sintonen S, et al.: Late cardiac effects of mediastinal radiotherapy in patients with Hodgkin's disease. *Cancer* 1987; 60: 331–337.
30. Lewis CL: Principles of radiation oncology. In Rosenthal S, Carignan JR, Smith BD: *Medical Care of the Cancer Patient*. WB Saunders: Philadelphia, 1987, p 76.
31. Buettner LL: *Personality Changes and Physiological Changes of a Personalized Fitness Enrichment Program for Cancer Patients*. Bowling Green, OH: Bowling Green State University, 1980. Thesis.
32. Young-McCaughan S, Sexton DL: Quality of life in women with breast cancer. *Oncol Nurs Forum* 1991; 18(4):751–757.
33. Winningham ML: *The Winningham Aerobic Interval Training (WAIT) Protocol Manual*. Columbus, OH. 1988. Available from author.
34. MacVicar MG, Winningham ML: Promoting the functional capacity of cancer patients. *Cancer Bull* 1986; 38(5):235–239.
35. Winningham ML, MacVicar MG: The effect of aerobic exercise on patient reports of nausea. *Oncol Nurs Forum* 1988; 15(4): 447–450.
36. MacVicar MG, Winningham ML, Nickel JL: Effects of aerobic interval training on cancer patients' functional capacity. *Nurs Res* 1989; 38(6):348–351.
37. Wood WC, et al.: *Cancer Manual*, ed 6. American Cancer Society, Mass Div: Boston, 1982, p 147.
38. Winningham ML, et al.: Effect of aerobic exercise on body weight and composition in breast cancer patients. *Oncol Nurs Forum* 1989; 16(5):683–689.
39. Nagle CE, Freitas JE: Radionuclide imaging of musculoskeletal injuries in athletes with negative radiographs. *Phys Sportsmed* 1987; 15(6):147–155.
40. McKirgan CC, Steingard PM: Bone tumors masquerading as traumatic injury. *Phys Sportsmed* 1989; 17(5):121–126.
41. Seyfried PL, et al.: A prospective study of swimming-related illness, I: Swimming-associated health risk. *Am J Public Health* 1985; 75(9):1068–1070.
42. Seyfried PL, et al.: A prospective study of swimming-related illness, II: Morbidity and the microbiological quality of water. *Am J Public Health* 1985; 75(9):1071–1075.

PART VII

Neuropsychological Disorders

CHAPTER 16

EXERCISE, EMOTIONS, AND TYPE A BEHAVIOR

CHARLES C. BENIGHT, PhD, and C. BARR TAYLOR, MD

Exercise has been credited with a variety of psychological benefits, ranging from improving one's overall sense of well-being to serving as an antianxiety and antidepressant treatment. Four areas concerned with psychological health and its relationship with physical activity are addressed in this chapter: (1) the use of exercise for the treatment of anxiety, (2) exercise as therapy for depression, (3) exercise to enhance one's general sense of well-being, and (4) the role of exercise in altering the coronary-prone (type A) behavior pattern.

Exercise and Anxiety

Discussing anxiety and its treatment requires differentiating between symptoms of anxiety and the clinical syndromes of anxiety (panic disorder, agoraphobia, and generalized anxiety). Although research on exercise as a therapeutic intervention has focused primarily on the symptom of anxiety, both will be discussed.

Anxiety is a universal emotion frequently experienced by most people, at least in minor degrees. Anxiety has been defined as ". . . a feeling of uneasiness and apprehension about some undefined threat. The threat is often physi-

319

cal with intimations of bodily harm or death, or psychological with threats to self-esteem and well-being. The feeling is diffuse and ineffable, and the indefinable nature of the feeling gives it a peculiarly unpleasant and intolerable quality.''[1]

Anxiety involves cognition (e.g., worrying), symptoms (e.g., palpitations), physiologic changes (e.g., increased heart rate), and behavior (e.g., pacing, fidgeting). Each of these interact in ways that often exacerbate one another. For instance, worrying may focus attention on symptoms that, when identified, further increase worry. Anxiety is increased under conditions of heightened arousal, threat, and lack of control. Symptoms of anxiety and clinical anxiety syndromes (e.g., panic disorder, agoraphobia, generalized anxiety disorder) differ in intensity, in the occurrence of additional symptoms (e.g., panic attacks), and in how individuals manage these symptoms.

A number of standardized, reliable, and valid self-report or interview-determined measures of anxiety have been developed.[2] The most common measures include the Taylor Manifest Anxiety Scale,[3] the Spielberger State–Trait Anxiety Scale,[4] the anxiety scale of the Profile of Mood States,[5] the SCL-90 anxiety scale,[6] and the Hamilton Anxiety Interview.[7] These measures are correlated. The literature differentiates between state anxiety—the level of anxiety at the time of measurement—and trait anxiety—a person's general level of anxiety over the past week or longer.

The neuroanatomy of anxiety is poorly understood. A variety of neuroanatomical structures and systems have been implicated (for a review, see Taylor and Arnow[1]). The locus ceruleus, noradrenergic and serotonergic neurotransmitters, and the so-called GABA–benzodiazepine system are important in the expression of anxiety.

EXERCISE AND SYMPTOMS OF ANXIETY

Uncontrolled studies on the effects of exercise on anxiety provide support for regular physical activity as a treatment for this disorder. It has been reported that joggers experience less anxiety than sedentary individuals,[8] and aerobically active young adults claim to be less anxious and depressed than nonactive students of the same age.[9] Various investigations have found that anxiety was decreased following a 12-minute run,[10] after 6 weeks of basic training,[11] and after approximately 40 minutes of intense exercise (80% VO_{2max}).[12] In contrast, no significant decrease in anxiety was reported for a group of elderly subjects who performed mild exercise.[13]

Several controlled trials lend further support that exercise lowers anxiety levels. Reductions in anxiety were found for students participating in an exercise class as compared to a control class.[14] Similarly, adults in fitness classes reported decreased anxiety as compared to volunteer controls from the community.[15,16] In Denmark, 64 unemployed men were randomized into either an exercise group, a placebo group, or a no-treatment control group.[17] The exercises consisted of either calisthenics, volleyball, or badminton, which was followed by swimming twice a week for 2 hours. The placebo group engaged in discussion of various topics led by a social worker. After 3 months, the exercise group was less anxious than the other two groups.

In another well-designed study,[18] 109 sedentary adult volunteers were randomized either to high-intensity aerobic training, moderate-intensity aerobic training, attention-placebo, or a waiting list. Curiously, the high, moderate, and attention-placebo groups all increased aerobic fitness as indexed by the Cooper 12-minute walk-run test. In this test, subjects are asked to walk or run as far as they can in 12 minutes. Changes in the attention-placebo group may have occurred because the group underwent strength, mobility, and flexibility exercises followed by discontinuous exercise for at least 30 minutes at an intensity that did not elevate heart rate above 50% of maximal. Only the moderate-intensity group exhibited a decrease in tension-anxiety, which differed significantly from the other two groups. A controlled study[19] of 120 sedentary men and women found no significant differences between the exercise and control groups on anxiety, even though the former showed significant improvement in fitness level as compared to the control group. However, the participants in this latter study were nonanxious individuals prior to training.

Mechanisms of Anxiety Reduction

Overall, regular exercise appears to reduce the symptom of anxiety in normal populations. Several mechanisms have been proposed for this change. One hypothesis is that exercise empowers the individual with a greater sense of personal control and self-efficacy, which can attenuate anxiety.[20] This sense of control would break anxiety's progression by changing the initial appraisal of the environment from one of constant threat to one of challenge. This change could improve one's belief in the ability to maintain control over anxiety-provoking thoughts. Supporting this hypothesis are training studies that have found increased levels of perceived self-efficacy or personal sense of control following aerobic conditioning.[21-24] In fact, after a 10-week walk-jog treatment, individuals continued to improve their perceptions of self-efficacy at a 12-week follow-up assessment.[22] Thus, habitual exercise might attenuate anxiety by instilling individuals with a greater sense of personal mastery.

Another hypothesis is that anxiety is reduced by distraction. This hypothesis is based on the premise that exercise creates a cognitive diversion from stressful stimuli.[25,26] The individual temporarily diverts his or her focus from the stimuli to the demands of exercise. There is tentative support for the diversion hypothesis. Seventy-five adult men were randomly assigned to one of three groups.[27] The groups consisted of 20 minutes of moderate exercise on a treadmill, relaxing using Benson's relaxation response strategy, or distraction that consisted of sitting quietly in a sound-filtered room. All three groups reported significant reductions in anxiety. The authors interpret these findings as evidence that exercise, just as meditation or cognitive diversion, distracts people from concentrating on anxiety-provoking stimuli. Other investigations[23,28,29] also have shown exercise to be as effective as other stress-management techniques such as yoga, progressive relaxation, and stress inoculation training. The interpretation is that exercise may have a time-out period in common with other stress-reducing activities. Possible contributing factors include social interaction and improved self-efficacy. These results suggest that effects of exercise on anxiety are not dependent on the acute or chronic physiologic changes with physical activity.

For acute exercise, it has been hypothesized that an anxious individual who has exercised will be unable to generate the physiologic reactivity that normally accompanies the experience of anxiety, and thus physically feels less anxious.[26] Other research has supplied evidence for the reduction of physiologic measures of anxiety (e.g., muscular tension) immediately following a bout of exercise.[30-32] Some studies[12,33] indicate that the anxiety reduction is contingent on acute, high-intensity aerobic exercise (e.g., between 60% and 80% VO_{2max}).

Habitual exercise improves cardiovascular functioning, resulting in lower overall sympathetic reactivity under stress[34] and quicker sympathetic recovery after exposure to stress.[24] Some research retrospectively separating subjects into fit and unfit categories reveals lower reported stress levels for the more fit,[35] aerobically conditioned,[36] and generally physically active individuals.[37] One study, after successfully manipulating aerobic fitness, found no differences in physiologic reactivity to an arithmetic laboratory stressor.[24] However, these negative findings were attributed to a ceiling effect caused by the high intensity of the laboratory stressor.

Dishman[38] suggests exercise might reduce anxiety through the social reinforcement and support involved in group participation, the most common format for exercising, rather than through the physical activity itself. Encouraging comments from group members might reduce anxious thoughts and improve one's sense of self-efficacy in controlling such thoughts.

In summary, exercise may mediate reduction in anxiety through a variety of mechanisms, which include (1) enhanced self-efficacy based on improved sense of personal control, (2) distraction from thoughts surrounding anxiety-producing stimuli, (3) improved physiologic response to stressful conditions, or (4) social support from other group members. Most likely, the effect of exercise involves a combination of these. Although scientific data are not conclusive, exercise appears to reduce symptoms of anxiety even in individuals without clinical anxiety.

EXERCISE AND CLINICAL ANXIETY SYNDROMES

Clinical anxiety is a collective term for eight different clinical syndromes identified in the latest American Psychiatric Association's *Diagnostic and Statistical Manual-III-R:*[39]

1. panic disorder, with agoraphobia and without
2. agoraphobia without panic
3. social phobia
4. simple phobia
5. obsessive–compulsive disorder
6. post-traumatic stress disorder
7. generalized anxiety disorder
8. anxiety disorder not otherwise specified.

To meet the criteria for a DSM-III-R diagnosis, the anxious symptoms must interfere with the patient's social, family, or work function and lead him or her to seek treatment or to use alcohol or illicit drugs to control the anxiety.[1]

Little research and no controlled studies[40] have focused on the role of exercise in reducing clinically diagnosed anxiety disorder. Results of the available nonexperimental investigations are equivocal. For example, one study[41] found that increased anxiety levels were reported retrospectively by both normal and DSM-III–diagnosed anxiety subjects during acute exercise. Two other researchers[42,43] reported that patients with panic disorder have evidence of poor physical fitness as measured by exercise stress testing, perhaps related to inactivity.

Based on the observation that some anxious patients have poor exercise tolerance and unusually high post-exercise blood lactate levels, Pitts and McClure[44] wondered if lactate, a metabolic product of exercise, might be associated with anxiety. They infused lactate into anxious patients and produced panic attacks. However, the specific role of lactate in producing panic remains unclear.[45] Although panic disorder patients may fear exercise, it is rare for patients to report having a panic attack during exercise. One group[43] reported that panic patients were able to undergo a symptom-limited treadmill test, which functioned both to disclose possible cardiovascular disease and to reassure them.

Several questions remain unanswered concerning exercise and clinical anxiety. How physical activity might differentially affect the various subdiagnoses of anxiety is still unknown, and whether exercise at various intensity levels may increase anxiety symptoms remains to be investigated. Finally, how exertion might influence state anxiety as opposed to more chronic anxiety is unclear. When used appropriately, we have found aerobic exercise to be useful, particularly for patients suffering from panic disorder with or without avoidance, agoraphobia without panic attacks, and generalized anxiety disorder. Group-based exercise programs can be useful for patients with social phobias.

CASE: A.G., a 37-year-old accountant, presented with a 6-month history of panic attacks. The first attack occurred about 2 months after he broke up with a girlfriend. It began with shortness of breath followed by increased heart rate, flushing, and dizziness. He worried that he was having a heart attack and went to an emergency room, where he was told he was having an "anxiety attack." At baseline he was having three to five severe panic attacks per week. He had a Hamilton Anxiety[7] rating of 20 and a Hamilton Depression[46] rating of 6, indicating severe anxiety but little depression.

The patient underwent an exercise stress test, which he completed to 10 metabolic equivalents (METs). He started jogging 2 to 3 miles per day, two to three times per week, in an attempt to reduce the panic attacks. He began therapy with imipramine 50 mg, which was increased over 3 months to 175 mg/d. While treated, he experienced no panic attacks and little anxiety, but he disliked the imipramine because of feeling an increased heart rate and decreased exercise tolerance. Therefore the drug therapy was discontinued. He remained free of panic attacks for the next 6 months.

Following a series of setbacks at work, his symptoms returned. He wanted to try to "live with the panic attacks" rather than restart therapy with imipramine, but felt he needed something more than exercise. Because he had continued jogging and found the activity useful as "self-improvement" time, we prepared a relaxation tape for him to use before and after exercising, and another tape that taught him how to control panic. He was instructed to use this tape while jogging. After 2 months, the panic attacks stopped. Six months later, he was no longer experiencing panic attacks, anxiety, or depression.

> **COMMENT:** This case demonstrates exercise as a vehicle for providing relaxation and cognitive interventions to reduce a patient's panic attacks.

Exercise and Depression

The research considering exercise as a therapeutic intervention for depression has focused on both depressive symptoms and clinical depression. To interpret the effects of exercise on these disorders, we present a brief overview of depression, its etiology, and its psychosocial consequences.

CONCEPTUALIZATION OF DEPRESSION

Depression is described as sadness, apathy, discouragement, and an overall feeling of hopelessness. Most people feel at least a little depression at one time or another. When these feelings become severe, a psychiatric diagnosis of mood disorder is made based on the diagnostic criteria outlined in the DSM-III-R.[39] Clinical depression or mood disorder is separated into dysthymic disorder and major depressive disorder. Dysthymic disorder refers to a more chronic yet less severe experience of depressed affect, whereas major depressive disorder is more severe, with reported symptoms of intense depression most of the day, weight loss, fatigue, and possibly suicidal ideation.

As with anxiety, standardized instruments have been developed to measure depression. The most widely used self-report instruments include the Beck Depression Inventory,[47] SCL-90 depression scale,[6] the depression scale of the Profile of Mood States,[5] and the Zung depression scale.[48] The Hamilton Depression Inventory,[46] a clinical interview, is used in many studies.

The etiology of clinical depression (and probably the more benign blues) is multivariate. Environmental events, genetic susceptibility, learning history, cognition, and individual changes in neurochemistry contribute to depressed mood. The clinical sequelae include reduced self-esteem, reduced social contact, negative cognitive interpretations, apathy, fatigue, and lethargy.[49] Once these clinical manifestations appear, a vicious cycle often keeps people from utilizing natural coping strategies to relieve their depressed state.

EXERCISE AND DEPRESSED MOOD IN NORMAL POPULATIONS

Research considering normal subjects, not randomly assigned to treatments, shows a moderate reduction in depressed mood or an improvement in mood following habitual exercise.[9,11,50,51] Randomized studies, however, have shown mixed results, with two finding significant differences between exercisers and controls,[18,52] and two that did not find any significant difference.[19,53] In these studies, the populations were not depressed, and thus were less likely to demonstrate a reduction in depression scores. On the other hand, there is evidence that exercise may benefit individuals with clinical depression.

EXERCISE AND CLINICAL DEPRESSION

Several uncontrolled or single-case subject trials with clinically depressed patients have found significant reductions in depression associated with exercise.[54,55] Four women suffering from major depression underwent regular aerobic exercise after an attention-placebo period. They exercised for 30 minutes four times a week for 6 weeks at 85% of predicted maximum heart rate on a stationary cycle. The women showed no changes during baseline but a major reduction in depression following exercise, an effect that persisted at 3 months' follow-up.[56]

Greist and colleagues[57] have undertaken several studies on depression. In an early investigation, clinically depressed outpatients were randomized to running therapy (walk-jog three times a week for 30 or 40 minutes of exercise for 10 weeks), individual psychotherapy for 10 sessions, or unlimited individual psychotherapy. At the end of treatment, depressive scores on the Depression Symptom Checklist were reduced as much in the running group as in the two psychotherapy groups. Although no statistical analysis of these data was reported and interpretation must be made with caution, the decrease in depressive symptoms was maintained at 12-month follow-up testing. Other investigators[58] randomized 60 depressed individuals to either running therapy, meditation–relaxation therapy, or cognitive–interpersonal psychotherapy. Individuals assigned to the running therapy group met twice a week for 45 minutes for walk-jog sessions. The drop-out rate was high for all three groups (56% for the running group), and there were no differences between groups after the end of treatment 12 weeks later. At 3 months' follow-up, however, both the running and meditation groups had greater reductions in depressive scores than the psychotherapy group.

An elegant experiment was undertaken by McCann and Holmes.[59] A group of 43 mildly depressed women were randomized to one of three groups: strenuous exercise (an aerobic dance class, jogging, and running) for 1 hour twice a week, a progressive muscle relaxation group or a wait-list control. The experimenters tried to control for subject expectation by telling them that the purpose of the experiment was to evaluate stress-management techniques.

After 10 weeks, the exercise group reported less depression than did subjects in the other two groups. A study in Norway[60] randomized 49 depressed individuals to either exercise or nonexercise. Although the findings could have been confounded, since more of the nonexercisers than exercisers took antidepressant medication, after 9 weeks the exercising group had higher fitness levels and significantly lower depression scores. In Canada, 30 community-dwelling, moderately depressed elderly men and women were randomly assigned to walking 20–40 minutes three times a week, to a social-contact control, or to a wait-list control. After 6 weeks, both exercise and social contact resulted in significant reductions in depressed mood.[61]

These studies suggest that exercise can have a significant impact on depression. In some cases, exercise appears to have immediate effects on alleviating depression, independent of achieving fitness. There is some evidence that exercise must be continued to remain effective. Exercise may be an appropriate adjunct to psychotherapy for both inpatients and outpatients. Although physical activity appears to help patients taking medication, the interaction of antidepressant medication and exercise should be monitored. Patients on certain tricyclic antidepressants should note their heart rate during peak exercise, as the anticholinergic effect of these medications significantly increases heart rate.

Antidepressant Mechanisms of Exercise

Exercise may alleviate depression through a number of mechanisms. First, exercise enhances self-confidence, improving self-efficacy and thereby reducing depression. Second, exercise might benefit those with depression by distraction, shifting attention away from negative ruminations and allowing positive affect to be introduced. And third, an improved network of social support could reduce depression. Unfortunately, other than research showing that exercise is related to improved self-confidence,[21,52,62,63] no studies have attempted to delineate these mechanisms specifically in relation to depression.

Since the biologic cause of depression is not well understood, any discussion of how exercise might alleviate depression through changes in biochemistry is speculative. Exertion appears to increase the levels of various neurotransmitters—dopamine and serotonin—in the same direction as do antidepressants.[64,65] However, limitations in the measurement of central catecholamine secretion during exercise have been noted.[66] Plasma or urine 3-methoxy-4-hydroxyphenyglycol can be used as a crude index, but since exercise itself causes large increases in catecholamines, these readings are not reliable. To date, the best measurement of central catecholamine activation is from cerebrospinal fluid (CSF), particularly increased levels of 5-hydroxyindole-acetic acid (5-HIAA).[66] Support for increased 5-HIAA levels following exercise is provided by a study[67] that found an increase in CSF levels of 5-HIAA following heightened psychomotor activity (e.g., running up and down the hospital corridor) in a group of nine subjects diagnosed with primary affective illness. However, other studies have failed to show such a connection or showed reduced CSF levels of 5-HIAA in depressed populations.[68] Exercise also appears to increase levels of beta-endorphins, which are also believed to be low in depressed individuals.[69] Further research is needed before conclusions can be drawn regarding the relationship between CSF metabolite levels, exercise, and depression.

CASE: R.W., a 45-year-old middle-management executive in a highly competitive electronics company, presented with a chief complaint of feeling depressed and angry. He had taken a leave of absence from work because he could not concentrate on his job assignments. Furthermore, he was sleeping excessively and found it nearly impossible to wake up and dress in time for work. He complained of lack of energy, tearfulness, and feeling depressed. He met all the DSM-III-R criteria for major depressive episode. Results of his examination were normal except for decreased pulmonary function secondary to 25 years of smoking two or more packs of cigarettes per day. His baseline Hamilton Depression Inventory was 25, indicating significant depression.

The patient reluctantly began imipramine 50 mg, which was increased to 200 mg/d. On this medication and with 10 sessions of weekly psychotherapy, he showed some improvement but still felt listless. He then began an exercise program, starting with walking three to four times per week, increasing intensity of activity to walk-jogging three to four times per week, 20 to 30 minutes each session. There was a slow but significant improvement in his affect associated with the exercise. Three months later, while he continued to exercise, medication was stopped, and he continued to feel much better. He returned to work with significantly improved work performance. On follow-up 2 years later, he continued to exercise regularly and has not had a recurrent depression. The patient attributes much of his improvement to the exercise.

COMMENT: This patient is typical of the use of exercise with depressed individuals. We strongly encourage depressed patients to exercise. Given the inertia associated with depression, however, it is often necessary to provide concrete guidance to help such patients get started in a program. After they agree to exercise, we ask patients to provide a date and time when they plan to exercise. Group programs are particularly recommended for depressed patients, as they provide the added benefit of group support.

Exercise and Emotional Well-Being

Well-being includes a sense of shape and appearance, health, fitness, safety, and perhaps even security. Although it is difficult to define and measure, investigations of individuals' sense of well-being have consistently found beneficial effects from exercise. Two Canadian general fitness surveys reported a positive association between exercise and well-being.[70,71] A recent review of the literature[72] reported that three quarters of the correlational studies identified significant relationships between exercise and positive mood.

Controlled studies have also shown an improvement in well-being. For example, 51 nonexercising volunteers from a university setting were randomized to 6 weeks of aerobic exercise or 6 weeks of low-level placebo exercise.[73] Those conditioning aerobically experienced significant improvement in well-being compared to the control group.

Exercise intensity may influence its effects on well-being. When 94 community volunteers were randomly assigned to a 10-week high-intensity aerobic training program, a moderate-intensity aerobic program, an attention–placebo control condition, or a wait-list control, only the moderate-intensity exercise group demonstrated benefits on variables related to well-being.[18] Others also have found lower-intensity exercise to enhance well-being.[74] In contrast, our study of 120 healthy, sedentary middle-aged men and women randomly assigned to either a 6-month home-based aerobic exercise program or to an assessment-only control condition found changes in satisfaction with shape or appearance, fitness, and weight, but not in well-being or mood.[19]

Collectively, the evidence suggests that regular exercise improves one's sense of well-being. Although the effect of training intensity, as well as the breadth of emotional benefit from physical activity, requires further investigation, moderate-intensity exercise seems to confer as much benefit as higher levels of exertion. Based on this evidence, exercise is advocated as a useful adjunct to make patients feel better. A recommendation to spend at least 2 to 3 hours a week walking or engaging in some other type of low-level activity is warranted. This achievable level of exercise would be useful to enhance emotional well-being for most individuals.

Exercise and the Coronary-Prone (Type A) Behavior Pattern

The coronary-prone behavior pattern (type A) is characterized by time urgency, competitiveness, hostility, and vigorous speech. Type A behavior is implicated as a major risk factor for the development of coronary heart disease.[75,76] Recent evidence[77-79] suggests that hostility, cynicism, and chronic anger are the factors of type A behavior specifically associated with coronary heart disease.

Limited research suggests that exercise reduces some aspects of type A behavior. Several investigations[80-83] have shown reductions in type A behavior and physiologic reactivity following habitual exercise, but two studies[84,85] failed to find such effects. Schaeffer and associates[86] found that a 9-month aerobic fitness program failed to reduce global type A ratings, as assessed by the Type A Structured Interview. On the other hand, they reported significantly greater reduction in hostility in the aerobic treatment group than in nontreatment controls.

In our clinic, exercise is prescribed for those with type A personality profiles as part of a stress-management program that also involves other techniques. Because type A individuals tend to overdo everything, they must be cautioned not to make the time to exercise yet another burden.

> **CASE:** M.G., a 55-year-old salesman, suffered an uncomplicated myocardial infarction (MI). Three weeks post–MI, he underwent a symptom-limited treadmill exercise test without complication. His maximum heart rate was 165 bpm, and he was prescribed exercise at a heart rate of 125 to 140 bpm, for 20 to 30 minutes three times per week. He joined a local YMCA cardiac therapy class to help structure his exercise. After 2 days, however, he decided to increase his exercise heart rate to 150 bpm and extend his jogging time by 15 minutes. He also engaged in spurts of fast interval running. He immediately established for himself a goal to decrease his lap time by 2 minutes each week. He also identified a jogger 6 months' post–MI whom he planned to beat within a month. During the first week of exercise, he ignored some mild chest pain. When the nurse called him at the end of the week to discuss his progress, he boasted that he was well ahead of the guidelines that she had set. Because the nurse suspected that he was prone to excessive competitive behavior, she not only reminded him of the guidelines, but also emphasized the dangers of exceeding them. She pointed out that he was not listening to his body (the chest pain) and that failure to do so might kill him. She asked him if this excessively competitive behavior was a problem for him in other areas. He assured her that his success in life was due to such behavior, and he was not willing to change it. However, he was willing to follow the guidelines, to stop exercising if he experienced chest pain, and to let her know if he had any further symptoms.
>
> Four months later, he continued to exercise, and by now had returned to work. It was apparent to the nurse that he had added exercise to his already busy schedule; he was now exercising four times a week for about 1 hour, usually from 6:00 to 7:00 PM, just before he went home. She spent time discussing the importance of making exercise fun rather than a burden, and giving up another activity rather than simply adding exercise to his schedule. Perhaps in part because of the exercise, he was

more receptive to this advice and began to change his priorities in ways that gave him more satisfaction without diminishing his accomplishments.

COMMENT: This case illustrates many aspects of providing an exercise program for patients with type A personality. They often exceed guidelines and may turn what can be a pleasant and helpful experience into a driven, perhaps dangerous, one. Most individuals with type A behavior are very compliant, willing to follow guidelines, and usually are the people who make the greatest changes in their lifestyle following an acute MI. These guidelines need to be explicit and monitored. How such people incorporate regular exercise into their lifestyle is often indicative of general problems they may have, and discussing it can be helpful in other areas. We ask patients to monitor their sense of irritability and anger—emotions that most people find unpleasant and would like to diminish—as a guide to help them determine if exercise benefits them in this area. Exercise without other stress-management procedures is rarely enough to make changes in a person's life, but it can be a useful component of such a program.

The Psychological Risks of Exercise

Much has been written about the negative psychological effects of exercise. The potential adverse consequences include using exercise to avoid other social, work, and family responsibilities, and becoming obsessed, even fanatical, about exercise, so that its interruption causes depression and irritability. There is no doubt that some become addicted to exercise and that certain clinical problems, primarily anorexia nervosa, are associated with excessive exercising, but such cases are rare.[40] Given the exposure of the population to exercising (over 30 million Americans have jogged at one time or another), the relatively few psychological problems that result show that it is very safe psychologically.

Physicians should be alert to the occasional patient who becomes obsessed with exercise. Clinical characteristics of "addicted" patients include training to the exclusion of other important activities, dysphoria or panic when the exercise schedule is disrupted, exercising against medical advice, and exercising to decrease or maintain an excessively low body weight. Overall, however, the challenge of achieving adherence to a regular exercise program far outweighs concern about the rare individual who becomes obsessed with habitual exertion.

Summary

Regular physical activity enhances psychological well-being. In addition, exercise appears useful for symptoms of anxiety and depression, and the syndrome of clinical anxiety. Physical conditioning also may contribute to a stress-management program for those with a type A personality. The mechanisms of these exercise benefits are not well-defined. Studies suggest that regular participation in low- to moderate-intensity activities, rather than a defined increment in aerobic capacity, is the factor that mediates benefits. The focus for benefits is on adherence to an enjoyed physical activity. Principles of achieving regular participation (as discussed in chapter 1) and involvement in group activities are important considerations when using exercise for its psychological benefits.

REFERENCES

1. Taylor CB, Arnow B: *The Nature and Treatment of Anxiety Disorders.* The Free Press: New York, 1988.
2. Tanaka-Matsumi J, Kameoka VA: Reliabilities and concurrent validities of popular self-report measures of depression, anxiety, and social disability. *J Clin Psychol* 1986; 54:328–333.
3. Taylor JA: A personality scale for manifest anxiety. *J Abnorm Psychol* 1953; 48: 285–290.
4. Spielberger CD: The measurement of state and trait anxiety: Conceptual and methodological issues. In Levi L, ed: *Emotions: Their Parameters and Measurement.* Raven Press: New York, 1975.
5. McNair DM, Lorr M, Droppleman LF: *Manual: Profile of Mood States.* Educational and Industrial Testing Services: San Diego, 1971.
6. Derogatis L, Lipman R, Cove L: The SCL-90: An outpatient psychiatric rating scale: Preliminary report. *Psychopharmacol Bull* 1973; 9:13–28.
7. Hamilton M: The assessment of anxiety states by rating. *Br J Med Psychol* 1959; 32: 50–55.
8. Francis K, Carter R: Psychological characteristics of joggers. *J Sports Med* 1982; 24: 69–74.
9. Hayden R, Allen G: Relationship between aerobic exercise, anxiety, and depression: Convergent validation by knowledgeable informants. *J Sports Med* 1984; 24:69–74.
10. Wood D. The relationship between state anxiety and acute physical activity. *Am Correct Ther J* 1977; 31:67–69.
11. Kowal D, Patton J, Vogel J: Psychological states and aerobic fitness of male and female recruits before and after basic training. *Aviat Space Environ Med* 1978; 49: 603–606.
12. Morgan W: Anxiety reduction following acute physical activity. *Psychiatr Ann* 1979; 9:141–147.
13. Molloy D, et al.: Acute effects of exercise on neuropsychological function in elderly subjects. *J Am Geriatr Soc* 1988; 36:29–33.
14. Lichtman S, Poser E: The effects of exercise on mood and cognitive functioning. *J Psychosom Res* 1983; 27:43–52.
15. Blumenthal JA, et al.: Psychological changes accompany aerobic exercise in healthy middle-aged adults. *Psychosom Med* 1982; 44:529–536.
16. Simons C, Birkimer J: An exploration of factors predicting effects of aerobic conditioning on mood state. *J Psychosom Res* 1988; 32:63–75.
17. Fasting K, Gronningsaeter H: Unemployment, trait anxiety, and physical exercise. *Scand J Sport Sci* 1986; 8:99–103.
18. Moses J, et al.: The effects of exercise training on mental well-being in the normal population: A controlled trial. *J Psychosom Res* 1989; 33:47–61.
19. King A, et al.: The influence of regular aerobic exercise on psychological health: A randomized, controlled trial of healthy middle-aged adults. *Health Psychol* 1989; 8: 305–324.
20. Bandura A: Self-efficacy conception of anxiety. *Anxiety Res* 1988; 1:77–98.
21. Jasnoski M, et al.: Exercise, changes in aerobic capacity, and changes in self-perceptions: An experimental investigation. *J Res Personality* 1981; 15:460–466.
22. Long B: Aerobic conditioning and stress inoculation: A comparison of stress-management interventions. *Cognitive Ther Res* 1984; 8:517–542.
23. Long B, Haney C: Coping strategies for working women: Aerobic exercise and relaxation interventions. *Behav Ther* 1988; 19:75–83.
24. Sinyor D, et al.: Experimental manipulation of aerobic fitness and response to psychosocial stress: Heart rate and self-report measures. *Psychosom Med* 1986; 48:324–337.
25. Hughes J: Psychological effects of habitual aerobic exercise: A critical review. *Prev Med* 1984; 13:66–78.
26. Morgan W: Effective beneficence of vigorous physical activity. *Med Sci Sports Exerc* 1985; 17:94–100.
27. Bahrke M, Morgan W: Anxiety reduction following exercise and meditation. *Cognitive Ther Res* 1978; 2:323–333.
28. Berger B, Owen D: Stress reduction and mood enhancement in four exercise modes: Swimming, body conditioning, hatha yoga, and fencing. *Res Q Exerc Sports* 1988; 59: 148–159.
29. Raglin J, Morgan W: Influence of exercise and quiet rest on state anxiety and blood pressure. *Med Sci Sports Exerc* 1987; 19: 456–463.
30. deVries H: Immediate and long-term effects of exercise upon resting muscle action potential level. *J Sports Med Phys Fitness* 1968; 8:1–11.
31. deVries H, Adams G: Electromyographic comparison of single doses of exercise and meprobamate as to effects on muscular relaxation. *Am J Phys Med* 1972; 51:130–141.
32. deVries H, et al.: Tranquilizer effect of exercise. *Am J Phys Med* 1981; 60:57–60.
33. Farrell P, et al.: Enkephalins, catecholamines, and psychological mood alterations:

Effects of prolonged exercise. *Med Sci Sports Exerc* 1987; 19:347–353.

34. Cantor J, Zillman D, Day K: Relationships between cardiorespiratory fitness and physiological responses to films. *Percept Motor Skills* 1978; 46:1123–1130.

35. Tucker L, Cole G, Friedman G: Physical fitness: A buffer against stress. *Percept Motor Skills* 1986; 63:955–961.

36. Roth D, Holmes D: Influence of physical fitness in determining the impact of stressful life events on physical and psychological health. *Psychosom Med* 1985; 47:164–173.

37. Brown J, Siegel J: Exercise as a buffer of life stress: A prospective study of adolescent health. *Health Psychol* 1988; 7:341–353.

38. Dishman R: Medical psychology in exercise and sport. *Med Clin North Am* 1985; 69: 123–143.

39. American Psychiatric Association: *Diagnostic and Statistical Manual III-R.* APA Press: Washington, DC, 1988.

40. Taylor CB, Sallis JF, Needle R: The relation of physical activity and exercise to mental health. *Public Health Rep* 1985; 100: 195–202.

41. Cameron O, Hudson C: Influence of exercise on anxiety level in patients with anxiety disorders. *Psychosom Med* 1986; 27: 720–723.

42. Gaffney F, et al.: Hemodynamic, ventilatory, and biochemical responses of panic patients and normal controls with sodium lactate infusion and spontaneous panic attacks. *Arch Gen Psychiat* 1988; 45:53–60.

43. Taylor DB, et al.: Treadmill exercise testing and ambulatory heart rate measures in patients with panic attacks. *Am J Cardiol* 1987; 60:48J–52J.

44. Pitts FM, McClure JN: Lactate metabolism in anxiety neurosis. *N Engl J Med* 1967; 277:1329–1336.

45. Margraf J, Ehlers A, Roth WT: Sodium lactate infusions and panic attacks: A review and critique. *Psychosom Med* 1986; 48: 23–51.

46. Hamilton M: A rating scale for depression. *J Neurol Neurosurg Psychiatr* 1960; 23:56–62.

47. Beck A, Steer R, Gabin M: Psychometric properties of the Beck Depression Inventory: Twenty-five years of evaluation. *Clin Psychol Rev* 1988; 8:77–100.

48. Zung WWK: A self-rating depression scale. *Arch Gen Psychiat* 1965; 12:63–70.

49. Beck A: *Cognitive Therapy and the Emotional Disorders.* International Universities Press: New York, 1976.

50. Berger B, Owen D: Mood alteration with swimming: Swimmers really do "feel better." *Psychosom Med* 1983; 45:425–433.

51. Brown R, Ramirez D, Taub J: The prescription of exercise for depression. *Phys Sportsmed* 1978; 6(Dec):34–49.

52. Folkins C: Effects of physical training on mood. *J Clin Psychol* 1976; 32:385–388.

53. Morgan W, Pollock M: Physical activity and cardiovascular health: Psychological aspects. In *Physical Activity and Human Well-being: A Collection of Formal Papers,* vol 1, book 1. Presented at the International Congress of Physical Activity Sciences, Quebec City, July 11–16, 1976. Symposia Specialties: Miami, 1976.

54. Kostrubala T: *The Joy of Running.* JB Lippincott: New York, 1976.

55. Lobstein D, Mosbacher B, Ismail A: Depression as a powerful discriminator between physically active and sedentary middle-aged men. *J Psychosom Res* 1983; 27:69–76.

56. Doyne E, Chambless E, Beutler L: Aerobic exercise as a treatment for depression in women. *Behav Ther* 1983; 24:434–440.

57. Griest J, et al.: Running as treatment for depression. *Compr Psychiat* 1979; 20:41–54.

58. Klein H, et al.: A comparative outcome study of group psychotherapy vs exercise treatments for depression. *Int J Mental Health* 1985; 13:148–177.

59. McCann I, Holmes D: The influence of aerobic exercise on depression. *J Pers Soc Psychol* 1984; 46:1142–1147.

60. Martinsen E: Exercise and medication in the psychiatric patient. In Morgan WP, Goldston SE, eds: *Exercise and Mental Health.* Hemisphere Publishing: Washington, DC, 1987.

61. McNeil JK, LeBlanc EM, Joyner M: The effect of exercise on depressive symptoms in moderately depressed elderly. *Psychol Aging* 1991; 6:487–488.

62. Martineck T, Cheffers J, Zaichkowsky L: Physical activity, motor development, and self-concept: Race and age differences. *Percept Motor Skills* 1978; 46:147–154.

63. McGowan R, Jarman B, Pedersen D: Effects of a competitive endurance training program on self-concept and peer approval. *J Psychol* 1974; 86:57–60.

64. Brown B, Van Huss W: Exercise and brain catecholamines. *J Appl Physiol* 1973; 34: 664–669.

65. Brown B, et al.: Chronic response to rat brain norepinephrine and serotonin levels of endurance training. *J Appl Psychol* 1979; 46:19–23.

66. Veale D: Exercise and mental health. *Acta Psychiat Scand* 1987; 76:113–120.

67. Post R, et al.: Psychomotor activity and cerebrospinal fluid amine metabolites in affective illness. *Am J Psychiat* 1973; 130: 67–72.

68. Papeschi R, McClure JD: Homovanillic acid and 5-hydroxyindoleacetic acid in cerebrospinal fluid of depressed patients. *Arch Gen Psychiat* 1971; 25:354–358.

69. Berk L, et al.: Beta-endorphin response to exercise in athletes and nonathletes (abstract). *Med Sci Sports Exerc* 1981; 13:134.

70. Statistics Canada: *Culture Statistics/Recreational Activities 1976.* Ottawa, 1980. Minister of Supply and Services Canada Catalogue No. 87-501, occasional.

71. *Canada Fitness Survey: Fitness and Lifestyle in Canada.* Fitness Canada: Ottawa, 1983.

72. Plante T, Rodin J: Physical fitness and enhanced psychological health. *Cur Psychol* 1990; 9(1):3–24.

73. Goldwater B, Collins M: Psychological effects of cardiovascular conditioning: A controlled experiment. *Psychosom Med* 1985; 47:174–181.

74. Steptoe A, Cox S: Acute effects of aerobic exercise on mood. *Health Psychol* 1988; 7:329–340.

75. Haynes S, et al.: The relationship of psychosocial factors in coronary heart disease in the Framingham Study. *Am J Epidemiol* 1978; 107:384–402.

76. Haynes S, Feinleib M, Kannel W: The relationship of psychosocial factors to coronary heart disease in the Framingham Study, III: Eight-year incidence of coronary heart disease. *Am J Epidemiol* 1980; 111:37–58.

77. Booth-Kewley S, Friedman H: Psychological predictors of heart disease: A quantitative review. *Psychol Bull* 1987; 101:343–362.

78. Dembroski T, et al.: Components of hostility as predictors of sudden death and myocardial infarction in the Multiple Risk Factor Intervention Trial. *Psychosom Med* 1989; 51:514–522.

79. Williams R: *The Trusting Heart.* Warner: New York, 1988.

80. Blumenthal J, et al.: Effects of exercise on the type A (coronary-prone) behavior pattern. *Psychosom Med* 1980; 42:289–296.

81. Blumenthal J, et al.: Exercise training in healthy type A middle-aged men: Effects on behavioral and cardiovascular responses. *Psychosom Med* 1988; 50:418–433.

82. Gillespie WJ, et al.: Changes in selected psychophysiological indicators of coronary risk in male corporate executives as a result of an aerobic exercise program (abstract). *Med Sci Sports Exerc* 1982; 14:116.

83. Lobitz W, et al.: Physical exercise and anxiety management training for cardiac stress management in a nonpatient population. *J Cardiovasc Rehab* 1983; 3:683–688.

84. Jasnoski M, Holmes DS: Influence of initial aerobic fitness, aerobic training, and changes in aerobic fitness on personality functioning. *J Psychosom Res* 1981; 25:553–556.

85. Roskies E, et al.: The Montreal Type A Intervention Project: Major findings. *Health Psychol* 1986; 5:45–69.

86. Schaeffer MA, Krantz DS, Weiss SM, et al.: Effects of occupational-based behavioral counseling and exercise interventions on Type A components and cardiovascular reactivity. *J Cardiol* 1988; 10:371–377.

Index

A "t" after a page number indicates a table; an "f" indicates a figure.